Eosinophilic Gastrointestinal Diseases

Guest Editors

GLENN T. FURUTA, MD
DAN ATKINS, MD

IMMUNOLOGY AND ALLERGY CLINICS OF NORTH AMERICA

www.immunology.theclinics.com

Consulting Editor
RAFEUL ALAM, MD, PhD

February 2009 • Volume 29 • Number 1

SAUNDERS an imprint of ELSEVIER, Inc.

W.B. SAUNDERS COMPANY
A Division of Elsevier Inc.

1600 John F. Kennedy Blvd., ● Suite 1800, ● Philadelphia, PA 19103-2899.
http://www.theclinics.com

IMMUNOLOGY AND ALLERGY CLINICS OF NORTH AMERICA Volume 29, Number 1
February 2009 ISSN 0889–8561, ISBN-13: 978-1-4377-0489-1, ISBN-10: 1-4377-0489-1

Editor: Patrick Manley

Immunology and Allergy Clinics of North America (ISSN 0889–8561) is published quarterly by Elsevier Inc., 360 Park Avenue South, New York, NY 10010-1710. Months of issue are February, May, August, and November. Business and Editorial Offices: 1600 John F. Kennedy Blvd., Suite 1800, Philadelphia, PA 19103-2899. Customer Service Office: 11830 Westline Industrial Drive, St. Louis, MO 63146. Periodicals postage paid at New York, NY and additional mailing offices. Subscription prices are $233.00 per year for US individuals, $366.00 per year for US institutions, $113.00 per year for US students and residents, $286.00 per year for Canadian individuals, $163.00 per year for Canadian students, $454.00 per year for Canadian institutions, $325.00 per year for international individuals, $454.00 per year for international institutions, $163.00 per year for international students. To receive student/resident rate, orders must be accompanied by name of affiliated institution, date of term, and the *signature* of program/residency coordinator on institution letterhead. Orders will be billed at individual rate until proof of status is received. Foreign air speed delivery is included in all *Clinics* subscription prices. All prices are subject to change without notice. **POSTMASTER**: Send address changes to *Immunology and Allergy Clinics of North America,* Elsevier Journals Customer Service, 11830 Westline Industrial Drive, St. Louis, MO 63146. **Customer Service: 1-800-654-2452 (US and Canada). From outside of the United States and Canada, call 1-314-453-7041. Fax: 1-314-453-5170. For print support, e-mail: JournalsCustomerService-usa@ elsevier.com. For online support, e-mail: JournalsOnlineSupport-usa@elsevier.com.**

Reprints. For copies of 100 or more, of articles in this publication, please contact the Commercial Reprints Department, Elsevier Inc., 360 Park Avenue South, New York, New York 10010-1710. Tel. (212) 633-3812, Fax: (212) 462-1935, e-mail: reprints@elsevier.com.

Immunology and Allergy Clinics of North America is covered in MEDLINE/PubMed (Index Medicus), Current Contents/Life Sciences, Science Citation Index, ISI/BIOMED, Chemical Abstracts, and EMBASE/Excerpta Medica.

Printed and bound by CPI Group (UK) Ltd, Croydon, CR0 4YY
Transferred to Digital Print 2011

Contributors

CONSULTING EDITOR

RAFEUL ALAM, MD, PhD
Veda and Chauncey Ritter Chair in Immunology, Professor, and Director, Division of
Immunology and Allergy, National Jewish Health; and University of Colorado Health
Sciences Center, Denver, Colorado

GUEST EDITORS

GLENN T. FURUTA, MD
Associate Professor of Pediatrics, University of Colorado Denver, School of Medicine;
and Director, Gastrointestinal Eosinophilic Disease Program, National Jewish Health,
The Children's Hospital Denver, Aurora, Colorado

DAN ATKINS, MD
Professor, Department of Pediatrics, Division of Pediatric Allergy and Immunology;
Medical Director, Pediatric Day Program; Head, Division of Ambulatory Pediatrics;
Co-Director, Gastrointestinal Eosinophilic Disease Program, National Jewish Health, The
Children's Hospital Denver; and Associate Professor of Pediatrics, University of Colorado
Denver School of Medicine, Denver, Colorado

AUTHORS

SEEMA S. ACEVES, MD, PhD
Assistant Adjunct Professor in Pediatrics and Medicine, Division of Allergy and
Immunology, Rady Children's Hospital; Department of Pediatrics, University of California;
and Department of Medicine, University of California, San Diego, California

STEVEN J. ACKERMAN, PhD
Professor, Department of Biochemistry and Molecular Genetics, The University of Illinois
at Chicago College of Medicine; and Department of Medicine (Hematology-Oncology),
The University of Illinois at Chicago, Chicago, Illinois

DAN ATKINS, MD
Professor, Department of Pediatrics, Division of Pediatric Allergy and Immunology;
Medical Director, Pediatric Day Program; Head, Division of Ambulatory Pediatrics,
National Jewish Health; Associate Professor, Department of Pediatrics, University of
Colorado Health Sciences Center, Denver, Colorado

CARINE BLANCHARD, PhD
Instructor of Pediatrics, Division of Allergy and Immunology, Department of Pediatrics,
Cincinnati Children's Hospital Medical Center, Cincinnati, Ohio

PETER A. L. BONIS, MD
Associate Professor of Medicine, Division of Gastroenterology, Tufts Medical Center,
Boston, Massachusetts; and Associate Professor of Medicine, Division of Clinical Care
Research, Tufts Medical Center, Boston, Massachusetts

TERRI A. BROWN-WHITEHORN, MD
Assistant Clinical Professor of Pediatrics, Division of Allergy and Immunology,
The Children's Hospital of Philadelphia, University of Pennsylvania School of Medicine,
Philadelphia, Pennsylvania

A. WESLEY BURKS, MD
Professor and Chief, Division of Allergy and Immunology, Department of Pediatrics,
Duke University Medical Center, Durham, North Carolina

MIRNA CHEHADE, MD
Pediatric Gastroenterology and Nutrition, Pediatric Allergy and Immunology, Mount Sinai
School of Medicine, New York, New York

SEAN P. COLGAN, PhD
Mucosal Inflammation Program, Division of Gastroenterology, University of Colorado
Denver School of Medicine, Aurora, Colorado

MARGARET H. COLLINS, MD
Professor of Pathology, Division of Pathology and Laboratory Medicine, Cincinnati
Children's Hospital Medical Center, University of Cincinnati, Cincinnati, Ohio

ELEONORA DEHLINK, MD, PhD
Division of Gastroenterology and Nutrition, Children's Hospital Boston, Harvard Medical
School, Boston, Massachusetts; and Department of Pediatrics and Adolescent Medicine,
Medical University of Vienna, Vienna, Austria

EDDA FIEBIGER, PhD
Division of Gastroenterology and Nutrition, Children's Hospital Boston, Harvard Medical
School, Boston, Massachusetts

SOPHIE FILLON, PhD
Section of Pediatric Gastroenterology, Hepatology, and Nutrition, University of Colorado
Denver School of Medicine, Aurora, Colorado

DAVID M. FLEISCHER, MD
Assistant Professor, Department of Pediatrics, Division of Pediatric Allergy and
Immunology, National Jewish Health, University of Colorado Health Sciences, Denver,
Colorado

JAMES P. FRANCIOSI, MD, MS, MSCE
Assistant Professor, Division of Gastroenterology, Hepatology, and Nutrition, Cincinnati
Children's Hospital Medical Center; and University of Cincinnati College of Medicine,
Cincinnati, Ohio

GLENN T. FURUTA, MD
Associate Professor of Pediatrics, University of Colorado Denver, School of Medicine;
and Director, Gastrointestinal Eosinophilic Disease Program, National Jewish Health,
The Children's Hospital Denver, Aurora, Colorado

ANGELA M. HAAS, MA, CCC-SLP
Speech-Language Pathologist; and Feeding Disorders Program Specialist, Audiology,
Speech Pathology, and Learning Services, Feeding and Swallowing Program,
The Children's Hospital Denver, Aurora, Colorado

SIMON P. HOGAN, PhD
Assistant Professor of Pediatrics, Division of Allergy and Immunology, Department of Pediatrics, Cincinnati Children's Hospital Medical Center, Cincinnati, Ohio

SOMA JYONOUCHI, MD
Fellow, Division of Allergy and Immunology, The Children's Hospital of Philadelphia, University of Pennsylvania School of Medicine, Philadelphia, Pennsylvania

ROHIT KATIAL, MD
Professor, Department of Medicine; Program Director, Division of Allergy and Immunology, Department of Medicine; and Director, Weinberg Clinical Research Unit, National Jewish Health, Denver, Colorado

MARY D. KLINNERT, PhD
Associate Professor, Department of Pediatrics, National Jewish Health, Denver, Colorado; and Associate Professor, Department of Psychiatry, University of Colorado Denver, Aurora, Colorado

CHRIS A. LIACOURAS, MD
Professor, Division of Gastroenterology, Hepatology, and Nutrition, The Children's Hospital of Philadelphia; and University of Pennsylvania School of Medicine, Philadelphia, Pennsylvania

NANCY CRESKOFF MAUNE, OTR
Occupational Therapist; and Clinical Training Coordinator, Department of Occupational Therapy, Feeding and Swallowing Program, The Children's Hospital Denver, Aurora, Colorado

EMILY McCLOUD, MS, RD
Clinical Dietician, National Jewish Health, Denver, Colorado

ANIL MISHRA, PhD
Assistant Professor, Department of Pediatrics, Division of Allergy and Immunology, Cincinnati Children's Hospital Medical Center, University of Cincinnati, Cincinnati, Ohio

PHILIP E. PUTNAM, MD, FAAP
Associate Professor of Pediatrics, Division of Pediatric Gastroenterology, Hepatology, and Nutrition, Cincinnati Children's Hospital Medical Center, Cincinnati, Ohio; and Medical Director, Cincinnati Center for Eosinophilic Disorders, University of Cincinnati, Cincinnati, Ohio

ZACHARY D. ROBINSON, MS
Section of Pediatric Gastroenterology, Hepatology, and Nutrition, University of Colorado Denver School of Medicine, Aurora, Colorado

MARC E. ROTHENBERG, MD, PhD
Professor of Pediatrics; Director, Cincinnati Center for Eosinophilic Disorders; Director, Division of Allergy and Immunology, Department of Pediatrics, Cincinnati Children's Hospital Medical Center, Cincinnati, Ohio

HUGH A. SAMPSON, MD
Pediatric Allergy and Immunology, Mount Sinai School of Medicine, New York, New York

CATHERINE M. SANTANGELO, RD
Pediatric Dietitian, Division of Gastroenterology/Nutrition, The Children's Hospital, Denver, Colorado

JONATHAN M. SPERGEL, MD, PhD
Associate Professor of Pediatrics, Division of Allergy and Immunology, The Children's Hospital of Philadelphia, University of Pennsylvania School of Medicine, Philadelphia, Pennsylvania

ALEX STRAUMANN, MD
Associate Professor of Medicine, Department of Gastroenterology, Kantonsspital Olten, Olten, Switzerland

POOJA VARSHNEY, MD
Fellow, Division of Allergy and Immunology, Department of Pediatrics, Duke University Medical Center, Durham, North Carolina

BARRY K. WERSHIL, MD
Professor of Pediatrics and Chief, Division of Pediatric Gastroenterology, Hepatology, and Nutrition, Children's Memorial Hospital; and Feinberg School of Medicine at Northwestern, Chicago, Illinois

Contents

> Children who have eosinophilic esophagitis require comprehensive evaluation before treatment and ongoing assessment during treatment. When completed at the appropriate times and under well-controlled circumstances, investigation yields the correct diagnosis, assures recognition of sequelae or recurrence of the inflammation, or confirms whether therapy has been effective. Proper management of each child depends on compulsive follow-up until all of the therapeutic goals have been achieved and the child is on a stable regimen without esophageal inflammation. This article summarizes the issues facing the patient and the physician during this process.

> Eosinophilic esophagitis (EoE) is a rapidly increasing, chronic, T helper 2–type inflammatory disease of the esophagus characterized by esophagus related symptoms and a dense esophageal eosinophilia, both of which are refractory to proton pump inhibitors. The adult patient presents with a typical history of dysphagia for solids and has often experienced food impactions. However the general appearance shows an apparently healthy individual; the physical examination is usually unremarkable. The endoscopic findings are often subtle and misleading. The diagnosis is therefore based on the histologic finding of a dense eosinophilic infiltration of the esophageal mucosa. In adult patients, topical and systemic corticosteroids, leukotriene receptor antagonists, immunomodulators, and dilation have proven efficacy, whereas therapy with diet is still under evaluation.

Eosinophilic esophagitis is specific disease that involves an isolated esophageal eosinophilic inflammation and clinical symptoms that do not respond to acid-suppression therapy or are associated with normal esophageal pH monitoring. To establish the diagnosis, upper endoscopy with esophageal biopsies is required. Referral to an allergist and food allergen testing is recommended. Dietary and topical corticosteroid therapies are commonly used and are effective in the majority of patients.

Eosinophilic esophagitis (EoE) is a newly recognized disease and is an emerging entity throughout developing and developed countries, including the United States. Therefore, understanding the causes, natural history, diagnosis, and management is important for future therapeutic interventions. The pathogenesis of EoE is still not clear, but a growing body of evidence has established that this condition represents a T-cell–mediated immune response involving several proinflammatory mediators and chemoattractants known to regulate eosinophilic accumulation in the esophagus, such as IL-4, IL-5, IL-3 and eotaxin-1, -2, and -3. Determining the mechanism or mechanisms through which human esophageal-derived factors ultimately induce the functional abnormalities observed, and to which antigens patients who have EoE are sensitized that lead to the manifestation of symptoms, is of significant interest.

The cause of eosinophilic esophagitis remains unknown, but its epidemiology and clinical features provide pieces to the puzzle. Eosinophilic esophagitis probably emerged in the 1950s or early 1960s, has an increasing incidence, occurs in most developed countries, is related to food allergies, affects adults and children, has a strong male predominance, clusters in families, and is commonly associated with other allergic and atopic disorders. Several theories have been proposed to explain its evolution, but none has been convincingly demonstrated.

Eosinophilic Gastrointestinal Diseases

This article focuses on the evaluation and management of eosinophilic gastrointestinal diseases other than eosinophilic esophagitis. Those diseases include eosinophilic gastritis, gastroenteritis, enteritis, and colitis. The diagnosis of eosinophilic gastrointestinal disease is primarily dependent on the clinical history and histopathology of multiple biopsy specimens after ruling out other causes of intestinal eosinophilia. The diagnosis of eosinophilic gastrointestinal diseases other than eosinophilic esophagitis is complicated by the lack of uniformly accepted diagnostic criteria. Treatment involves evaluation for food sensitivity, elimination diets, and the use of anti-allergy and anti-inflammatory medications with varying degrees of success. Little is known about the natural history of eosinophilic gastrointestinal diseases, underscoring the need for long-term follow-up studies of patients with these disorders.

Feeding issues may affect many aspects of a child's health, development, growth, nutrition and overall well-being. There is a developmental continuum for the acquisition of feeding skills, which includes motor skills, sensory systems, behavioral/emotional components and communication. Food refusal, dysphagia, reduced volume and reduced variety of intake are common complaints associated with eosinophilic gastrointestinal diseases in children. As the understanding of this disease process evolves, clinicians are recognizing that feeding difficulties are a prevalent characteristic of children with eosinophilic gastrointestinal disease and the difficulties can disrupt a child's progress along the typical developmental feeding continuum. Despite effective medical treatment, the residual effects on feeding can persist and need to be addressed. Collaboration regarding the medical, nutritional, and developmental plan of care optimizes outcomes for the well-being of children and families affected by this disease.

Over the past decade, eosinophilic esophagitis has become increasingly prevalent in the United States. One of the effective treatment approaches is dietary management, which aims to eliminate exposure to food allergens. Approaches to dietary management include the use of elemental diets, elimination diets, and tailored elimination diets, each of which poses potential nutrition risks. The benefits and potential downsides of each treatment are discussed in detail. Regardless of the diet therapy selected, a complete nutrition assessment by a registered dietitian with expertise in the management of food allergies is recommended for all patients diagnosed with eosinophilic esophagitis.

segments. EGIDs have multiple possible etiologies. Pathologists must avoid overdiagnosis of EGIDs by applying site-specific criteria for eosinophil density to mucosal biopsy specimens. Gastroenterologists must avoid contributing to overdiagnosis by submitting biopsy samples from each segment of the gastrointestinal tract separately, especially from the colon where the maximum mucosal eosinophil density in the right side normally exceeds that of the more distal colon. More studies of normal tissue and tissue from patients who are known or suspected to have EGIDs, with clinicopathologic correlations, are required to more fully define the spectrum of histopathology in EGIDs.

Eosinophilic gastrointestinal diseases (EGIDs) encompass a variety of disorders including eosinophilic esophagitis (EE), eosinophilic gastroenteritis (EG), and eosinophilic colitis. Although the pathogenesis of EGIDs is still poorly understood, dietary food antigens have been shown to cause EGIDs through several short-term clinical studies. The relationship of EGIDs with food allergy points to a potential breach of oral tolerance in EGIDs and to a potentially important role played by lymphocytes in responding to the oral food antigens. This article discusses the concept of oral tolerance, the available evidence for the role that lymphocytes play in the induction and pathogenesis of EGIDs, and the evidence for a potential breach in oral tolerance in EGIDs.

Primary eosinophilic gastrointestinal diseases (EGIDs) are a heterogeneous group of diseases including eosinophilic esophagitis, eosinophilic gastritis, eosinophilic gastroenteritis, eosinophilic enteritis, and eosinophilic colitis. The unifying hallmark and diagnostic marker of EGIDs is an eosinophil-rich inflammatory infiltrate of the GI mucosa, in the absence of known causes for eosinophilia. The etiology of EGIDs is not yet fully understood. The pathogenesis however seems to involve a complex interplay of genetic predisposition, exposure to food- and environmental allergens and IgE-mediated activation of the immune system. Accumulating evidence relates EGIDs to the group of T-helper (Th) 2 mediated immune disorders, like IgE-mediated allergy. In this article we discuss a possible role of IgE-mediated immune-activation via the high affinity receptor for IgE, FcεRI, in the pathogenesis of primary EGIDs. Beyond its defined role in type I allergic reactions, we here hypothesize that activation of tetrameric FcεRI on mast cells and basophils as well as trimeric FcεRI on human eosinophils and antigen presenting cells in the gastrointestinal mucosa is critically involved in the pathology of EGIDs. We also discuss how IgE-independent triggering of FcεRI could be a mechanisms responsible for activation of the immune system in patients with EGID.

Eosinophilic gastrointestinal diseases (EGIDs) are characterized by a wide variety of gastrointestinal symptoms that occur in conjunction with increased numbers of eosinophils in intestinal tissues. With the precise role or roles of eosinophils in gastrointestinal dysfunction incompletely understood, this subject remains an area of intense investigation. Most studies suggest that the intimate anatomic association of eosinophils with the intestinal epithelium implicates participation in the pathophysiology of EGIDs. This article reviews the limited evidence suggesting that the epithelium and eosinophils interact in the gastrointestinal tract and in other organ systems and describes how the epithelium and eosinophils might participate in gastrointestinal inflammatory diseases.

Pooja Varshney and A. Wesley Burks

Although the precise link is not completely understood, eosinophilic gastrointestinal diseases have been shown to be highly associated with atopy. Oral tolerance describes the specific suppression of immune responses to an antigen by prior administration of the antigen by the oral route. Like other allergic gastrointestinal diseases, eosinophilic gastrointestinal disorders may result from a loss of oral tolerance or a failure in the induction of tolerance. Further study to clarify the role of tolerance in the development of eosinophilic gastrointestinal diseases can help identify potential prevention strategies and therapeutic targets.

Barry K. Wershil

The mast cell plays a critical role in allergic responses in the gastrointestinal tract and other sites. Emerging evidence indicates that mast cells also participate in the pathogenesis of eosinophilic esophagitis, although their precise role has not been defined. This article reviews the biology of mast cells and examines the potential involvement of the cell as an effector of the inflammatory response and tissue remodeling, and as a cell that has the potential to function as an immunomodulator and limit inflammation.

Seema S. Aceves and Steven J. Ackerman

The clinical and pathologic features of eosinophilic esophagitis (EE) include extensive tissue remodeling. Increasing evidence supports a key role for the eosinophil in multiple aspects of the esophageal remodeling and fibrosis seen in this allergic disease. This article reviews the clinical implications of esophageal remodeling and fibrosis in EE and discusses the possible pathogenic mechanisms inducing and regulating these responses. The focus is specifically on eosinophil and cytokine interactions with the esophageal epithelium, vascular endothelium, resident fibroblasts, and smooth muscle. Current and potential therapeutic interventions are discussed that may impact the development or resolution of chronic esophageal remodeling and fibrosis in EE.

THE CLINICS ARE NOW AVAILABLE ONLINE!

Access your subscription at:
www.theclinics.com

Foreword

What Do Eosinophils Do in the Gastrointestinal Mucosa?

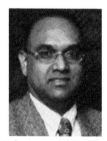

Rafeul Alam, MD, PhD
Consulting Editor

Low levels of eosinophils reside in the lower gastrointestinal (GI) mucosa. The physiologic relevance of this gut homing of eosinophils remains a mystery. The gut homing plays an important role in educating T cells for a specialized and well-tempered immune response to a multitude of food and microbial antigens that are present in the GI tract. Whether eosinophils undergo a similar training is unknown. Eosinophils clearly have the capacity to work as a team player with T cells in a variety of immunologic conditions. Eosinophils have been shown to selectively produce Th1 or Th2 cytokines, depending upon the prevailing immune response in the milieu. The role of eosinophils in defense against helminth infection is well known. Recent studies have demonstrated that eosinophils are involved in the defense against viruses and bacteria. Eosinophils are rich in RNAses and are therefore specially suited to fight RNA viruses. Eosinophils release microtraps of mitochondrial DNA when they encounter bacteria. The mitochondrial DNA has direct antibacterial effects. Thus, eosinophils possess a variety of tools and ammunition to defend the host and also to aid the other cells of the immune system. Why and when this host defense evolves into a host disease remains a daunting challenge.

Similar to allergic diseases, the incidence of eosinophilic disorders of the GI tract is on the rise. Is it all related to increased allergic sensitivity? What is the connection between food allergy and eosinophilic esophagitis? Why the esophagus, since most of the food absorption takes place in other parts of the GI tract? What is the relationship between respiratory allergy and eosinophilic esophagitis? To get answers to some of these questions, we have invited an allergist and a gastroenterologist to be coeditors for this issue. Drs. Fred Atkins and Glen Furuta are leaders in their respective fields.

Supported by NIH grants RO1 AI059719 and AI68088, PPG HL 36577, and N01 HHSN272200700048C.

doi:10.1016/j.iac.2008.11.001   immunology.theclinics.com

They have solicited an outstanding series of articles that address the basic and clinical science of eosinophilic gastrointestinal diseases. This is a timely and very important topic for allergy-immunology specialists and gastroenterologists.

Rafeul Alam, MD, PhD
Division of Allergy and Immunology
National Jewish Health
University of Colorado Denver Health Sciences Center
1400 Jackson Street
Denver, CO 80206, USA

E-mail address:
alamr@njc.org (R. Alam)

Preface

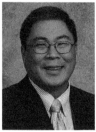 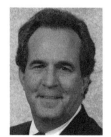

Glenn T. Furuta, MD   Dan Atkins, MD
Guest Editors

The emergence of eosinophilic esophagitis over the past decade as an increasingly recognized clinicopathologic entity has rekindled interest in a topic of common concern among allergists, immunologists, and gastroenterologists: namely, the roles of the eosinophil in gastrointestinal (GI) health and disease. This renewed interest has chemotaxed beyond the esophagus, which is normally devoid of eosinophils, to encompass the remainder of the GI tract, where varying numbers of eosinophils are normally encountered. This issue raises questions about when the presence of eosinophils should be considered pathologic and how best to evaluate, accurately diagnose, and manage this group of rarer disorders (eosinophilic gastritis, gastroenteritis, colitis) that present with common GI complaints. Although rarely life-threatening, the unpleasant myriad of symptoms and comorbid conditions associated with more distal eosinophilic GI diseases (EGIDs), in addition to their chronicity and complexity, extend beyond the gut, significantly reducing the quality of life of the affected patients and underscoring the need for a coordinated multidisciplinary approach to evaluation and long-term management. In fact, the opportunity to interact with and learn from our colleagues from different specialties is one of the rewards of working with patients who have these diseases. Thus, it is fitting that a gastroenterologist and allergist collaborate as coeditors of this issue, with articles contributed by a host of dedicated, experienced, and highly regarded allergists, gastroenterologists, pathologists, immunologists, basic scientists, dieticians, speech and occupational therapists, and psychosocial clinicians.

The intended goal of this issue is to provide a multilayered examination of the current state of knowledge that can serve as a reference for future discussions and research concerning EGIDs. Accordingly, this issue begins with articles that summarize a current approach to the evaluation and management of eosinophilic esophagitis (EoE) and a review of the potential pathogenic mechanisms involved. The remainder of the issue focuses on the less often encountered, but equally challenging, diseases associated with abnormal accumulations of eosinophils throughout the remainder of the GI tract. An approach to the evaluation and management of EGIDs is provided, along with articles that focus on the role of environmental influences and the association

Immunol Allergy Clin N Am 29 (2009) xix–xx
doi:10.1016/j.iac.2008.11.002
0889-8561/08/$ – see front matter

of these disorders with other allergic diseases. Additional articles discuss the features of feeding dysfunction observed in a subpopulation of affected children, nutritional issues requiring consideration, and the substantial psychosocial impact of these disorders. The remaining articles review the potential role of individual cells (eosinophils, lymphocytes, mast cells, and epithelial cells), receptors, and chemotactic factors in eosinophilic inflammation in the gut, while other articles explore the relationship between eosinophilic inflammation and fibrosis and the role of faulty oral tolerance in the development of EGIDs. An articles that discusses the biomarkers of allergic disease as they might pertain to the GI tract is included, as a means of monitoring disease other than by endoscopic procedures with biopsies is sorely needed.

As coeditors of this issue of *Immunology and Allergy Clinics of North America*, we feel especially privileged to be associated with the outstanding group of colleagues who authored these articles and remain indebted to them for their laudable efforts in bringing this issue to fruition. In addition, we remain indebted to our patients and their families who, through the sharing of their stories, continue to teach and encourage us to do more. As a result, we dedicate this issue to our patients for their courage, our colleagues for their efforts in promoting this field and, finally, to our families—Mary, Michael, Lauren, Henry and Ellie—for their unyielding love and support. Our combined hope is that this issue will serve as a catalyst for stimulating further interest in this area, leading to new observations, new insights, and, ultimately, more effective therapies or cures.

Glenn T. Furuta, MD
Gastrointestinal Eosinophilic Disease Program
National Jewish Health
The Children's Hospital Denver
13123 East 16th Avenue, Aurora, CO 80045, USA

Dan Atkins, MD
Department of Pediatrics
Division of Pediatric Allergy and Immunology
National Jewish Health
The Children's Hospital Denver
University of Colorado Denver School of Medicine
1400 Jackson Street
Denver, CO 80206, USA

E-mail addresses:
Furuta.Glenn@tchden.org (G.T. Furuta)
atkinsd@njc.org (D. Atkins)

Evaluation of the Child who has Eosinophilic Esophagitis

Philip E. Putnam, MD, FAAP

KEYWORDS

• Eosinophilic esophagitis • Pediatrics • Clinical evaluation

Children who have eosinophilic esophagitis (EoE) require comprehensive evaluation before treatment and ongoing assessment during treatment. When completed at the appropriate times and under well-controlled circumstances, investigation yields the correct diagnosis, assures recognition of sequelae or recurrence of the inflammation, or confirms whether therapy has been effective. Proper management of each child depends on compulsive follow-up until all of the therapeutic goals have been achieved and the child is on a stable regimen without esophageal inflammation. This article summarizes the issues facing the patient and the physician.

HISTORY AND PHYSICAL EXAMINATION

No universally applicable description of a child who has EoE exists and no features of the history uniformly permit the diagnosis to be made, because the main manifestations of EoE are otherwise nonspecific. As such, clinicians must include EoE in the differential diagnosis across the pediatric age range in light of a multitude of symptoms.

Pain, vomiting, and dysphagia are the most common symptoms of EoE in children. The primary complaint varies by age, as described by Noel and colleagues.[1,2] Feeding disorders, manifest as gagging, choking, and refusal, are among the most frequent presenting features of EoE in infants and toddlers. These symptoms can be manifestations of gastroesophageal reflux disease (GERD) at that age, so the clinician must be alert to the possibility of EoE, particularly when the symptoms fail to respond to appropriate antireflux therapy, or when the gastrointestinal symptoms are associated with eczema, overt food allergies, or reactive airways. Similarly, the onset of vomiting with the introduction of solids in the second half of the first year of life, especially in an atopic child, should raise concern for EoE or food allergy, rather than GERD. Vomiting and abdominal pain are more prominent presenting complaints in school-aged children who are diagnosed ultimately with EoE, but the symptoms are nonspecific and do not have characteristic features that distinguish EoE from other conditions.

Division of Pediatric Gastroenterology, Hepatology, and Nutrition, Cincinnati Children's Hospital Medical Center, 3333 Burnet Avenue, ML 2010, Cincinnati, OH 45229, USA
E-mail address: phil.putnam@cchmc.org

Immunol Allergy Clin N Am 29 (2009) 1–10
doi:10.1016/j.iac.2008.09.013
0889-8561/08/$ – see front matter © 2009 Elsevier Inc. All rights reserved.

Dysphagia tends to develop in early adolescence and is the predominant symptom reported by adults who have EoE.[1]

Although not diagnostic in and of itself at presentation, the history serves several major functions. It should be used to establish the present status of the child with regard to symptoms that could be attributable to esophageal inflammation; past and present medication use for the symptoms of interest (and their effectiveness); and diet; and to elicit symptoms that would be concerning for structural or nutritional complications of the disease (such as severe dysphagia or failure to gain weight). The history may also elicit the presence of symptoms that should arise only from gastrointestinal disease distal to the esophagus (eg, lower quadrant abdominal pain or diarrhea) or other systemic disease, which would then warrant additional investigation and consideration of an alternative diagnosis.

Two thirds of the children who have EoE have a history of asthma, eczema, food allergies, environmental allergies, or chronic rhinitis.[3,4] As a result of the food allergy or eczema, many of these children have undergone extensive revision of their diet before presentation. Understanding how the patient arrived at his/her present diet requires tabulating those foods which caused an overt adverse reaction, along with the nature of the reaction the antigen elicits, and the timing of the response after ingestion. Prior to diagnosis, food antigen elimination based on symptoms of obvious immediate hypersensitivity (eg, hives) or consistent adverse response (eg, vomiting) is common. Other foods may have been empirically eliminated, not because the patient experienced symptoms from that food consistently, but because the child's symptoms generally were thought to be of an allergic nature and because that food is among the foods to which adverse reactions are common (eg, cow milk). Foods may also have been eliminated inappropriately because of misinterpretation of symptoms that were inconsistently present after ingestion, or because of symptoms that did not have an immunologic basis (eg, osmotic diarrhea after apple juice).

For patients already on an elimination diet, great care must be taken to understand the duration and degree of compulsion with which the elimination is maintained by the child and the family. Clues that a diet is being compulsively controlled include a precise list of foods that are avoided and ingested that the parent (and child) can recite, evidence for educated label reading by the primary shopper/meal preparer, avoidance of eating out (or having questioned the wait staff and chef at a select restaurant for information before ordering), and careful control of the available food when a child is not under the direct observation of the parent (eg, at school or with relatives or friends). In the absence of the preceding, one must be wary that the diet is not well controlled. Additional clues that a diet is probably not being adhered to include statements like, "We try to limit food X," or, "He really doesn't eat it, he just chews it up and spits it out;" the presence of a sympathetic parent/sibling/grandparent who "just lets him/her have a little once in a while;" and any school-aged child who cannot list the foods he/she is supposed to avoid.

Nutritional assessment is also a crucial part of the evaluation of children who have EoE at presentation and during treatment. Normal progression of linear growth and weight gain must be maintained or restored for children who have allergic gastrointestinal disease, including EoE. Planned and empiric dietary antigen eliminations may conflict with the need to provide balanced, complete nutrition. Severe dietary restrictions pose significant risk for protein-calorie or micronutrient inadequacy if a supplement is not offered and accepted. Similarly, after diagnosis, dietary antigen elimination based on allergy testing can preclude adequate nutrition when many nutritionally important foods are removed from the diet simultaneously, unless support is provided. It is essential to have an evaluation by a dietician who has expertise in evaluating the quality of the existing diet, and who can suggest alternatives that are antigen specific to avoid contamination of the diet by foods that would promote recurrent or persistent esophagitis.

PHYSICAL EXAMINATION

No known abnormalities on physical examination establish a diagnosis of EoE, but associated findings such as atopic dermatitis, rhinitis, allergic shiners, and reactive airways in a child who has suspicious gastrointestinal symptoms should promote a careful search for EoE.

EOSINOPHILS IN THE ESOPHAGUS: ENDOSCOPIC AND HISTOLOGIC DIAGNOSIS

The diagnosis of EoE remains the responsibility of the gastrointestinal endoscopist and the pathologist because confirmatory endoscopic biopsies from esophageal mucosa are still the only means of establishing the diagnosis and assessing the effectiveness of treatment. A minimum criterion for the pathologist is at least 15 eosinophils/high-power field in an affected area. This consensus criterion was developed during the First International Gastrointestinal Eosinophil Research Symposium (FIGERS) and allows the pathologist to make a histologic diagnosis when sufficient mucosal eosinophilia exists, although the clinical diagnosis requires additional features to be present, as will be discussed later.[5] Basal cell layer expansion (measured as a proportion of the epithelial thickness) is a frequent finding in EoE, but the lack of it does not preclude the diagnosis.

The normal esophageal mucosa is devoid of eosinophils. Unfortunately, eosinophils participate with neutrophils, lymphocytes, or mast cells in various inflammatory conditions, making the presence of eosinophils necessary, but not sufficient, for a clinical diagnosis of EoE. Acid-induced esophagitis as a manifestation of GERD is the most frequent confounding diagnosis because reflux esophagitis may coexist with clinical EoE or mimic it histologically on hematoxylin- and eosin-stained sections.[6] Few mast cells are present in reflux esophagitis, which may help in discriminating reflux esophagitis from EoE at presentation if special stains are applied to identify them because they are not distinguishable on hematoxylin- and eosin-stained sections.[7]

Because the range of eosinophil numbers in GERD and EoE varies considerably, the potential exists for esophagitis with more than 15 eosinophils/high-power field in the esophageal mucosa to respond completely to antireflux therapy. In that setting, the clinical diagnosis is therefore "GERD with reflux esophagitis," despite the appropriate histologic diagnosis of EoE. The number of eosinophils in reflux esophagitis is typically fewer than 7/high-power field,[6] but recent reports of children who have large numbers of eosinophils consistent with EoE that responded to antireflux therapy compels us to be careful in assigning a clinical diagnosis only when additional information supports the diagnosis.[8]

The issue is further confounded by the presence of eosinophils in the inflammatory infiltrate in other conditions, such as Crohn's disease, celiac disease (concurrent with EoE), and infections.[9] The correct clinical diagnosis in each case requires thoughtful evaluation taking into consideration the other conditions.

The clinical circumstances at the time of the biopsy are critical to interpretation of the result. Biopsies obtained after 2 months of twice-daily PPI that still have active eosinophilic inflammation establish the diagnosis of EoE.[5] After the esophagitis has come under control, subsequent biopsies taken after food challenge or after a change in pharmacotherapy determine the adequacy of therapy and direct future treatment.

ESOPHAGEAL HISTOLOGY

Endoscopic biopsies are small fragments of tissue that are often not placed on the slide correctly for true cross-sectional analysis. Morphometry can be challenging at the least and impossible at times. Even the counting of eosinophils can be problematic. Because they often layer just under the luminal surface of the esophagus in EoE, the number may be underestimated from a poorly oriented section in which the immediate subluminal area is off the slide.

The eosinophilia in EoE can be remarkably patchy, particularly during treatment. It is not unusual to have an abnormal biopsy specimen taken millimeters from another specimen that is completely normal. Studies in adults who have EoE have established that six biopsies from the esophagus assure diagnosis.[10] Taking fewer biopsies risks missing the diagnosis because of sampling error.

Up to 30% of individuals who have histologic EoE have endoscopically normal mucosa, making histology the only reliable diagnostic criterion.[3] Nevertheless, one series of endoscopic findings should alert the endoscopist that EoE is a likely diagnosis. Longitudinal furrowing or vertical lines along the length of the esophagus, thickening of the mucosa resulting in loss of translucency and the ability to see the submucosal vessels, and exudate (visible as small adherent white specks) are common endoscopic findings in children who have EoE.[5] Long-standing disease tends to create a ringed appearance, which is more common in the adult population who have EoE. In addition, strictures, diffuse narrowing (so-called "small-caliber esophagus"), and remarkable friability of the epithelium such that it tears longitudinally just with passage of the scope (tissue paper mucosa) can be features of EoE.

LABORATORY EVALUATION

At this time, laboratory evaluation does not offer testing on which to make a diagnosis of EoE. Mild peripheral eosinophilia is present in fewer than one half of children who have EoE, and is nonspecific. To date, no other biomarkers have proved to have sufficient positive and negative predictive value either to be used as initial screening or to monitor patients over time during treatment. Correlations between various blood and tissue cytokines have been investigated and, although statistical correlations have been demonstrated, the correlation is not strong enough to supplant histology.[11–13] As such, no current recommendation exists for routine screening of patients for biomarkers related to EoE.

ALLERGY EVALUATION

Allergy evaluation is important for children who have EoE but by itself does not offer insight into the presence or absence of eosinophilic inflammation in the esophagus. Once the diagnosis has been confirmed histologically, food allergy testing to discover evidence of adverse immune responsiveness to particular foods has been used to identify potentially offending foods as objectively as possible.[5,14,15] Standard skin prick testing has been performed most commonly, and skin patch testing has also been promoted. The results of CAP-FEIA to foods have not correlated well enough with the histologic result of antigen elimination to use those tests on a routine basis to guide diet changes. Unfortunately, the positive and negative predictive value of skin prick and skin patch testing is also less than perfect for individual foods. As such, clinical response (symptoms) and histologically proved recurrent esophagitis on ingestion are still the only reliable indicators of reaction to a particular food.

Nevertheless, allergy skin testing provides a rough guide on which to base the initial elimination of selected foods in response to a positive result. Whether a single positive skin test is clinically a false-positive test awaits actual ingestion of the food as a trial. When the esophagitis is active and the intention is to manage the child by eliminating food antigens, all offending foods must be removed simultaneously because the esophagitis will persist even if one offending food remains in the diet.

RADIOGRAPHY AND MANOMETRY IN EOSINOPHILIC ESOPHAGITIS

Barium esophagogram may identify radiographic evidence of esophageal abnormalities that result from EoE. Narrow-caliber esophagus, stricture, Schatzki ring, or the rippled appearance of the concentric rings in the "trachealized" esophagus may be evident, although confirmation of the diagnosis will still rest on histologic evidence of eosinophil-predominant inflammation. Only selected patients will warrant this radiographic evaluation (eg, when the history of dysphagia is concerning for an anatomic obstruction) because it is valuable to have the radiographic images before endoscopy.

Case series reporting the results of esophageal manometry in adult patients who have EoE provide insight into the nature of the dysmotility that leads to dysphagia, but manometry is not indicated in the routine evaluation of patients who have EoE.[16] Similarly, endoscopic ultrasound has been performed in children who have EoE and demonstrates panmural thickening that is not otherwise evident by routine endoscopy, but it is not required for the evaluation of otherwise uncomplicated children who have EoE.[17]

THERAPEUTIC TRIAL: ELEMENTAL DIET

Total dietary antigen elimination (ie, the use of an amino acid–based formula to provide total diet replacement with a nonallergenic formula) is often used as a therapeutic trial to determine whether dietary antigens are solely responsible for initiating the esophagitis. It is also used in highly allergic children who have adverse reactions to a plethora of dietary substances and for whom an elimination diet is inadequate (either nutritionally or because of persistent EoE).[3,18,19] If the esophagitis resolves when all dietary antigens are eliminated, confirming that food antigen exposure was responsible for triggering the immune response leading to the esophagitis, sequential reintroduction of dietary antigens with interval endoscopic follow-up effectively establishes the safety of individual foods for that child. Nutritional support from the formula is necessary until an adequate diet has been established and confirmed to not cause recurrent esophagitis.

At the same time, if the esophagitis does not resolve with compulsive and exclusive use of an amino acid–based formula, the child's EoE phenotype is further clarified as having some other, as yet unidentified, factor generating the esophagitis. Failure of the esophagitis to respond to an elemental diet does not exclude food antigens as triggers, but establishes, at a minimum, that something besides food also promotes eosinophilic inflammation.

An amino acid–based formula is also used to augment nutritional intake for a child on a restricted diet that would not otherwise offer adequate nutrition for growth and development. Because cow and soy milk proteins are frequent contributors to EoE, transition to more traditional (and less expensive and more palatable) milk- or soy-based formula is only possible when the child is tolerant of them. Although it may seem illogical to have a child on an elemental formula plus solid food, it is often the case that the available alternatives to cow and soy milk (such as rice milk) are nutritionally inadequate or offer offending antigens that cause the esophagitis to flare, so that an elemental formula is the only means of broadly augmenting the nutritional quality of the diet, at least temporarily.

EVALUATION DURING TREATMENT

The goals of therapy are to control symptoms, normalize the histology, and prevent complications from untreated inflammation. The ideal approach for each child who has active, food-allergic, EoE would be the immediate withdrawal of all offending foods simultaneously, while assuring perfect nutrition for normal growth and development. The success of this "directed elimination diet" would depend on a perfect ability to test each affected child in a manner that identifies each offending food antigen without false-negative or false-positive results to every relevant antigen in the diet. It would also require that the remaining available foods would provide complete and balanced nutrition, and that the child would consume those alternate foods. Unfortunately, clinical experience suggests that no therapy for EoE is universally successful or universally acceptable, skin testing is imperfect, and patient compliance varies.

An alternative to dietary antigen elimination is the use of "topical" steroids (fluticasone or budesonide) as primary, secondary, or adjunctive treatment of EoE. Fluticasone is delivered from a metered dose inhaler into the mouth without inhaling (and without an aerochamber) and swallowed. Budesonide, on the other hand, is administered from a spoon after the contents of a vial (originally intended for use in a nebulizer but which can be taken orally) are mixed with an artificial sweetener to increase the viscosity and presumably slow transit over the esophageal lining for local anti-inflammatory effect.[20] These medications are popular because of the limited side effects, ease of administration, and the notion that they impact less on quality of life than does a severely restricted diet. However, they are not always effective, particularly in children who have food antigen–driven EoE who are still ingesting offending foods.[21,22]

TREATMENT APPROACHES AND DECISION MAKING

Once the clinical diagnosis of EoE is established, the options for therapy are reviewed with the patient and family. The algorithm shown in **Fig. 1** displays the author's schema for patient management. The decision as to which path to take after diagnosis rests heavily on the history and allergy evaluation, and should be devised in a fashion that does not repeat prior failed therapies and that will be most accepted by the patient, thereby increasing the likelihood of compliance.

Repeat endoscopy at the appropriate interval is needed to determine whether or not the inflammation has completely abated, irrespective of the therapy initiated. Symptoms can resolve in 2 to 4 weeks, regardless of the type of treatment, but are an unreliable measure of inflammation because the absence of symptoms does not assure the absence of histologic inflammation.[23] Histologic response to topical steroids is generally complete in 4 to 12 weeks. Histologic response to dietary antigen elimination can be seen in 4 to 8 weeks but is remarkably variable, having taken more than 4 months in some individuals. Evidence-based guidelines as to the frequency of follow-up endoscopy have not been published, and clinical practice varies. The author's practice is to repeat the endoscopy 12 weeks after any diet or medication change, which allows ample time for as complete a response to develop as possible. Incomplete responses are difficult to interpret and often require extension of the trial and another endoscopy to comprehend the impact of therapy fully before making changes.

Successful therapy does result in complete resolution of the inflammation. Partial responses are recognized, at which time a judgment must be made as to the necessity of more aggressive or alternative therapy (and often, better compliance), which depends on the degree of remaining inflammation. In the author's practice, resolution

Treatment Flow for EE Patients at the CCED

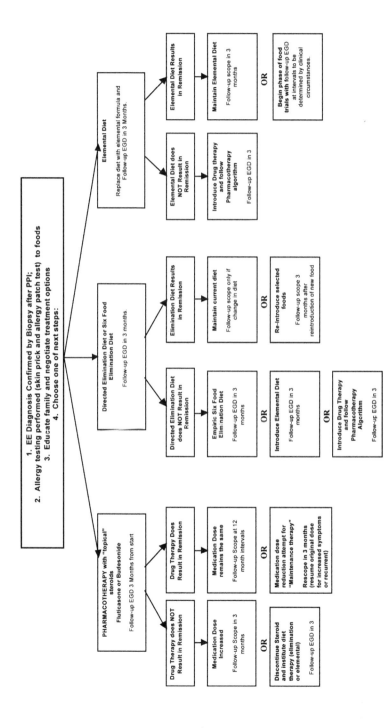

Fig. 1. The scheme followed by the multidisciplinary team within the Cincinnati Center for Eosinophilic Disorders for the management of children who have EoE. EGD, esophagogastroduodenoscopy.

of basal cell layer hyperplasia and a minimal or patchy residual eosinophilia (2–6 eosinophils/high-power field) without symptoms or lamina propria fibrosis is considered acceptable control, although that view is admittedly unencumbered by data.

The time from diagnosis to stable therapy is variable for children who have EoE and depends on many factors. To date, an evidence-based recommendation for follow-up once an effective dose of medication has been proved has not been publicly recommended. In the authors' clinical practice, yearly endoscopy in children on a maintenance dose of topical steroid has been enlightening. Otherwise unsuspected recurrent esophagitis due to noncompliance or inadequate dose due to growth has been observed. Occasional yeast infections have also been discovered.

Children managed with dietary elimination typically undergo several endoscopies in the process of identifying those foods which cause an adverse histologic response. From an elemental diet to a final stable diet, the number of endoscopies is variable, depending on the number of foods attempted and the success rate. As is the case for pharmacotherapy, no formal recommendation exists for periodic surveillance in children who have arrived at a stable elimination diet, but issues of compliance with ongoing restrictions and the development of esophagitis in response to previously tolerated foods have been concerns.

Because EoE is a chronic disease, recurrent esophagitis has been nearly uniform among patients when either therapy (ie, topical steroids or dietary antigen elimination) is withdrawn.[3] Cessation of topical steroid therapy or resumption of offending food antigens has led to either return of symptoms or active histologic esophagitis, or both. Occasional patients who have the food allergies have ultimately developed tolerance and have been able to resume all foods without recurrent disease, but the number of patients so described is small.[3] As such, after any change in diet or medication, careful endoscopic re-evaluation of children is necessary to assess the impact of the change and direct future therapy.

Chronic active EoE is associated with tissue remodeling manifest as deposition of dense collagen in the lamina propria, risking the development of small-caliber esophagus and strictures, both of which have been observed as consequences of EoE in children and adults.[24–27] Assuring that esophageal histology has returned to normal is an essential part of the management of each child, to prevent further injury to the esophagus.

SUMMARY

EoE is a chronic inflammatory condition with symptoms mimicking other esophageal disorders. In children, it is most often a manifestation of adverse immune response to dietary constituents, and can be managed by avoidance of those antigens that elicit the response. After GERD has been excluded, clinical evaluation by history, formal and thorough food allergy testing, and endoscopic biopsies are necessary to establish the diagnosis. Endoscopic re-evaluation after diet or medication change determines whether a specific therapy has achieved a complete histologic response and forms the basis for future management, with the goal of maintaining clinical and histologic remission to avoid long-term complications such as esophageal stricture formation.

REFERENCES

1. Noel RJ, Putnam PE, Rothenberg ME. Eosinophilic esophagitis. N Engl J Med 2004;351(9):940–1.
2. Pentiuk SP, Miller CK, Kaul A. Eosinophilic esophagitis in infants and toddlers. Dysphagia 2007;22(1):44–8.

3. Liacouras CA, Spergel JM, Ruchelli E, et al. Eosinophilic esophagitis: a 10-year experience in 381 children. Clin Gastroenterol Hepatol 2005;3(12):1198–206.
4. Assa'ad AH, Putnam PE, Collins MH, et al. Pediatric patients with eosinophilic esophagitis: an 8-year follow-up. J Allergy Clin Immunol 2007;119(3):731–8.
5. Furuta GT, Liacouras CA, Collins MH, et al. Eosinophilic esophagitis in children and adults: a systematic review and consensus recommendations for diagnosis and treatment; First International Gastrointestinal Eosinophil Research Symposium (FIGERS) Subcommittees. Gastroenterology 2007;133(4):1342–63.
6. Ruchelli E, Wenner W, Voytek T, Brown K, Liacouras. Severity of esophageal eosinophilia predicts response to conventional gastroesophageal reflux therapy. Pediatr Dev Pathol 1999;2(1):15–8.
7. Kirsch R, Bokhary R, Marcon MA, et al. Activated mucosal mast cells differentiate eosinophilic (allergic) esophagitis from gastroesophageal reflux disease. J Pediatr Gastroenterol Nutr 2007;44(1):20–6.
8. Ngo P, Furuta GT, Antonioli DA, et al. Eosinophils in the esophagus–peptic or allergic eosinophilic esophagitis? Case series of three patients with esophageal eosinophilia. Am J Gastroenterol 2006;101(7):1666–70.
9. Ooi CY, Day AS, Jackson R, et al. Eosinophilic esophagitis in children with celiac disease. J Gastroenterol Hepatol 2007 Dec 5, Epub ahead of print.
10. Gonsalves N, Policarpio-Nicolas M, Zhang Q, et al. Histopathologic variability and endoscopic correlates in adults with eosinophilic esophagitis. Gastrointest Endosc 2006;64(3):313–9.
11. Konikoff MR, Blanchard C, Kirby C, et al. Potential of blood eosinophils, eosinophil-derived neurotoxin, and eotaxin-3 as biomarkers of eosinophilic esophagitis. Clin Gastroenterol Hepatol 2006;4(11):1328–36, Epub 2006 Oct 23.
12. Gupta SK, Fitzgerald JF, Kondratyuk T, et al. Cytokine expression in normal and inflamed esophageal mucosa: a study into the pathogenesis of allergic eosinophilic esophagitis. J Pediatr Gastroenterol Nutr 2006;42(1):22–6.
13. Straumann A, Kristl J, Conus S, et al. Cytokine expression in healthy and inflamed mucosa: probing the role of eosinophils in the digestive tract. Inflamm Bowel Dis 2005;11(8):720–6.
14. Spergel JM, Andrews T, Brown-Whitehorn TF, et al. Treatment of eosinophilic esophagitis with specific food elimination diet directed by a combination of skin prick and patch tests. Ann Allergy Asthma Immunol 2005;95(4):336–43.
15. Spergel JM, Brown-Whitehorn T, Beausoleil JL, et al. Predictive values for skin prick test and atopy patch test for eosinophilic esophagitis. J Allergy Clin Immunol 2007;119(2):509–11.
16. Lucendo AJ, Pascual-Turrión JM, Navarro M, et al. Endoscopic, bioptic, and manometric findings in eosinophilic esophagitis before and after steroid therapy: a case series. Endoscopy 2007;39(9):765–71.
17. Fox VL, Nurko S, Teitelbaum JE, et al. High-resolution EUS in children with eosinophilic "allergic" esophagitis. Gastrointest Endosc 2003;57(1):30–6.
18. Markowitz JE, Spergel JM, Ruchelli E, et al. Elemental diet is an effective treatment for eosinophilic esophagitis in children and adolescents. Am J Gastroenterol 2003;98(4):777–82.
19. Kelly KJ, Lazenby AJ, Rowe PC, et al. Eosinophilic esophagitis attributed to gastroesophageal reflux: improvement with an amino acid-based formula. Gastroenterology 1995;109(5):1503–12.
20. Aceves SS, Bastian JF, Newbury RO, et al. Oral viscous budesonide: a potential new therapy for eosinophilic esophagitis in children. Am J Gastroenterol 2007; 102(10):2271–9.

21. Konikoff MR, Noel RJ, Blanchard C, et al. A randomized, double-blind, placebo-controlled trial of fluticasone propionate for pediatric eosinophilic esophagitis. Gastroenterology 2006;131(5):1629–31.
22. Noel RJ, Putnam PE, Collins MH, et al. Clinical and immunopathologic effects of swallowed fluticasone for eosinophilic esophagitis. Clin Gastroenterol Hepatol 2004;2(7):568–75.
23. Pentiuk SP, Putnam PE, Collins MH, et al. Dissociation between symptoms and histological severity in pediatric eosinophilic esophagitis. J Pediatr Gastroenterol Nutr, in press.
24. Khan S, Orenstein SR, Di Lorenzo C, et al. Eosinophilic esophagitis: strictures, impactions, dysphagia. Dig Dis Sci 2003;48(1):22–9.
25. Vasilopoulos S, Murphy P, Auerbach A, et al. The small-caliber esophagus: an unappreciated cause of dysphagia for solids in patients with eosinophilic esophagitis. Gastrointest Endosc 2002;55(1):99–106.
26. Aceves SS, Newbury RO, Dohil R, et al. Esophageal remodeling in pediatric eosinophilic esophagitis. J Allergy Clin Immunol 2007;119(1):206–12.
27. Cohen MS, Kaufman AB, Palazzo JP, et al. An audit of endoscopic complications in adult eosinophilic esophagitis. Clin Gastroenterol Hepatol 2007;5(10):1149–53.

Clinical Evaluation of the Adult who has Eosinophilic Esophagitis

Alex Straumann, MD

KEYWORDS

- Eosinophilic esophagitis • Physical examination
- Laboratory abnormalities • Endoscopic signs
- Histologic findings

Eosinophilic esophagitis (EoE) may affect individuals at any age, and similar genotypic abnormalities are found in children and in adults, thereby indicating that the disorder is one single entity. However, some phenotypic manifestations of EoE are highly age dependent and justify a different management. The clinical evaluation of adult patients who have EoE entails the exceptional feature that treating physicians typically encounter apparently healthy individuals.[1] EoE cannot be described as an overt disease, nor is it, except for episodic complications, spectacular or dramatic. This characteristic is firstly due to the anatomic location of the esophagus, hidden deep within the chest cavity and, secondly, because in adults, EoE rarely evokes systemic effects, such as fatigue, fever, wasting, or severe pain. This presentation contrasts sharply with pediatric EoE, whereby general symptoms, such as food refusal, failure to thrive, and pain, alert family members and physicians early during the course of the disease.[2,3] This unimpressive adult presentation may explain the fact that after symptoms commence in the adult, some 4 to 5 years usually pass before EoE is finally diagnosed.[4] Nevertheless, gastroenterologists are familiar with this pattern of clinical appearance from other chronic gastrointestinal inflammatory diseases (eg, Crohn's disease or microscopic colitis). Despite the absence of a dramatic appearance, EoE is a relevant burden for most affected individuals, substantially impairing the patient's quality of life[5] and associated with several relevant risks.[6–9]

In summary, the clinical evaluation of an adult patient who has suspected EoE requires a deep probing into the issue, firstly, by taking a thorough medical and family history and secondly, by using invasive examinations, even beyond the frontiers of the endoscope, using histologic and immunohistologic methods.

Department of Gastroenterology, Kantonsspital Olten, Roemerstrasse 7, CH-4600 Olten, Switzerland
E-mail address: alex.straumann@hin.ch

Immunol Allergy Clin N Am 29 (2009) 11–18
doi:10.1016/j.iac.2008.09.007   immunology.theclinics.com
0889-8561/08/$ – see front matter © 2009 Elsevier Inc. All rights reserved.

DEFINITION

EoE is defined in adults, adolescents, and children as a clinicopathologic disease characterized by upper intestinal symptoms and dense esophageal eosinophilia, both of which persist despite prolonged treatment with proton pump inhibitors (PPI). Eosinophilic inflammation is absent in the stomach, small intestine, and colon.[1] The diagnosis of EoE is not based on one single marker (eg, number of eosinophils in the esophagus), but rather, on several clinical and pathologic features. This comprehensive definition is the guideline for the diagnostic work-up and for the choice of the diagnostic procedures in a patient who has suspected EoE.

EPIDEMIOLOGIC FEATURES AND DEMOGRAPHIC CHARACTERISTICS

Previously considered a rare curiosity, the startling prevalence of adult EoE has reached almost epidemic proportions. One prospective long-term study performed in Switzerland showed that the prevalence of adult EoE increased during a 19-year period from an initial 2, to a final 43, patients per 100,000 inhabitants. These data illustrate that EoE is indeed of general relevance because about 1 individual in 2500 is affected. In addition, the actual incidence in this area is 2.39 newly diagnosed cases per 100,000 inhabitants per year[10] (personal experience). But is this a true rise in the incidence or simply an increased awareness of the disease? Because this study was conducted in a demographically stable, well-defined indicator area, under population-based conditions and unchanged recording practices, the data likely reflect an actual increase in EoE cases, and not just an enhanced awareness of the disease.

EoE shows a strong predilection for the male gender; among the reported cases, more than 70% involve men.[11] In a national database analysis, Katzka and colleagues[11] demonstrated that EoE occurs in all age groups; their patients ranged in age from 1 to 98 years, but the disease tended to peak in the fifth decade of life.

PRESENTING SYMPTOMS IN ADULTS WHO HAVE EOSINOPHILIC ESOPHAGITIS

Important clues can be found by taking a careful history that focuses on esophageal-related and upper abdominal symptoms, atopic diseases, and family history of both. As in many other diseases, the presenting symptoms have age-related differences. In contrast to children who experience food refusal, failure to thrive, and pain, EoE in adolescents and adults causes a rather narrow spectrum of symptoms, with the typical complaint being dysphagia for solids.[12,13] In some patients, difficulty with swallowing occurs occasionally and then increases over time, whereas others report an abrupt onset of symptoms. Patients can often locate precisely the critical, most affected segment of the esophagus. In general, symptoms are more prominent and the swallowing disturbances more pronounced when the ingested food's consistency is dry or rough, or when the patient eats quickly. The dependency of the dysphagia on the food consistency indicates a probable mechanical problem with bolus transport through the affected esophagus, and not an immediate allergic reaction or spasm induced by the release of eosinophil granule proteins.

During the course of the disease, more than one third of untreated patients who have EoE will experience long-lasting food impaction that will require endoscopic bolus removal.[9] In a recent report from a private practice setting, Desai[14] found that 17 of 31 (55%) adults presenting with food impaction were found to have EoE. EoE is most likely the leading cause of food impaction, at least in younger male patients.

A few patients experience retrosternal pain that is either spontaneously occurring, or induced by ingesting alcohol (eg, white wine) or acidic liquids (eg, orange juice) (author's personal experience). EoE retrosternal pain more closely resembles that described for vigorous achalasia than for gastroesophageal reflux disease (GERD): it is neither ascending nor related to reflux of acidic or gastric contents. Typical GERD symptoms may appear during the long-term course of EoE as a result of the insufficient lower esophageal sphincter (LES) evoked by the chronic inflammation.[15] Many adults have symptoms, including recurrent food impactions, for years (an average of 4 to 5) before a diagnosis of EoE is finally made.[4]

More than 70% of adults who have EoE have a history of atopic disease, mainly allergic diseases of the airways, such as seasonal rhinoconjunctivitis and asthma.[1] Finally, a family history may provide further information: Noel and coworkers[16] found that in their series of 103 patients who had EoE, 73.5% had a positive family history for atopic diseases and 6.8% for EoE, and 9.7% had undergone esophageal dilation.

PHYSICAL EXAMINATION

In contrast to the conspicuous medical history, the physical examination of adult patients who have EoE is usually unremarkable[1] because of the anatomic inaccessibility of the esophagus during the physical examination and because EoE in adults seldom provokes systemic manifestations.

LABORATORY ANALYSES

Laboratory analyses of a patient who has EoE have no more than a complementary value. Unfortunately, we still do not have reliable, noninvasive markers, either for establishing the diagnosis or for monitoring the disease.[1] However, two routine laboratory methods may prove informative: Between 5% and 50% of adults who have EoE have a mild eosinophilia on their differential blood count,[17] although values seldom exceed 1500 eosinophils /mm^3. A differential blood count may therefore provide supporting evidence for the presence of EoE, but it is by no means diagnostic. Whether the degree of the eosinophilia correlates with the disease activity is not yet elucidated. Furthermore, approximately 70% of patients who have EoE have elevated total IgE values.[1,17] To date, no studies have been able to document whether total IgE can serve as a surrogate marker for disease progression or resolution, but some evidence indicates that, when compared with patients having normal levels, those who have high total IgE levels respond less well to corticosteroid treatment.[18]

ENDOSCOPIC FINDINGS

Although neither a pathognomonic endoscopic sign nor a typical pattern of abnormalities is associated with EoE, upper endoscopy is the first diagnostic step in the evaluation of an individual who has dysphagia.[19] Many different endoscopic features are associated with EoE, the leading ones being longitudinal furrowing, white exudates, edema, longitudinal shearing, friability, crêpe paper mucosa, small-caliber esophagus, Schatzki ring, corrugated or ringed esophagus, and solitary rings.[15] These signs usually appear in random combination in any given patient.[20] White exudates and longitudinal furrowing likely reflect acute inflammation, whereas crêpe-paper mucosa, corrugated rings, and strictures are likely a consequence of the chronic eosinophilic inflammation. All these signs are suggestive of the diagnosis of EoE, but the endoscopic suspicion requires histologic confirmation. Some early studies report normal-appearing mucosa in EoE.[12] However, as experience is gained in endoscopic identification of EoE, more endoscopists will be able to identify those subtle mucosal changes that were likely overlooked previously.

HISTOLOGIC FEATURES AND DIAGNOSTIC CRITERIA

Considering EoE as a clinicopathologic entity and according to its definition, diagnosis requires histologic confirmation: the esophageal biopsy shows a marked eosinophilic infiltration.[1] Under healthy conditions, the human esophagus is devoid of eosinophils.[21,22] Despite the fact that an eosinophilic infiltration of the esophagus is a nonspecific sign that can be found in several other conditions,[23] finding a relevant number of eosinophils in the esophageal mucosa is highly suspicious for EoE. Experts still dispute the precise density of eosinophils required to confirm the diagnosis[24] because the infiltration seen in EoE is of a patchy nature and may even fluctuate during the course of the disease. Using an arithmetic model, Gonsalves and colleagues[25] have demonstrated that the selected threshold value (peak number of eosinophils per high-power field) and the number of biopsies taken for analysis determine the sensitivity of the combined "endoscopy–histology" method. Today, most experts agree that diagnosis of EoE can be established if a peak infiltration of at least 15 eosinophils per high-power field is found in combination with other subsidiary histologic findings and typical symptoms.[1] The additional histologic abnormalities suggestive for EoE include eosinophilic microabscesses, superficial layering, basal zone hyperplasia, and increased papillary size.[1] EoE exclusively involves the esophagus; gastric and duodenal biopsies are normal.

NATURAL HISTORY AND COMPLICATIONS OF EOSINOPHILIC ESOPHAGITIS

Despite the fact that our understanding of the natural history of EoE is still limited, it has become clear that this is a chronic disease whose course may be either chronic persistent or chronic relapsing.[5] So far, no case of EoE with a superimposed premalignant condition or with a malignancy has been reported, but long-term follow-up is required to confirm this observation. The main concern is that a long-standing, untreated eosinophilic inflammation would evoke irreversible structural alterations of the esophagus, leading to fibrosis and angiogenesis, and result in thickening of the wall with abnormal fragility.[5,26] Strictures are rarely reported in children, suggesting that this complication requires years of unbridled eosinophilic inflammation.[3] This so-called "esophageal remodeling" may provoke several complications.

Acute food impactions are the leading complication of untreated EoE. Indeed, EoE was diagnosed in about 60% of adult patients referred for a diagnostic work-up of food impaction.[14] During the course of their disease, more than one third of adult patients will experience long-lasting food impactions that require endoscopic removal.[9] The risk for impaction depends primarily on the consistency of the food, and particularly problematic are dry rice and fibrous meat (eg, chicken or beef). This extremely disagreeable and frightening form of dysphagia is a sword of Damocles hanging permanently over almost all patients who have EoE. Food impactions are often the trigger for patients to consult a physician to perform a diagnostic work-up of long-lasting dysphagia. These unforeseeable events harbor several risks, such as retching-induced esophageal rupture (Boerhaave syndrome) or procedure-related perforation,[9] which has the practical consequence that, in patients who have a long history of dysphagia, invasive procedures (eg, removal of impacted food or dilations) must be performed most delicately.

In addition to the leading symptom of "dysphagia," typical reflux symptoms that respond to pharmacologic acid suppression may appear during the long-term course of EoE. In their case series, Remedios and colleagues[15] found that among 26 adult patients who had EoE, 10 (38%) had coexisting reflux disease previously confirmed by pH monitoring. Furthermore, based on motility studies, the investigators found that 8 of the 10 patients with coexisting reflux also had a reduced pressure in the LES. These findings suggest that, in EoE, the chronic inflammation can lead to an LES dysfunction, and thus to a clinically relevant, secondary reflux disease. However, our knowledge of the natural history of EoE is still fragmentary and further studies are urgently needed. Finally, it is only with a precise understanding of the natural course of a disease, including its inherent complications, that an informed decision for possible therapeutic interventions can be made. The natural course of EoE still awaits cracking.

THERAPEUTIC PRINCIPLES FOR ADULTS WHO HAVE EOSINOPHILIC ESOPHAGITIS

At least three reasons exist to treat an adult patient presenting with clinically and histologically confirmed active EoE: (1) to alleviate the diminished quality of life that the dysphagia evokes; (2) to prevent acute food impactions and their associated risks; and (3) to protect the esophagus from long-term sequelae. Nevertheless, just what the optimal treatment is for EoE has yet to be defined, and experience has been limited mostly to case series and small controlled trials.[18,27] In adult patients who have EoE, topical and systemic corticosteroids, leukotriene receptor antagonists, immunomodulators, and dilation have proven efficacy, and PPI can reduce the often-present GERD-like symptoms,[1] whereas therapy with diet is still under evaluation.[28] To fulfill the diagnostic criteria for EoE, a treatment attempt with PPI acid suppression is considered almost mandatory. Although PPI may be useful for patients who have established EoE who have symptoms due to concomitant or EoE-induced GERD, it cannot be considered a primary therapeutic option for EoE.

Several clinical trials and many case series have demonstrated that systemic and topical corticosteroids are highly effective in resolving symptoms and signs of active EoE.[17,18] A comparison of topical with systemic corticosteroids has shown no significant difference in the efficacy of these two forms.[27] In general, topical corticosteroids are used as first-line medications. They are well tolerated and, in most patients, clinical and histologic resolution is achieved within a few weeks. The drugs, either fluticasone propionate (Flonase, Veramyst) or budesonide (Rhinocort Aqua), are administered by mouth and can be divided into twice or four-times-daily doses. Most experts recommend starting with a high-dose induction treatment followed by a low-dose maintenance therapy. With the exception of oropharyngeal candidiasis, topical corticosteroids are almost free of side effects.[18] However, when topical or systemic corticosteroids are discontinued, the disease generally recurs within a few months.[3,18,27] The long-term management is still not defined and further studies are urgently needed to clarify treatment schedules and pharmacokinetic properties of topical corticosteroid treatment. The use of systemic corticosteroids should be limited to patients who have persistent symptoms and inflammation despite adequate dosage and correct application of topical corticosteroids.

At high dosages, leukotriene receptor antagonists, (eg, montelukast, Singulair), have been shown to induce symptomatic relief. However, their use has not been shown to affect the underlying esophageal eosinophilia significantly.[29] Like so much with EoE, the use of this drug for the treatment of EoE requires further investigation.

Novel biologic agents, such as monoclonal antibodies directed against interleukin-5 (eg, mepolizumab)[30] or tumor necrosis factor-alpha blocking agents (eg, infliximab, Remicade),[31] present a unique opportunity for patients who have severe EoE refractory to standard therapies. However, these molecules await larger clinical trials and cannot be recommended for routine use at the present time.

Esophageal dilation is useful for patients whose symptoms do not respond adequately to medical therapy, mainly patients presenting with a functional narrowing of the esophagus.[32] This condition may occur as a sequela of the chronic, untreated eosinophilic inflammation. Dilation encompasses a certain risk for mucosal tearing and frank perforation.[9] Because the responsiveness of strictures cannot be predicted based on endoscopic findings, a therapeutic attempt with topical corticosteroids before performing dilation is highly recommended. With respect to the abnormal fragility of the EoE mucosa, an inspection of the esophagus should be done following dilation to assess the extent of possible laceration. Because dilation in patients who have EoE has to be performed subtly and less aggressively than in non-EoE stenoses, several sessions may be required before the patient reaps benefits from this therapy.

OUTLOOK

Even though our understanding of EoE has increased enormously during the last decade, many issues remain unresolved. Indeed, our understanding of EoE's natural history is still limited and we have no predictive factors to identify patients who are at risk for developing esophageal remodeling. We need indicators for distinguishing between pure EoE and GERD-associated esophageal eosinophilia, and we need non-invasive markers for monitoring disease activity. Future efforts must focus on defining long-term medical management and the still-controversial managing of patients refractory to standard therapies. Should one treat asymptomatic patients who have esophageal eosinophilia? Further joint efforts between clinical researchers and basic scientists addressing these issues are urgently needed to improve the lives of those ever-increasing numbers of individuals affected with EoE.

ACKNOWLEDGMENTS

We would like to thank our Swiss gastroenterology colleagues for referring their patients who have EoE to our institution, and Kathleen Bucher for her competent editorial work.

REFERENCES

1. Furuta GT, Liacouras C, Collins MH, et al. Eosinophilic esophagitis in children and adults: a systematic review and consensus recommendations for diagnosis and treatment. Gastroenterology 2007;133:1342–63.
2. Orenstein SR, Shalaby TH, DiLorenzo C, et al. The spectrum of pediatric eosinophilic esophagitis beyond infancy: a clinical series of 30 children. Am J Gastroenterol 2000;95:1422–30.
3. Liacouras CA, Spergel JM, Ruchelli E, et al. Eosinophilic esophagitis: a 10-year experience in 381 children. Clin Gastroenterol Hepatol 2005;3:1198–206.
4. Portmann S, Heer P, Bussmann CH, et al. Epidemiology of eosinophilic esophagitis: data from a community-based longitudinal study [abstract]. Gastroenterology 2007;132:A609.
5. Straumann A, Spichtin HP, Grize L, et al. Natural history of primary eosinophilic esophagitis: a follow-up of 30 adult patients for up to 11.5 years. Gastroenterology 2003;125:1660–9.
6. Riou PJ, Nicholson AG, Pastorino U. Esophageal rupture in a patient with idiopathic eosinophilic esophagitis. Ann Thorac Surg 1996;62:1854–6.

7. Cohen MS, Kaufmann A, DiMarino AJ, et al. Eosinophilic esophagitis presenting as spontaneous esophageal rupture (Boerhaave's syndrome). Clin Gastroenterol Hepatol 2007;5 [image of the month].
8. Morrow JB, Vargo JJ, Goldblum JR, et al. The ringed esophagus: histological features of GERD. Am J Gastroenterol 2001;96:984–9.
9. Straumann A, Bussmann C, Zuber M, et al. Eosinophilic esophagitis: analysis of food impaction and perforation in 251 adolescent and adult patients. Clin Gastroenterol Hepatol 2008;6:598–600.
10. Straumann A, Simon HU. Eosinophilic esophagitis: escalating epidemiology? J Allergy Clin Immunol 2005;115:418–9.
11. Kapel RC, Miller JK, Torres C, et al. Eosinophilic esophagitis: a prevalent disease in the United States that affects all age groups. Gastroenterology 2008;134:1316–21.
12. Attwood SE, Smyrk TC, Demeester TR, et al. Esophageal eosinophilia with dysphagia. A distinct clinicopathologic syndrome. Dig Dis Sci 1993;38:109–16.
13. Straumann A, Spichtin HP, Bernoulli R, et al. Idiopathic eosinophilic esophagitis: a frequently overlooked disease with typical clinical aspects and discrete endoscopic findings. [in German with English abstract]. Schweiz Med Wochenschr 1994;124:1419–29.
14. Desai TK, Stecevic V, Chang CH, et al. Association of eosinophilic inflammation with esophageal food impaction in adults. Gastrointest Endosc 2005;61:795–801.
15. Remedios M, Campbell C, Jones DM, et al. Eosinophilic esophagitis in adults: clinical, endoscopic, histologic findings, and response to treatment with fluticasone proprionate. Gastrointest Endosc 2006;63:3–12.
16. Noel RJ, Putnam PE, Rothenberg ME. Eosinophilc esophagitis. N Engl J Med 2004;351:940–1.
17. Arora AS, Yamazaki K. Eosinophilic esophagitis: asthma of the esophagus? Clin Gastroenterol Hepatol 2004;2:523–30.
18. Konikoff MR, Noel RJ, Blanchard C, et al. A randomized double-blind, placebo-controlled trial of fluticasone proprionate for pediatric eosinophilic esophagitis. Gastroenterology 2006;131:1381–91.
19. Varadarajulu S, Eloubeidi MA, Patel RS, et al. The yield and the predictors of esophageal pathology when upper endoscopy is used for the initial evaluation of dysphagia. Gastrointest Endosc 2005;61:804–8.
20. Straumann A, Spichtin HP, Bucher KA, et al. Eosinophilic esophagitis: red on microscopy, white on endoscopy. Digestion 2004;70:109–16.
21. Kato M, Kephart GM, Talley NJ, et al. Eosinophil infiltration and degranulation in normal human tissue. Anat Rec 1998;252:418–25.
22. Lowichik A, Weinberg AG. A quantitative evaluation of mucosal eosinophils in the pediatric gastrointestinal tract. Mod Pathol 1996;9:110–4.
23. Steiner SJ, Gupta SK, Croffie JM, et al. Correlation between number of eosinophils and reflux index on same day esophageal biopsy and 24 hour esophageal pH monitoring. Am J Gastroenterol 2004;99:801–5.
24. Dellon ES, Aderoju A, Woosley JT, et al. Variability in diagnostic criteria for eosinophilic esophagitis: a systematic review. Am J Gastroenterol 2007;102:1–14.
25. Gonsalves N, Policarpio-Nicolas M, Zhang Q, et al. Histopathologic variability and endoscopic correlates in adults with eosinophilic esophagitis. Gastrointest Endosc 2006;64:313–9.
26. Aceves SS, Newbury RO, Dohil R, et al. Esophageal remodeling in pediatric eosinophilic esophagitis. J Allergy Clin Immunol 2007;119:206–12.

27. Schaefer ET, Fitzgerald JF, Molleston JP, et al. Comparison of oral prednisone and topical fluticasone in the treatment of eosinophilic esophagitis: a randomized trial in children. Clin Gastroenterol Hepatol 2008;6:165–73.

28. Gonsalves N, Ritz S, Yang G, et al. A prospective clinical trial of allergy testing and food elimination diet in adults with eosinophilic esophagitis. Gastroenterology 2007;132:A6 [abstract].

29. Attwood SE, Lewis CJ, Bronder CS, et al. Eosinophilic oesophagitis: a novel treatment using Montelukast. Gut 2003;52:181–5.

30. Stein ML, Collins MH, Villanueva JM, et al. Anti-IL-5 (mepolizumab) therapy for eosinophilic esophagitis. J Allergy Clin Immunol 2006;118:1312–9.

31. Straumann A, Bussmann Ch, Conus S, et al. A monoclonal antibody to TNF-alpha for severe eosinophilic esophagitis in adults: a prospective, translational pilot-study [abstract]. Gastroenterology 2008;134:A105.

32. Schoepfer AM, Gschossmann J, Scheurer U, et al. Esophageal strictures in eosinophilic esophagitis: dilation is an effective and safe therapeutic alternative after failure of topical corticosteroids. Endoscopy 2008;40:161–4.

Eosinophilic Esophagitis

James P. Franciosi, MD, MS, MSCE[a],*, Chris A. Liacouras, MD[b]

KEYWORDS

- Eosinophilic esophagitis • Diagnosis • Treatment

Eosinophilic esophagitis (EoE) is a clinicopathologic diagnosis that involves a localized eosinophilic inflammation of the esophagus. Our understanding and recognition of EoE has evolved over the past 30 years from isolated case reports of patients with esophageal eosinophilia to a well-defined clinical disorder with the first consensus recommendations published in 2007.[1] This disease has been given several names, including eosinophilic esophagitis, allergic esophagitis, primary eosinophilic esophagitis, and idiopathic eosinophilic esophagitis. Other recognized causes of esophageal eosinophilia should be excluded before making the diagnosis (**Box 1**). Currently, there are no pathognomonic symptoms, physical examination findings, serologic markers, or visual endoscopic findings. Esophageal endoscopic biopsies are required to establish the diagnosis. On endoscopic mucosal biopsies, EoE is defined as 15 or more eosinophils per high-powered field isolated to the esophagus and associated with characteristic clinical symptoms, which either do not respond to acid-blockade medication or are associated with normal pH monitoring of the distal esophagus.

CLINICAL MANIFESTATIONS

Although current reports suggest that patients with EoE are predominantly young Caucasian males, EoE can occur at any age and in either sex.[2] Manifestations of EoE may be protean or even clinically silent, but typical symptoms tend to correlate with age at presentation. In most children, predominant symptoms include, but are not limited to, abdominal pain, chest pain, symptoms like those of gastroesophageal reflux disease, vomiting, and, rarely, isolated nausea. Adolescents and adults frequently present with

This work was not supported by any institutional, National Institutes of Health, or industry grant.

[a] Division of Gastroenterology, Hepatology and Nutrition, Cincinnati Children's Hospital Medical Center and University of Cincinnati College of Medicine, 3333 Burnet Avenue, ML 2010, Cincinnati, OH 45229, USA

[b] Division of Gastroenterology, Hepatology and Nutrition, The Children's Hospital of Philadelphia, and University of Pennsylvania School of Medicine, 324 South 34th Street, Philadelphia, PA 19104-4399, USA

* Corresponding author.

E-mail address: james.franciosi@cchmc.org (J.P. Franciosi).

Box 1
Differential diagnosis of esophageal eosinophilia

Food allergy

Gastroesophageal reflux

Candida esophagitis

Eosinophilic gastroenteritis

Inflammatory bowel disease

Celiac disease

Parasitic infection

Connective tissue disease

Drug allergy

Hypereosinophilic syndrome

Autoimmune enteropathy

Viral esophagitis (herpes or cytomegalovirus)

Churg-Strauss syndrome

---

dysphagia and esophageal food impaction. Infants and young children may present with feeding refusal, feeding intolerance, and, less commonly, failure to thrive. Therefore, in evaluations of feeding disorders, it is important that the treatment teams have an understanding of EoE and make the appropriate referral to a gastroenterologist.

Symptom severity can be highly variable, ranging from minimal or no clinical symptoms in a minority of patients, to intermittent symptoms of dysphagia in teenagers, to frequent and severe symptoms of abdominal pain or vomiting in others. Because many EoE patients may compensate for their dysphagia, a careful history should be obtained with regard to particular food avoidance, eating slowly, excessive chewing, and having to drink after each bite of food.[3] EoE should be strongly considered in those patients who have severe or medically refractory symptoms of gastroesophageal reflux or with any history of esophageal food impaction. Personal or family history of atopic disease (asthma, eczema, rhinitis) and either environmental or food allergies is particularly important and demonstrated in up to 75% of patients.[1]

EPIDEMIOLOGY

Incidence and prevalence estimates of EoE in children up to 19 years of age are 1.25 and 4.3 per 10,000 children respectively.[4] Current literature makes clear that the prevalence of the diagnosis of EoE is increasing. Given that EoE is a chronic, nonfatal condition, a rise in the prevalence (total number cases in a given time period) is to be expected. However, there is debate as to whether the incident (new) cases being diagnosed represent a true increase in the number of cases or rather increased recognition of latent disease. As EoE is often regarded as an allergic, inflammatory disorder of the esophagus, a true rise in the incidence of EoE in parallel with the rising incidence of asthma and inflammatory bowel disease would not be surprising.[5] However, esophageal endoscopic biopsies are currently required to establish the diagnosis of EoE. Therefore, changes in referral patterns to gastroenterologists, acid-suppression medication prescribing practices, indications for upper endoscopy, and endoscopy practices may all bias epidemiologic studies. Possibly many EoE cases are missed because esophageal biopsies are not routinely performed today for adult esophagas-troduodenoscopy. Meanwhile, esophageal biopsies are only now beginning to be im-plemented for the evaluation of dysphagia. A study by Ronkainen and colleagues[6–8] has cast doubt on the use of endoscopic procedures as a basis for disease prevalence rates. In this study, investigators looked at results from a random sample of people who electively underwent esophageal endoscopy with biopsy without any clinical indication from endoscopic procedures. Investigators compared those results with those from other epidemiologic studies with prevalence rates based on patients referred to a gastroenterologist and where the number of esophageal biopsies was at the discretion of the endoscopist. The study found that the rate of disease preva-lence in the general population may be 10 times that extrapolated from studies based on referred patients. Further population-based studies are needed to investigate the prevalence of EoE using current definitions and noninvasive markers of disease.

PATHOPHYSIOLOGY

Clinical experience and experimental animal models support the strong association between EoE and allergic disease. EoE is believed to be a Th2-mediated disease in the context of genetically predisposed individuals and an inciting environmental trig-ger.[9] An important discovery has been the identification of a conserved EoE gene tran-script signature with overexpression of the chemokine eotaxin-3.[10] IL-5 and IL-13 are key Th2 cytokines that represent only part of a complex cellular and molecular cas-cade of interactions between Th2 cells, mast cells, and eosinophils.[11]

With regard to environmental etiologies, EoE is believed to be a mixed IgE- and non-IgE–mediated allergic response to food antigens, with non-IgE cell-mediated re-sponses predominating. In 1995, Kelly and colleagues[12] published a sentinel paper on EoE with a case series of 10 pediatric patients who demonstrated symptomatic and histologic improvement on an elemental diet (resolution in 8 patients; improve-ment in 2). Upon reintroduction of foods, all patients reverted to previous symptoms. Successful symptomatic and histologic improvement with elemental diets and food-elimination diets with return of symptoms and esophageal eosinophilia upon food re-introduction support food antigens as an important component in the pathophysiology of this disorder. Experimental and case report data have also suggested that aeroal-lergens may play a role in the development of EoE, albeit to a much lesser extent.[13] A current working hypothesis is that EoE subjects have an underlying genetic predispo-sition in combination with an environmental trigger, resulting in an esophageal eosin-ophilic inflammatory response. Whether the food antigenic reaction identified in a majority of patients is the manifestation of (1) a cross-reaction to various exposed esophageal epitopes secondary to mucosal injury, (2) increasingly hygienic popula-tions with lack of environmental sensitization, or (3) principally non-IgE–mediated food allergies presenting with previously unrecognized and misclassified gastrointes-tinal symptoms remains to be determined.

ENDOSCOPY

Currently, upper endoscopy with esophageal biopsies is the only way to diagnose EoE. Although linear furrowing, concentric esophageal rings. white surface exudate, Schatzki ring, small-caliber esophagus, and linear tears ("rents") have all been described as visual endoscopic findings in EoE patients, a visually normal esophageal appearance does not preclude the finding of significant esophageal eosinophilia on histology (**Figs. 1–3**). EoE has also been described as a patchy disease, and at least four esoph-ageal biopsies are required to obtain a sensitivity of at least 94% to detect EoE.[14]

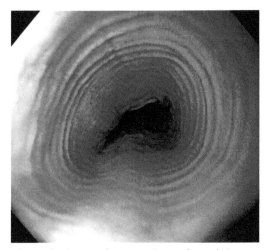

Fig. 1. Esophageal endoscopic picture of concentric esophageal rings.

ALLERGY TESTING

Food and environmental allergen testing is an important component to the evaluation of EoE patients. To identify both respective IgE-based and non-IgE–based causative food allergens, a combination of skin prick testing (SPT) and atopy patch testing (APT) is recommended. SPT is commercially available for a variety of foods (panels ranging from 13 to 42 foods) and environmental allergens. Results have been described in a cohort of 786 EoE patients from aggregated case series data.[1] In EoE patients, SPT most frequently identifies positive reactions to egg, milk, and soy (as well as to wheat, peanuts, beans, rye, and beef) among other various foods. The mean number of foods identified is reported to be 2.7 ($\pm$ 3.6) to 6 ($\pm$ 4.2) foods and at least one food identified in two thirds of patients. Theoretically, APT should be a better tool for identifying food allergens in EoE patients that are predominately non-IgE mediated. However, unlike SPT, which has been standardized and is commercially available, APT preparations,

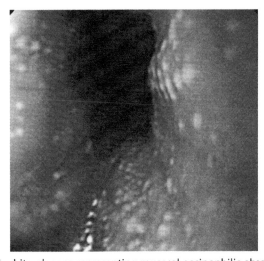

Fig. 2. Esophageal white plaques representing mucosal eosinophilic abscesses.

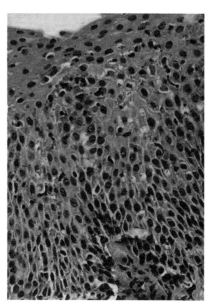

Fig. 3. Magnification of esophageal mucosa demonstrating numerous tissue eosinophils and an expanded basal cell layer.

methodologies, and results are highly variable among different practices. Therefore, there has not been widespread use of APT. The most common foods identified by APT are corn, soy, and wheat.[15] Resolution of esophageal eosinophilia has been reported in 67% of patients, and histologic improvement in 82% of patients using a combination of SPT- and APT-directed dietary elimination.[16]

Serum IgE levels, peripheral eosinophilia, and radio-allergo-sorbent testing are not sensitive indicators of the presence of isolated esophageal eosinophilic disease or disease activity. Biomarkers, such as eosinophil-derived neurotoxin and eotaxin-3, are under investigation.[17]

PERSPECTIVES FOR MANAGEMENT
Dietary Therapy

Although there have been no randomized clinical trials on dietary therapy for EoE, case series data from several centers in both adults and children support a 92% to 98% patient response to amino acid–based elemental formula with both symptomatic and histologic improvement.[16,18] Exclusive elemental formula is administered either orally or via nasogastric tube. A repeat esophagastroduodenoscopy is then performed after a period of 4 to 6 weeks to determine histologic improvement. Foods are then reintroduced in a sequential fashion beginning with least allergenic (fruits and vegetables) to highly antigenic (dairy, soy, egg, wheat, beef, peanut, and corn) in a sequential reintroduction of one new food per week and endoscopic surveillance after five to seven new foods (**Table 1**). Although highly effective, the psychosocial impact and quality-of-life issues on the patient and family as well as the number of endoscopies performed must be strongly considered when using this approach.

Directed elimination diets are often employed before considering an elemental diet, and have been shown to be effective in approximately 70% of patients.[16,19] From these directed elimination diets, the most common foods associated with EoE food allergy response include dairy, soy, egg, wheat, beef, peanut, and corn. However,

Table 1
Food introduction following an elemental diet

Diet A	Diet B	Diet C	Diet D
Vegetables (non-legume)	Other fruits	Peas	Milk
Carrots	Apples	White potatoes	
Squash	Bananas		Corn
Sweet potatoes	Kiwis	Grains	
Spinach	Pineapples	Rice	Peanuts
Broccoli	Mangos	Oats	
Lettuce	Watermelons	Barley	Wheat
	Honeydew melons	Rye	
Fruit	Cantaloupes		Beef
Grapes	Papayas	Meat[a]	
Pear	Guavas	Lamb	Soy
Peaches	Avocados	Chicken	
Plums		Turkey	Eggs
Apricots	Legumes	Pork	
Cherries	Lima beans		
Oranges	Chickpeas	Fish/Shellfish	
Grapefruit	White/black/red beans		
Lemons	String beans	Tree nuts	
Limes		Almonds	
Cherries		Walnuts	
Strawberries		Hazelnuts	
Blueberries		Brazil nuts	
		Pecans	

[a] Progress from well-cooked to increasingly rare

currently, results based on SPT and APT are center-specific and standardization of APT is sorely needed. Given the limitations of APT with regard to generalizability of results across centers, another dietary approach has been the empiric elimination of the most common cited allergenic foods. In a cohort of 35 EoE patients, Kawgawalla and colleagues[20] showed that approximately 74% responded symptomatically and histologically to the removal of the six most likely foods that cause EoE: dairy, soy, egg, wheat, peanut, and fish/shellfish. Although empiric diets are effective, strict amino acid–based diets demonstrate a significantly greater histologic and clinical improvement.

Pharmacologic Therapy

According to current diagnostic criteria put forth by the First International Gastrointestinal Eosinophilic Research Symposium Consensus Statement in 2007 for EoE, an empiric 6- to 8-week trial of acid-suppression therapy is needed before performing a diagnostic upper endoscopy with biopsy.[1] Therefore, without the use of high-dose acid-suppression therapy (proton pump inhibitor therapy of 2 mg/kg/d divided twice a day to a maximum of 40 mg twice a day) before endoscopy, patients cannot be confirmed to have EoE because gastroesophageal reflux disease is still a possibility. Acid-suppression therapy also has a role in established EoE patients as these patients often have reflux symptoms secondary to chronic esophageal inflammation and altered esophageal motility.

Among the first medical treatments for EoE shown to be effective were systemic corticosteroids, which improved both symptoms and esophageal histology in approximately 95% of patients.[21] However, upon discontinuation of corticosteroids, 90% have had recurrence of symptoms. When symptoms of EoE are severe enough to consider hospitalization or have led to the development of esophageal stricture formation, short-term systemic corticosteroids may be indicated (average dose 1.5 mg/kg/d; maximum dose 60 mg/d). However, the long-term use of systemic corticosteroids is associated with various adverse effects, including bone abnormalities, poor growth, mood abnormalities, and adrenal suppression.

In contrast to systemic corticosteroids, swallowed corticosteroid therapy is a mainstay of EoE therapy in adults and children. A randomized clinical trial comparing systemic corticosteroids (2 mg/kg/d, maximum 60 mg/d) with swallowed fluticasone proprionate (880 μg/d for ages 1–10 years and 1760 μg/day for ages 11 years or older)) demonstrated both histologic and symptomatic improvement in excess of 90% of patients in each groups.[22] Therefore, high-dose swallowed corticosteroids may be as effective as systemic corticosteroids with less toxicity. In the only randomized, double-blind, placebo-control trial of swallowed fluticasone (880-μg/d dosage in all ages 3–30 years old) in patients with active EoE, 50% of the fluticasone-treated patients achieved complete histologic remission compared with 9% of patients who received placebo.[23] The discrepancy between the two clinical studies may be related to fluticasone dosing and different study methodologies.

Oral viscous budesonide is another steroid preparation that has been used with some success in pediatric EoE patients. Aceves and colleagues[24] reported an 80% histologic response and an improvement in symptoms in a case series of 20 pediatric EoE patients (1 mg/d in children ages 1–10 and 2 mg/d in children over 10 years of age; 0.5 mg Pulmicort Respule with 5 g [packets] of sucralose [Splenda]). The advantage of using topical steroids is that their side effects are less severe than those seen with systemic steroids. The disadvantages include incomplete treatment of the disease (the disease generally recurs when the treatment is discontinued) and the development of possible side effects, including esophageal candidiasis. When using topical, swallowed corticosteroids, patients do not eat, drink, or rinse their mouth for 20 to 30 minutes after using the medication. Allergic rhinitis and environmental allergies should also be controlled with medication as these environmental allergies may have some role in EoE.

Additional atopic therapies, such as cromolyn sodium and leukotriene receptor antagonists, have also been used to treat EoE without success.[2] A case series of three adult EoE patients did not show efficacy of infliximab with regard to histologic symptomatic response.[25] Finally, other biologic agents that target the eosinophilic inflammatory cascade are currently in clinical trials or in various stages of development. Anti–IL-5 therapy is a particularly promising agent that has shown some efficacy in an open-label phase II study by Stein and colleagues.[26] Investigators performed an open-label phase safety and efficacy study of anti–IL-5 in four adult patients with EoE who had chronic dysphagia and esophageal strictures. Patients each received three infusions of anti–IL-5. The levels of plasma IL-5, peripheral blood eosinophils, and CCR3+ cells in blood, quality-of-life measurements, and histologic analysis of esophageal biopsies were determined before treatment and 1 month after treatment. The study showed a decrease in peripheral blood eosinophilia and CCR3+ cells as well as a significant decrease in esophageal eosinophils and a reduction in clinical symptoms. Currently, two pediatric studies using anti–IL-5 therapy are underway in patients with EoE.

Endoscopic Therapy

Although esophageal endoscopic dilation is a mainstay for peptic strictures, such dilation should be avoided for most EoE patients because of higher rates of esophageal perforation reported among such patients.[27] Dilation of the esophagus is useful to achieve immediate improvement in symptomatology for food impaction in those patients who have significant anatomic esophageal abnormalities. In patients with EoE, dilatation is not recommended as first-line therapy secondary to concerns of significant side effects (pain, bleeding, perforation) and not addressing the underlying pathogenesis. For example, a 17-year-old who presented with food impaction and long-segment esophageal stenosis developed minor bleeding and perforation of her esophagus postoperatively. Esophageal biopsy at the time revealed more than 100 eosinophils per high-power field and her perforation developed as a complication of dilation.[27] While dilatation has been associated with esophageal perforation, Schoepfer[28] recently reported the successful use of esophageal dilatation in a subset of EoE patients. As a rule, whenever possible, other modes of therapy should be used before performing dilatation.

SUMMARY

EoE is specific disease that involves an isolated esophageal eosinophilic inflammation and clinical symptoms that do not respond to proton pump inhibitor therapy. Upper endoscopy with esophageal biopsies is required to establish the diagnosis. Referral to an allergist and food allergen testing is recommended. Dietary and topical corticosteroid therapies are commonly used and are effective in the majority of patients.

REFERENCES

1. Furuta GT, Liacouras CA, Collins MH, et al. Eosinophilic esophagitis in children and adults: a systematic review and consensus recommendations for diagnosis and treatment. Gastroenterology 2007;133(4):1342–63.
2. Liacouras CA, Spergel JM, Ruchelli E, et al. Eosinophilic esophagitis: a 10-year experience in 381 children. Clin Gastroenterol Hepatol 2005;3(12):1198–206.
3. Putnam PE. Eosinophilic esophagitis in children: clinical manifestations. Gastroenterol Clin North Am 2008;37(2):369–81, vi.
4. Noel RJ, Putnam PE, Rothenberg ME. Eosinophilic esophagitis. N Engl J Med 2004;351(9):940–1.
5. Bach JF. The effect of infections on susceptibility to autoimmune and allergic diseases. N Engl J Med 2002;347(12):911–20.
6. Attwood SE. Eosinophilic oesophagitis is common: a difficult message to swallow? Int J Clin Pract 2008;62(7):978–9.
7. Basavaraju KP, Wong T. Eosinophilic oesophagitis: a common cause of dysphagia in young adults? Int J Clin Pract 2008;62(7):1096–107.
8. Ronkainen J, Talley NJ, Aro P, et al. Prevalence of oesophageal eosinophils and eosinophilic oesophagitis in adults: the population-based Kalixanda study. Gut 2007;56(5):615–20.
9. Rothenberg ME, Mishra A, Collins MH, et al. Pathogenesis and clinical features of eosinophilic esophagitis. J Allergy Clin Immunol 2001;108(6):891–4.
10. Blanchard C, Wang N, Stringer KF, et al. Eotaxin-3 and a uniquely conserved gene-expression profile in eosinophilic esophagitis. J Clin Invest 2006;116(2):536–47.
11. Blanchard C, Mingler MK, Vicario M, et al. IL-13 involvement in eosinophilic esophagitis: transcriptome analysis and reversibility with glucocorticoids. J Allergy Clin Immunol 2007;120(6):1292–300.
12. Kelly KJ, Lazenby AJ, Rowe PC, et al. Eosinophilic esophagitis attributed to gastroesophageal reflux: improvement with an amino acid–based formula. Gastroenterology 1995;109(5):1503–12.

13. Spergel JM. Eosinophilic oesophagitis and pollen. Clin Exp Allergy 2005;35(11): 1421-2.
14. Gonsalves N, Policarpio-Nicolas M, Zhang Q, et al. Histopathologic variability and endoscopic correlates in adults with eosinophilic esophagitis. Gastrointest Endosc 2006;64(3):313-9.
15. Spergel JM, Brown-Whitehorn T, Beausoleil JL, et al. Predictive values for skin prick test and atopy patch test for eosinophilic esophagitis. J Allergy Clin Immunol 2007;119(2):509-11.
16. Spergel JM, Andrews T, Brown-Whitehorn TF, et al. Treatment of eosinophilic esophagitis with specific food elimination diet directed by a combination of skin prick and patch tests. Ann Allergy Asthma Immunol 2005;95(4):336-43.
17. Konikoff MR, Blanchard C, Kirby C, et al. Potential of blood eosinophils, eosinophil-derived neurotoxin, and eotaxin-3 as biomarkers of eosinophilic esophagitis. Clin Gastroenterol Hepatol 2006;4(11):1328-36.
18. Markowitz JE, Spergel JM, Ruchelli E, et al. Elemental diet is an effective treatment for eosinophilic esophagitis in children and adolescents. Am J Gastroenterol 2003; 98(4):777-82.
19. Spergel JM, Shuker M. Nutritional management of eosinophilic esophagitis. Gastrointest Endosc Clin N Am 2008;18(1):179-94, xi.
20. Kagalwalla AF, Sentongo TA, Ritz S, et al. Effect of six-food elimination diet on clinical and histologic outcomes in eosinophilic esophagitis. Clin Gastroenterol Hepatol 2006;4(9):1097-102.
21. Liacouras CA, Wenner WJ, Brown K, et al. Primary eosinophilic esophagitis in children: successful treatment with oral corticosteroids. J Pediatr Gastroenterol Nutr 1998;26(4):380-5.
22. Schaefer ET, Fitzgerald JF, Molleston JP, et al. Comparison of oral prednisone and topical fluticasone in the treatment of eosinophilic esophagitis: a randomized trial in children. Clin Gastroenterol Hepatol 2008;6(2):165-73.
23. Konikoff MR, Noel RJ, Blanchard C, et al. A randomized, double-blind, placebo-controlled trial of fluticasone propionate for pediatric eosinophilic esophagitis. Gastroenterology 2006;131(5):1381-91.
24. Aceves SS, Dohil R, Newbury RO, et al. Topical viscous budesonide suspension for treatment of eosinophilic esophagitis. J Allergy Clin Immunol 2005;116(3):705-6.
25. Straumann A, Bussmann C, Conus S, et al. Anti-TNF-alpha (infliximab) therapy for severe adult eosinophilic esophagitis. J Allergy Clin Immunol 2008;122(2):425-7.
26. Stein ML, Collins MH, Villanueva JM, et al. Anti-IL-5 (mepolizumab) therapy for eosinophilic esophagitis. J Allergy Clin Immunol 2006;118(6):1312-9.
27. Eisenbach C, Merle U, Schirmacher P, et al. Perforation of the esophagus after dilation treatment for dysphagia in a patient with eosinophilic esophagitis. Endoscopy 2006;38:E43-4.
28. Schoepfer AM, Gschossmann J, Scheurer U, et al. Esophageal strictures in adult eosinophilic esophagitis: dilation is an effective and safe alternative after failure of topical corticosteroids. Endoscopy 2008;40(2):161-4.

Mechanism of Eosinophilic Esophagitis

Anil Mishra, PhD

KEYWORDS

- Esophagus • Eosinophils • Eotaxin • Interleukin • Mast cells
- Remodeling

The esophagus is the only segment in the gastrointestinal (GI) tract that is devoid of eosinophils, whereas most of the other leukocytes reside in the esophagus at baseline in a healthy state.[1,2] The esophagus is lined with mucous membrane and muscles that act with peristaltic action to move swallowed food down to the stomach. The epithelium of the esophagus is squamous but not keratinized like skin; therefore, keratinocytes are directly exposed to the esophageal content, which indicates that the esophageal epithelium may have a significant role in the induction of esophageal inflammation. The accumulation of eosinophils in the esophageal mucosa is the cardinal pathologic finding that occurs secondary to several unrelated diseases and is reported in several esophageal diseases, such as hypereosinophilic syndrome, eosinophilic gastroenteritis, drug reactions, fungal/parasitic infections, gastroesophageal reflux disease (GERD), and eosinophilic esophagitis (EoE).[1-11] EoE is a commonly observed medical problem and is well documented in pediatric patients, but the adult form has only recently gained recognition as a distinct entity. EoE is characterized by an increase in esophageal eosinophilia, basal cell hyperplasia, and several other esophageal abnormalities that include furrows, the formation of fine concentric mucosal rings (corrugated esophagus), and esophageal strictures (narrowing),[3-9] associated with extensive tissue remodeling and fibrosis.[10,11]

CLINICAL CHARACTERISTICS OF EOSINOPHILIC ESOPHAGITIS

Esophageal eosinophils are not pathognomonic for EoE because eosinophil infiltration in the esophagus occurs in various states, including GERD. Differentiating EoE from other esophageal disorders, specifically GERD, is often a challenge.[12] Patients who have primary EoE commonly report symptoms that include difficulty feeding, vomiting, chest pain, dysphagia, and food impaction;[13-16] these symptoms appear to occur

This work was supported by National Institutes of Health RO1 DK067255.
Department of Pediatrics, Division of Allergy and Immunology, 3333 Burnnet Avenue, Cincinnati Children's Hospital Medical Center, University of Cincinnati, Cincinnati, OH 45229, USA
E-mail address: anil.mishra@cchmc.org

Immunol Allergy Clin N Am 29 (2009) 29–40
doi:10.1016/j.iac.2008.09.010   immunology.theclinics.com

sequentially as the disease progresses from infancy into adulthood.[17] Dysphagia and food impaction are commonly observed in adult patients who have EoE.[18–20] However, longitudinal studies from childhood into adulthood are not yet available. Patients who have EoE are predominantly young men[13,14] and have high levels of eosinophils in the esophageal mucosa, extensive epithelial hyperplasia, and a high rate of atopic disease compared with patients who have GERD.[21,22] In particular, esophageal eosinophil levels of greater than 24/high-power field have been reported to correlate with lack of responsiveness to anti-GERD therapy;[23,24] these concentrations may be diagnostic of EoE rather than GERD, especially in patients already on anti-GERD therapy. A recent expert panel established as part of the First International Group of EoE Researchers recommended that a cutoff of 15 eosinophils/high-power field is sufficient for the diagnosis of EoE, provided that GERD has been eliminated as the diagnosis;[25] for research purposes a higher threshold level was recommended. Additionally, esophageal biopsies from EoE demonstrate a thickened mucosa with basal layer hyperplasia and papillary lengthening. Radiographic and endoscopic studies have shown many findings, including small-caliber esophagus, strictures, mucosal rings, ulcerations, whitish papules, and polyps.[8,15,16,26–28] EoE has been found to be associated with esophageal dysmotility but the cause of the motor disturbances is unclear. The eosinophil and mast cell activation and degranulation have been postulated as a possible cause of EoE pathogenesis.[29–31]

FOOD AND ENVIRONMENTAL ALLERGENS ARE LINKED TO EOSINOPHILIC ESOPHAGITIS

Food allergies affect an estimated 6% of children and 3.7% of adults in the United States and during the past decade, food allergies and their manifestations have substantially increased.[32,33] Food allergies can be classified into those that are IgE-mediated and those that are non–IgE-mediated. IgE-mediated reactions develop when food-specific IgE antibodies residing on mast cells and basophils come into contact with, and bind to, circulating food allergens and activate the cells to release potent mediators and cytokines. In non–IgE-mediated food allergic disorders, multiple inflammatory cells and their mediators play a role in immunopathogenesis. Most patients who have EoE (90%) have evidence of food and aeroallergen hypersensitivity, yet only a subset (10%–30%) has a history of food anaphylaxis.[34] Recent literature on pediatric patients who have EoE confirms that nearly all patients respond to an elemental diet, with resolution of symptoms and normalization of biopsies;[34] reintroduction of foods causes symptoms and esophageal eosinophilia to return.[35] Patients who have EoE have also been reported to exhibit seasonal variations in their symptoms and changes in their esophageal eosinophil levels. The mucosal eosinophil counts were elevated during the spring and summer and were suppressed during the winter,[36] indicating a role for aeroallergens. Studies of animal models have also linked EoE to aeroallergens and allergic diseases.[37] These findings indicate that sensitization pathways could occur in human EoE, and antigen-presenting cells may play an important role in the pathogenesis of EoE. An average of three to six foods per patient were directly linked to the development of esophageal eosinophilia and the common foods identified were milk, egg, soy, chicken, wheat, beef, corn, and peanuts.[34,35] Taken together, this finding provides supportive evidence that food and aeroallergen sensitization is causally involved in EoE (**Fig. 1**).

CELLULAR MEDIATORS THAT INFLUENCE THE OCCURRENCE OF EOSINOPHILIC ESOPHAGITIS

The current understanding of the pathophysiology of EoE comes from basic immunologic studies and clinical observation and treatment. Many eosinophils were detected

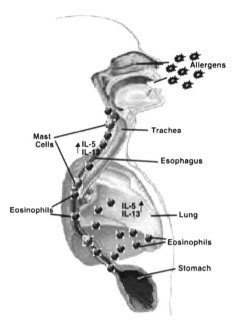

Fig. 1. Allergen-induced accumulation of inflammatory cells in the lung and esophagus. Food or aeroallergen exposure promotes eosinophilia and mastocytosis in the allergic lung and esophagus. Induced eosinophilia or mastocytosis is not observed in the stomach or small intestine. Allergen-induced Th2 cytokine (IL-5 and IL-13) induction is implicated in the induction of tissue eosinophilia.

in the esophagus following induction of EoE in humans and in an experimental mouse model of EoE. These eosinophils contain several toxic granular proteins. Eosinophil granules contain a crystalloid core composed of major basic protein (MBP-1 and -2), and a matrix composed of eosinophil cationic protein (ECP), eosinophil-derived neurotoxin (EDN), and eosinophil peroxides (EPO).[38,39] These cationic proteins share certain proinflammatory properties but differ in other ways. The MBP, EPO, and ECP have cytotoxic effects on epithelium and ECP and EDN possess anti-viral and ribonuclease activity.[40] MBP directly increases smooth muscle reactivity[41] and also triggers degranulation of mast cells and basophils.[42] Indeed, evidence is emerging that mast cells and eosinophils are both involved in EoE pathogenesis.[43,44] Several studies have shown that mast cells are present in the normal esophagus and their number increases in esophageal biopsies of patients who have EoE.[43,44] Mast cell gene (like tryptase or carboxypeptidase's 3)–induced expression is noticed in the esophageal biopsies of patients who have EoE.[43] Mast cells are known to release mediators (such as histamine and proteases) and on activation, they cause patho-physiologic alterations in tissues.[45,46] Evidence indicates that eosinophils and mast cells are present in an activated state in patients who have EoE.[31,43,47] Activated eosinophils and mast cells generate lipid mediators that stimulate smooth muscle contraction, increased vascular permeability, and mucus secretion.[48] Moreover, the leukotrienes released by these cells can also recruit inflammatory cells from the circu-lation, which would be an indirect pathway affecting the inflammatory response. Eosinophils and mast cells are also the source of transforming growth factor (TGF)-β that may induce tissue fibrosis. The amount of TGF-β is increased in the esophagus of human and mouse models of experimental EoE; therefore, induced TGF-β is capable of modifying clinical symptoms in the esophagus of patients who have EoE.

SIGNIFICANCE OF EOSINOPHIL-SPECIFIC RECEPTORS AND CHEMOKINES IN EOSINOPHILIC ESOPHAGITIS PATHOGENESIS

Eosinophil accumulation often occurs in the absence of infiltration by other inflammatory cells. As a result, a considerable amount of research has focused on identifying eosinophil-specific chemoattractants.[32] Eosinophils respond to various chemoattractants, including lipids and complement degradation products, and various chemokines, including eotaxin; regulated on activation, normal T expressed and secreted (RANTES); and monocyte chemoattractant proteins (MCPs). Eotaxin was originally identified as the predominant eosinophil chemoattractant and a potent activator of eosinophils.[33] The specificity of eotaxin for eosinophils is the result of the exclusive signaling of eotaxin through its receptor, chemokine receptor 3 (CCR3), which is expressed predominantly on human and mouse eosinophils.[32,49–52] Eosinophils express several chemokine receptors, but CCR3 is expressed at the highest level per cell.[49,50,53] CCR3 appears to function as the predominant chemokine receptor because CCR3 ligands are generally the most potent eosinophil chemoattractants. Consistent with the expression of CCR3, eosinophils respond to macrophage inflammatory protein (MIP)-1α, RANTES, MCP-2, MCP-3, MCP-4, eotaxin-1, eotaxin-2, and eotaxin-3. Eotaxin-2 and -3 have 30% homology to eotaxin-1.[44,54,55] Recently, the author and colleagues reported that eotaxin-3 is a signature gene for EoE, which is also a powerful eosinophil-activating protein.[44,55,56] Eotaxin-3 is induced in patients of all ages who have EoE, regardless of gender and the allergic status of the patient, and is completely distinct from the gene expression in patients who have reflux esophagitis. Eotaxin-3 is a chemoattractant for eosinophils, and esophageal epithelium is a rich source of eotaxin-3 in patients who have EoE,[44] which indicates that eotaxin-3 has a critical role in the accumulation of eosinophils in the esophageal mucosa of patients who have EoE. The author and colleagues recently showed that an eotaxin-3 gene single nucleotide polymorphism is associated with EoE.[44] Furthermore, the significance of eotaxin-3 is supported by their previous work demonstrating that mice with genes targeted for the eotaxin receptor, CCR3, were protected from the development of experimental EoE.[44]

MOLECULES INVOLVED IN THE PATHOGENESIS OF EOSINOPHILIC ESOPHAGITIS

Interleukin (IL)-5 is the most specific cytokine for eosinophil growth, differentiation, activation, and survival, and primes eosinophils to respond to chemoattractants such as eotaxin, an eosinophil-selective CC chemokine.[57–59] IL-5 also facilitates eosinophil migration from bone marrow to the blood.[60] Recent experiments have demonstrated that IL-5 is overexpressed in the esophagus of patients who have EoE.[61] Additionally, systemic overexpression of IL-5 (by way of pharmacologic or transgenic approaches) promotes eosinophil trafficking to the esophagus in mice,[62] and neutralizing anti–IL-5 (TRFK5) treatment in a murine model of EoE restricts eosinophil trafficking to the lung and esophagus.[37] Determining the role of IL-5 in EoE is of importance because two different studies have shown an improvement in the clinical and pathologic symptoms of EoE after anti–IL-5 treatment.[63] Animal studies have documented that dietary and environmental antigens, such as enteric-coated ovalbumin or Aspergillus antigen-induced esophageal eosinophilia,[37,64] were ablated in mice deficient in IL-5.[37,64] Interestingly, transgenic mice overexpressing IL-5 had constitutively elevated number of esophageal eosinophils.[65] Eosinophils also produce IL-5; therefore, it is important to understand whether local induction of IL-5 has a role in EoE pathogenesis. The author and colleagues recently showed that local expression of IL-5 is required for the induction of esophageal remodeling in human and experimental EoE.

IL-13 has also been implicated in various allergic conditions, including asthma,[66] atopic dermatitis,[31,67,68] and allergic rhinitis.[69–71] The overexpression of IL-13 by pharmacologic administration or transgenic approaches induces multiple features of asthma, including eosinophilia, mucus overproduction, and airway hyperresponsiveness.[72,73] Based on the importance of IL-13 in allergic diseases and the high concordance between asthma and EoE in humans, the author and colleagues delivered IL-13 to the lung by intratracheal administration (**Fig. 2**). Their experimentation established that pulmonary inflammation, triggered by IL-13, is associated with the development of EoE. In humans, IL-13–induced lung and esophageal eosinophilia was reduced by pretreatment with human neutralizing IL-13 (CAT-354) antibody.[74] Use of experimental models in mice has established that T helper 2 (Th2) signaling is required for induction of experimental EoE,[37] which will be further proved by the author's finding that STAT6 gene-deficient mice are protected from allergen– and IL-13–induced experimental EoE.[75,76] The emerging clinical and experimental data support a central role for IL-5 and IL-13 in EoE pathogenesis.[65,75] Furthermore, a clinical report indicated that stimulation with food and environmental aeroallergens induced Th2 cytokine (IL-5 and IL-13) production by peripheral blood mononuclear cells in adult patients who had EoE.[77] Collectively, these findings demonstrate that not only external allergic triggers but also intrinsic Th2 cytokines and eosinophil effector function are critical in EoE pathogenesis. The intimate connection between the lung and the esophagus has been shown in experimental models of EoE; however, recent findings indicate that allergen-induced EoE is independent of the lung inflammation.[78] Following intranasal allergen challenge, esophageal eosinophilic inflammation is induced in CD_4 gene-

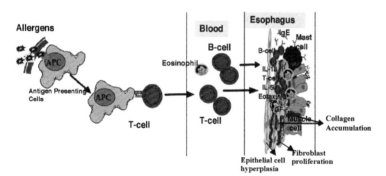

Fig. 2. Paradigm of allergen-induced esophageal accumulation of eosinophils, mast cells, and tissue remodeling in EoE. Antigen-presenting cells (APCs) process the allergen and present antigen to the T cells. These T cells home to the esophagus by way of blood circulation and, on activation, release eosinophil-specific cytokines (IL-5 and IL-13), which induce chemokines (eotaxin -1, -2, and -3) in the esophageal epithelium that attract eosinophils into the esophagus. Additionally, in response to allergens, B cell and mast cell numbers increase in the esophagus. B cells synthesize IgE locally or systemically, which may activate mast cells, because IgE is detected on the surface of mast cells in patients who have EoE. The activated eosinophil and mast cells are a rich source of TGF-β, which may play a critical role in the disease pathogenesis, including esophageal remodeling.

deficient mice without inducing eosinophilic lung inflammation,[78] although lung and esophageal inflammation is a T-cell–dependent process.[78] This finding indicates that a different mechanism is operational in the induction of esophageal and lung eosinophilic inflammation, which requires further research to provide a better understanding of the mechanistic pathway of the induction of EoE and its relationship to other allergic diseases.

PATHOPHYSIOLOGIC ABNORMALITIES DEVELOP IN EOSINOPHILIC ESOPHAGITIS

Recently, the author and others showed that eosinophil recruitment to the esophagus induces esophageal remodeling, specifically in the lamina propria in the pediatric EoE population.[10,11] An impressive collagen accumulation in the epithelial and subepithelial mucosa, increased vascularity, basal cell hyperplasia, and vascular activation, along with increased expression of TGF-β, VCAM-1, SMAD2/3, MUC5AC, and IL-5 genes was observed in esophageal biopsies of patients who had EoE.[10] The induced gene expression of TGF-β and its signaling molecule, SMAD2/3, in the esophagus of human and experimental EoE indicates that the TGF-β pathway may play a critical role in the development of esophageal pathophysiologic abnormalities, including the formation of esophageal rings and strictures in patients who have EoE. By using mouse models of EoE, the author and colleagues demonstrated that local IL-5 expression–induced esophageal eosinophilia is critical in the development of esophageal remodeling.[11] Fibroblast proliferation is observed in the esophageal biopsies of patients who have EoE, and eosinophil–fibroblast interactions generate subepithelial fibrosis in tissue in inflammatory states. The author's recent observation that local expression of IL-5 is critical for esophageal remodeling is in accordance with a previous report showing that IL-5 induces fibroblast to myofibroblast transdifferentiation and the expression of α-smooth muscle actin and induced extracellular matrix.[79] Although a few recent reports indicate that esophageal remodeling and fibrosis occurs in EoE, the mechanism of the induction of esophageal fibrogenesis remains unclear. To define the changes in esophageal epithelial cells, fibroblast proliferation and differentiation, extracellular matrix accumulation, and smooth muscle hyperplasia in EoE, more experimental studies are needed.

DIAGNOSIS AND THERAPIES FOR EOSINOPHILIC ESOPHAGITIS

EoE is a newly recognized disease and is an emerging entity throughout developing and developed countries, including the United States.[5,6,13,21,23,29,80–87] Therefore, understanding the causes, natural history, diagnosis, and management is important for future therapeutic interventions for EoE. The diagnosis of EoE is generally made by performing an esophageal biopsy, with evidence of eosinophils infiltrating the esophageal mucosa. Once EoE is diagnosed, an allergist will typically perform extensive allergy testing, looking for evidence of food and environmental allergen sensitization. Currently, therapy for esophageal inflammation is based on antigen-elimination trials, anti-inflammatory approaches, and physical dilatation when strictures are present. The last approach, which has been the strategy reported for adults, temporarily reduces symptoms of dysphagia; however, it involves the significant risk for rupture and hemorrhage, needs to be repeated regularly, and does not reduce the underlying inflammation.[88] An antigen-elimination approach in sensitized individuals (eg, aeroallergen avoidance and food elimination diets) is typically unsatisfactory or practically difficult (when patients are sensitized to many allergens), probably because the current allergen-sensitization tests (skin prick and patch tests, and allergen-specific plasma IgE levels) are not optimal for detecting sensitization. A diet consisting exclusively of an elemental (amino acid–based) formula frequently improves symptoms and normalizes esophageal pathology.[89–91] However, this approach is often not tolerated (especially in older individuals), frequently requires a feeding tube, and can be expensive. Systemic steroids are used for acute exacerbations, whereas topical glucocorticoids are used to provide long-term control.[92,93] Glucocorticoid treatment shows significant effect in reducing esophageal eosinophilia. Newer glucocorticoids with decreased systemic effect may improve the care of patients who have EoE. Although some treatments are effective in EoE, the molecular mechanisms involved in the remission have still not been established. Humanized antibody therapy designed to block IL-5 and IL-13 is currently in testing and has demonstrated great promise. Recent reports indicate that anti–IL-5 therapy has a significant effect on EoE in patients, and CAT-354, an IL-13–blocking antibody, has been shown to prevent lung and esophageal eosinophilia in mice.[63,74] The anti–IL-5 therapeutic trials have been conducted in a few patients and more extensive studies are needed. The development of an experimental model of EoE is the most useful tool for dissecting the molecular mechanisms involved in remission or resistance to therapy. The current knowledge suggests that targeting IL-5, IL-13, and eotaxin-3 may be promising therapeutic strategies for the treatment of EoE.

SUMMARY

EoE is linked to allergic responses to food or aeroallergens, but cases have also been reported in which patients have EoE without detectable food allergies by patch or prick skin testing. This finding indicates that EoE could also be associated with immune dysregulation and these tests might not reflect hypersensitivity driven by discrete antigens. The pathogenesis of EoE is still not clear, but a growing body of evidence has established that this condition represents a T cell–mediated immune response involving several proinflammatory mediators and chemoattractants known to regulate eosinophilic accumulation in the esophagus, such as IL-4, IL-5, IL-13, and eotaxin-1, -2, and -3. Recent findings indicate that the most highly expressed gene in patients who have Eoe is eotaxin-3, whereas eotaxin-1 and -2 are modestly increased. In addition, esophageal eosinophilia correlates with eotaxin-3 mRNA and protein levels in esophageal biopsies of patients who have EoE. It has recently been reported that the esophageal epithelium from esophageal biopsies of patients who have EoE expresses eotaxin-3, and exposure of esophageal epithelial cells to IL-13 induces eotaxin-3. These data indicate that IL-5, IL-13, and eotaxin-3 are the major mediators that regulate eosinophil numbers in the esophagus. Determining the mechanism or mechanisms through which human esophageal cell–derived factors ultimately induce the functional abnormalities observed, and to which antigens patients who have EoE are sensitized that lead to the manifestation of symptoms, is of significant interest. Esophageal dysmotility is a recognized complication of GERD, but has not yet been studied in EoE. Therefore, experimental models need to be designed to identify and evaluate the key factors in the inflammatory pathways of EoE that are directly responsible for altered smooth muscle contractility and eventually, clinical symptoms. These studies will lead to a better understanding of the mechanisms of the development of EoE and will likely provide further treatment options.

REFERENCES

1. Mishra A, Hogan SP, Lee JJ, et al. Fundamental signals that regulate eosinophil homing to the gastrointestinal tract. J Clin Invest 1999;103:1719–27.
2. DeBrosse CW, Case JW, Putnam PE, et al. Quantity and distribution of eosinophils in the gastrointestinal tract of children. Pediatr Dev Pathol 2006;9:210–8.

3. White RJ, Zhang Y, Morris GP, et al. Esophagitis-related esophageal shortening in opossum is associated with longitudinal muscle hyperresponsiveness. Am J Physiol Gastrointest Liver Physiol 2001;280:G463–9.
4. Paterson WG. Role of mast cell-derived mediators in acid-induced shortening of the esophagus. Am J Physiol 1998;274:G385–8.
5. Cantu P, Velio P, Prada A, et al. Ringed oesophagus and idiopathic eosinophilic oesophagitis in adults: an association in two cases. Dig Liver Dis 2005;37:129–34.
6. Croese J, Fairley SK, Masson JW, et al. Clinical and endoscopic features of eosinophilic esophagitis in adults. Gastrointest Endosc 2003;58:516–22.
7. Mann NS, Leung JW. Pathogenesis of esophageal rings in eosinophilic esophagitis. Med Hypotheses 2005;64:520–3.
8. Zimmerman SL, Levine MS, Rubesin SE, et al. Idiopathic eosinophilic esophagitis in adults: the ringed esophagus. Radiology 2005;236:159–65.
9. Ruigomez A, Alberto Garcia Rodriguez L, Wallander MA, et al. Esophageal stricture: incidence, treatment patterns, and recurrence rate. Am J Gastroenterol 2006;101:2685–92.
10. Aceves SS, Newbury RO, Dohil R, et al. Esophageal remodeling in pediatric eosinophilic esophagitis. J Allergy Clin Immunol 2007;119:206–12.
11. Mishra A, Wang M, Pemmaraju VR, et al. Esophageal remodeling develops as a consequence of tissue specific IL-5-induced eosinophilia. Gastroenterology 2008;134:204–14.
12. Dahms BB. Reflux esophagitis: sequelae and differential diagnosis in infants and children including eosinophilic esophagitis. Pediatr Dev Pathol 2004;7:5–16.
13. Orenstein SR, Shalaby TM, Di Lorenzo C, et al. The spectrum of pediatric eosinophilic esophagitis beyond infancy: a clinical series of 30 children. Am J Gastroenterol 2000;95:1422–30.
14. Walsh SV, Antonioli DA, Goldman H, et al. Allergic esophagitis in children: a clinicopathological entity. Am J Surg Pathol 1999;23:390–6.
15. Liacouras CA, Ruchelli E. Eosinophilic esophagitis. Curr Opin Pediatr 2004;16:560–6.
16. Sant'Anna AM, Rolland S, Fournet JC, et al. Eosinophilic esophagitis in children: symptoms, histology and pH probe results. J Pediatr Gastroenterol Nutr 2004;39:373–7.
17. Noel RJ, Putnam PE, Rothenberg ME. Eosinophilic esophagitis. N Engl J Med 2004;351:940–1.
18. Straumann A, Spichtin HP, Grize L, et al. Natural history of primary eosinophilic esophagitis: a follow-up of 30 adult patients for up to 11.5 years. Gastroenterology 2003;125:1660–9.
19. Vasilopoulos S, Murphy P, Auerbach A, et al. The small-caliber esophagus: an unappreciated cause of dysphagia for solids in patients with eosinophilic esophagitis. Gastrointest Endosc 2002;55:99–106.
20. Potter JW, Saeian K, Staff D, et al. Eosinophilic esophagitis in adults: an emerging problem with unique esophageal features. Gastrointest Endosc 2004;59:355–61.
21. Rothenberg ME, Mishra A, Collins MH, et al. Pathogenesis and clinical features of eosinophilic esophagitis. J Allergy Clin Immunol 2001;108:891–4.
22. Ruchelli E, Wenner W, Voytek T, et al. Severity of esophageal eosinophilia predicts response to conventional gastroesophageal reflux therapy. Pediatr Dev Pathol 1999;2:15–8.
23. Cury EK, Schraibman V, Faintuch S. Eosinophilic infiltration of the esophagus: gastroesophageal reflux versus eosinophilic esophagitis in children—discussion on daily practice. J Pediatr Surg 2004;39:e4–7.

24. Rothenberg ME. Eosinophilia. N Engl J Med 1998;338:1592–600.
25. Furuta GT, Liacouras CA, Collins MH, et al. Eosinophilic esophagitis in children and adults: a systematic review and consensus recommendations for diagnosis and treatment. Gastroenterology 2007;133:1342–63.
26. Fox VL, Nurko S, Furuta GT. Eosinophilic esophagitis: it's not just kid's stuff. Gastrointest Endosc 2002;56:260–70.
27. Liacouras CA, Wenner WJ, Brown K, et al. Primary eosinophilic esophagitis in children: successful treatment with oral corticosteroids. J Pediatr Gastroenterol Nutr 1998;26:380–5.
28. Vasilopoulos S, Shaker R. Defiant dysphagia: small-caliber esophagus and refractory benign esophageal strictures. Curr Gastroenterol Rep 2001;3:225–30.
29. Attwood SE, Smyrk TC, Demeester TR, et al. Esophageal eosinophilia with dysphagia. A distinct clinicopathologic syndrome. Dig Dis Sci 1993;38:109–16.
30. Tottrup A, Fredens K, Funch-Jensen P, et al. Eosinophil infiltration in primary esophageal achalasia. A possible pathogenic role. Dig Dis Sci 1989;34:1894–9.
31. Justinich CJ, Ricci A Jr, Kalafus DA, et al. Activated eosinophils in esophagitis in children: a transmission electron microscopic study. J Pediatr Gastroenterol Nutr 1997;25:194–8.
32. Gao JL, Sen AI, Kitaura M, et al. Identification of a mouse eosinophil receptor for the CC chemokine eotaxin. Biochem Biophys Res Commun 1996;223:679–84.
33. Elsner J, Hochstetter R, Kimmig D, et al. Human eotaxin represents a potent activator of the respiratory burst of human eosinophils. Eur J Immunol 1996;26: 1919–25.
34. Spergel JM. Eosinophilic esophagitis in adults and children: evidence for a food allergy component in many patients. Curr Opin Allergy Clin Immunol 2007;7:274–8.
35. Spergel JM, Andrews T, Brown-Whitehorn TF, et al. Treatment of eosinophilic esophagitis with specific food elimination diet directed by a combination of skin prick and patch tests. Ann Allergy Asthma Immunol 2005;95:336–43.
36. Rothenberg SJ, Kondrashov V, Manalo M, et al. Seasonal variation in bone lead contribution to blood lead during pregnancy. Environ Res 2001;85:191–4.
37. Mishra A, Hogan SP, Brandt EB, et al. An etiological role for aeroallergens and eosinophils in experimental esophagitis. J Clin Invest 2001;107:83–90.
38. Gleich GJ, Adolphson CR. The eosinophilic leukocyte: structure and function. Adv Immunol 1986;39:177–253.
39. Gleich GJ, Frigas E, Loegering DA, et al. Cytotoxic properties of the eosinophil major basic protein. J Immunol 1979;123:2925–7.
40. Slifman NR, Loegering DA, McKean DJ, et al. Ribonuclease activity associated with human eosinophil-derived neurotoxin and eosinophil cationic protein. J Immunol 1986;137:2913–7.
41. Jacoby DB, Gleich GJ, Fryer AD. Human eosinophil major basic protein is an endogenous allosteric antagonist at the inhibitory muscarinic M2 receptor. J Clin Invest 1993;91:1314–8.
42. O'Donnell MC, Ackerman SJ, Gleich GJ, et al. Activation of basophil and mast cell histamine release by eosinophil granule major basic protein. J Exp Med 1983;157:1981–91.
43. Kirsch R, Bokhary R, Marcon MA, et al. Activated mucosal mast cells differentiate eosinophilic (allergic) esophagitis from gastroesophageal reflux disease. J Pediatr Gastroenterol Nutr 2007;44:20–6.
44. Blanchard C, Wang N, Stringer KF, et al. Eotaxin-3 and a uniquely conserved gene-expression profile in eosinophilic esophagitis. J Clin Invest 2006;116: 536–47.

45. Tung HN, Schulze-Delrieu K, Shirazi S. Infiltration of hypertrophic esophageal smooth muscle by mast cells and basophils. J Submicrosc Cytol Pathol 1993; 25:93–102.
46. Sommerhoff CP. Mast cell tryptases and airway remodeling. Am J Respir Crit Care Med 2001;164:S52–8.
47. Straumann A, Kristl J, Conus S, et al. Cytokine expression in healthy and inflamed mucosa: probing the role of eosinophils in the digestive tract. Inflamm Bowel Dis 2005;11:720–6.
48. Lewis RA, Austen KF, Soberman RJ. Leukotrienes and other products of the 5-lipoxygenase pathway. Biochemistry and relation to pathobiology in human diseases. N Engl J Med 1990;323:645–55.
49. Ponath PD, Qin S, Post TW, et al. Molecular cloning and characterization of a human eotaxin receptor expressed selectively on eosinophils. J Exp Med 1996;183:2437–48.
50. Daugherty BL, Siciliano SJ, DeMartino JA, et al. Cloning, expression, and characterization of the human eosinophil eotaxin receptor. J Exp Med 1996;183: 2349–54.
51. Post TW, Bozic CR, Rothenberg ME, et al. Molecular characterization of two murine eosinophil beta chemokine receptors. J Immunol 1995;155:5299–305.
52. Alkhatib G, Combadiere C, Broder CC, et al. CC CKR5-a RANTES, MIP-1-alpha, MIP-1-beta receptor as a fusion cofactor for macrophage-tropic HIV-1. Science 1996;272:1955–8.
53. Combadiere C, Ahuja SK, Murphy PM. Cloning and functional expression of a human eosinophil CC chemokine receptor. J Biol Chem 1995;270:16491–4.
54. Forssmann U, Uguccioni M, Loetscher P, et al. Eotaxin-2, a novel CC chemokine that is selective for the chemokine receptor CCR3, and acts like eotaxin on human eosinophil and basophil leukocytes. J Exp Med 1997;185:2171–6.
55. Kitaura M, Suzuki N, Imai T, et al. Molecular cloning of a novel human CC chemokine (eotaxin-3) that is a functional ligand of CC chemokine receptor 3. J Biol Chem 1999;274:27975–80.
56. Blanchard C, Mingler MK, Vicario M, et al. IL-13 involvement in eosinophilic esophagitis: transcriptome analysis and reversibility with glucocorticoids. J Allergy Clin Immunol 2007;120:1292–300.
57. Sanderson CJ. Interleukin-5, eosinophils, and disease. Blood 1992;79:3101–9.
58. Collins PD, Marleau S, Griffiths-Johnson DA, et al. Cooperation between interleukin-5 and the chemokine eotaxin to induce eosinophil accumulation in vivo. J Exp Med 1995;182:1169–74.
59. Rothenberg SJ, Manalo M, Jiang J, et al. Blood lead level and blood pressure during pregnancy in South Central Los Angeles. Arch Environ Health 1999;54: 382–9.
60. Paul CC, Tolbert M, Mahrer S, et al. Cooperative effects of interleukin-3 (IL-3), IL-5, and granulocyte-macrophage colony-stimulating factor: a new myeloid cell line inducible to eosinophils. Blood 1993;81:1193–9.
61. Straumann A, Bauer M, Fischer B, et al. Idiopathic eosinophilic esophagitis is associated with a T(H)2-type allergic inflammatory response. J Allergy Clin Immunol 2001;108:954–61.
62. Mishra A, Hogan SP, Brandt EB, et al. Enterocyte expression of the eotaxin and interleukin-5 transgenes induces compartmentalized dysregulation of eosinophil trafficking. J Biol Chem 2002;277:4406–12.
63. Stein ML, Collins MH, Villanueva JM, et al. Anti-IL-5 (mepolizumab) therapy for eosinophilic esophagitis. J Allergy Clin Immunol 2006;118:1312–9.

64. Hogan SP, Mishra A, Brandt EB, et al. A pathological function for eotaxin and eosinophils in eosinophilic gastrointestinal inflammation. Nat Immunol 2001;2: 353–60.
65. Mishra A, Hogan SP, Brandt EB, et al. IL-5 promotes eosinophil trafficking to the esophagus. J Immunol 2002;168:2464–9.
66. Barata LT, Ying S, Grant JA, et al. Allergen-induced recruitment of Fc epsilon RI+ eosinophils in human atopic skin. Eur J Immunol 1997;27:1236–41.
67. Akdis M, Akdis CA, Weigl L, et al. Skin-homing, CLA+ memory T cells are activated in atopic dermatitis and regulate IgE by an IL-13-dominated cytokine pattern: IgG4 counter-regulation by CLA-memory T cells. J Immunol 1997;159: 4611–9.
68. Katagiri K, Itami S, Hatano Y, et al. In vivo expression of IL-4, IL-5, IL-13 and IFN-gamma mRNAs in peripheral blood mononuclear cells and effect of cyclosporin A in a patient with Kimura's disease. Br J Dermatol 1997;137:972–7.
69. Pawankar RU, Okuda M, Hasegawa S, et al. Interleukin-13 expression in the nasal mucosa of perennial allergic rhinitis. Am J Respir Crit Care Med 1995; 152:2059–67.
70. Pawankar R, Okuda M, Yssel H, et al. Nasal mast cells in perennial allergic rhinitics exhibit increased expression of the Fc epsilonRI, CD40L, IL-4, and IL-13, and can induce IgE synthesis in B cells. J Clin Invest 1997;99:1492–9.
71. Al Ghamdi K, Ghaffar O, Small P, et al. IL-4 and IL-13 expression in chronic sinusitis: relationship with cellular infiltrate and effect of topical corticosteroid treatment. J Otolaryngol 1997;26:160–6.
72. Elias JA, Zhu Z, Chupp G, et al. Airway remodeling in asthma. J Clin Invest 1999; 104:1001–6.
73. Kim CH, Qu CK, Hangoc G, et al. Abnormal chemokine-induced responses of immature and mature hematopoietic cells from motheaten mice implicate the protein tyrosine phosphatase SHP-1 in chemokine responses. J Exp Med 1999; 190:681–90.
74. Blanchard C, Mishra A, Saito-Akei H, et al. Inhibition of human interleukin-13-induced respiratory and oesophageal inflammation by anti-human-interleukin-13 antibody (CAT-354). Clin Exp Allergy 2005;35:1096–103.
75. Mishra A, Rothenberg ME. Intratracheal IL-13 induces eosinophilic esophagitis by an IL-5, eotaxin-1, and STAT6-dependent mechanism. Gastroenterology 2003;125:1419–27.
76. Akei HS, Mishra A, Blanchard C, et al. Epicutaneous antigen exposure primes for experimental eosinophilic esophagitis in mice. Gastroenterology 2005;129: 985–94.
77. Yamazaki K, Murray JA, Arora AS, et al. Allergen-specific in vitro cytokine production in adult patients with eosinophilic esophagitis. Dig Dis Sci 2006;51: 1934–41.
78. Mishra A, Schlotman J, Wang M, et al. Critical role for adaptive T cell immunity in experimental eosinophilic esophagitis in mice. J Leukoc Biol 2007;81:916–24.
79. Tanaka H, Komai M, Nagao K, et al. Role of interleukin-5 and eosinophils in allergen-induced airway remodeling in mice. Am J Respir Cell Mol Biol 2004;31: 62–8.
80. Fujiwara H, Morita A, Kobayashi H, et al. Infiltrating eosinophils and eotaxin: their association with idiopathic eosinophilic esophagitis. Ann Allergy Asthma Immunol 2002;89:429–32.
81. Munitiz V, Martinez de Haro LF, Ortiz A, et al. Primary eosinophilic esophagitis. Dis Esophagus 2003;16:165–8.

82. Lucendo AJ, Carrion G, Navarro M, et al. Eosinophilic esophagitis in adults: an emerging disease. Dig Dis Sci 2004;49:1884–8.
83. Straumann A, Spichtin HP, Bucher KA, et al. Eosinophilic esophagitis: red on microscopy, white on endoscopy. Digestion 2004;70:109–16.
84. Straumann A. [What is your diagnosis? Primary eosinophilic esophagitis]. Schweiz Rundsch Med Prax 2004;93:795–6.
85. Furuta GT. Eosinophils in the esophagus: acid is not the only cause. J Pediatr Gastroenterol Nutr 1998;26:468–71.
86. Straumann A. [Eosinophilic esophagitis: a novel entity?]. Schweiz Rundsch Med Prax 2006;95:191–5.
87. Furuta GT. Clinicopathologic features of esophagitis in children. Gastrointest Endosc Clin N Am 2001;11:683–715, vii.
88. Nostrant TT. Esophageal dilation/dilators. Curr Treat Options Gastroenterol 2005; 8:85–95.
89. Liacouras CA, Spergel JM, Ruchelli E, et al. Eosinophilic esophagitis: a 10-year experience in 381 children. Clin Gastroenterol Hepatol 2005;3:1198–206.
90. Markowitz JE, Liacouras CA. Eosinophilic esophagitis. Gastroenterol Clin North Am 2003;32:949–66.
91. Kelly KJ, Lazenby AJ, Rowe PC, et al. Eosinophilic esophagitis attributed to gastroesophageal reflux: improvement with an amino acid-based formula. Gastroenterology 1995;109:1503–12.
92. Faubion WA Jr, Perrault J, Burgart LJ, et al. Treatment of eosinophilic esophagitis with inhaled corticosteroids. J Pediatr Gastroenterol Nutr 1998;27:90–3.
93. Arora AS, Perrault J, Smyrk TC. Topical corticosteroid treatment of dysphagia due to eosinophilic esophagitis in adults. Mayo Clin Proc 2003;78:830–5.

Putting the Puzzle Together: Epidemiological and Clinical Clues in the Etiology of Eosinophilic Esophagitis

Peter A.L. Bonis, MD[a,b],*

KEYWORDS

- Eosinophilic esophagitis • Epidemiology • Pathogenesis
- Pesticides • Hygiene hypothesis • Food allergy

The cause of eosinophilic esophagitis (EoE) is unknown, but its epidemiology and clinical features provide pieces to the puzzle. EoE appears to have emerged after World War II (possibly in the 1950s or early 1960s), has an increasing incidence, occurs in most developed countries, is related to food allergies, affects adults and children, has a strong male predominance, clusters in families, and is commonly associated with other allergic and atopic disorders.

A comprehensive understanding of the pathogenesis of EoE requires that its immunobiology be reconciled with these observations. Some authorities have categorized EoE as another example of the rising incidence of allergic and atopic diseases observed in the last several decades, suggesting that these disorders share an underlying cause. A unifying theory that explains this phenomenon has yet to be convincingly established, although several have been proposed.

EOSINOPHILIC ESOPHAGITIS LIKELY BEGAN AFTER WORLD WAR II

An understanding of the timetable in the onset of EoE is incomplete at best, but indirect evidence points toward its origins sometime after World War II, possibly in the

[a] Division of Gastroenterology, Tufts Medical Center, 750 Washington Street, Boston, MA 02111, USA
[b] Division of Clinical Care Research, Tufts Medical Center, 750 Washington Street, Boston, MA 02111, USA
* UpToDate Inc, 95 Sawyer Road Waltham, MA 02453.
E-mail address: pbonis@uptodate.com

Immunol Allergy Clin N Am 29 (2009) 41–52
doi:10.1016/j.iac.2008.09.005 immunology.theclinics.com
0889-8561/08/$ – see front matter © 2009 Elsevier Inc. All rights reserved.

1950s or 1960s. A hallmark of EoE is the corrugated ringed esophagus that has been described repeatedly in older children and adults.[1–4] The rings are seen easily on endoscopy and barium studies of the esophagus. The characteristic radiologic pattern was reported throughout the 1980s and 1990s, although it was believed to be due to congenital causes or gastroesophageal reflux disease.[5–8] The finding was first reported in the mid-1970s,[9,10] more than 20 years after the first description of a Schatzki's ring.[11] Barium radiography was used routinely in the evaluation of dysphagia, making it unlikely that this finding would have gone unreported had it been present in earlier decades.

An earlier report in 1966 described a 46-year-old man who presented in 1965 with midesophageal rings on barium studies, a history of dysphagia since 1945, and pain after dilation, all features compatible with EoE.[12] However, on esophagoscopy, the rings appeared to be thin, membranous webs (not characteristic of EoE). Two other midesophageal webs were described in a series of 58 patients in a report from 1958, but neither had clinical features suggestive of EoE.[13]

The decade in which EoE began would have to account for the latency period from the onset of EoE to the development of the ringed esophagus. Clinical observations and histologic studies suggest that the rings evolve from longstanding eosinophilic inflammation and associated subepithelial fibrosis.[14,15] The proportion of patients destined to develop rings, associated risk factors, and rate of progression remain unclear. However, assuming a latency period of 10 to 15 years, available reports and clinical experience suggest that EoE began sometime in the 1950s or early 1960s.

THE INCIDENCE IS RISING

More patients with EoE are being identified, but the extent to which this can be attributed to increased recognition versus a true rise in the incidence has been debated until recently. For example, one study, based upon analysis of a pathology database in Iowa, found that the prevalence of EoE was similar in recent years to that of the early 1990s, indicating that the rising incidence is attributable to increased recognition.[16] Similar findings have been reported by others.[17]

However, other single-center reports and at least five population-based studies have reached conclusions that suggest the rising incidence is not fully explained by increasing recognition.[2,18–22] As an example, one report (published as an abstract) examined the incidence of EoE in Olmsted County, Minnesota, over a 30-year period.[21] Between 1976 and 1985 at least five population-based studies have concluded that the incidence was estimated to be 1 per 100,000 population compared with approximately 4 per 100,000 between 1986 and 1995 and 9 per 100,000 between 1996 and 2005. The prevalence was estimated to be 105 per 100,000 population in 2007. These trends persisted even when using relatively stringent definitions of EoE to avoid misclassification, albeit one of the generally accepted diagnostic criteria (persistence of esophageal eosinophilia despite a proton-pump inhibitor[23]) was not systematically applied. A prospective database maintained in Ohio in which the diagnostic criteria have been uniform shows a similar increase in recent years (Marc Rothenberg, personal communication, 2008).[20]

Not all of these studies used the same definition of EoE. Thus the disease may have been misclassified in some patients.[24] Nevertheless, considered together, these data appear to have settled the issue of recognition versus a true rising incidence, suggesting that both are occurring, at least in some regions.

The increasing incidence of EoE suggests that whatever factors led to its evolution in the mid-20th century continue to exist today. This epidemiologic pattern is consistent with an ongoing (perhaps intensifying) environmental cause.

GEOGRAPHIC DISTRIBUTION

EoE has been reported in several countries, including Chile, Denmark, Sweden, Belgium, Greece, France, Spain, Germany, Switzerland, Japan, England, Italy, the Netherlands, New Zealand, Australia, and the United States.[23] EoE has not been reported in Africa, an observation that is potentially important because it is consistent with the hygiene hypothesis of allergy (see below).

A detailed understanding of the distribution of EoE within countries or geographic regions could be important for understanding environmental causes. For example, clustering in urban environments (which has been demonstrated in some studies of asthma) could suggest a role for specific environmental pollutants. Alternatively, a decrease in disease burden in farming or agricultural environments could support the hygiene theory. A north-south gradient could support the vitamin D hypothesis related to decreased sunlight exposure in northern climates (see below).

The available evidence regarding geographic distribution is substantially incomplete. A pathology database study in the United States suggested the disease is present in most states but could not determine geographic clustering.[25] Another study (presented as an abstract) in both an urban and a rural setting found that EoE was being increasingly recognized but also found that patients in the rural setting were more likely to have refluxlike symptoms, while those in the urban setting were more likely to have a history of food allergy and atopy.[26] The question of whether these observations have a bearing on pathogenesis requires more study.

AN ETIOLOGIC THEORY HAS TO EXPLAIN THE OBSERVED CLINICAL FEATURES

A comprehensive theory that explains the origin of EoE has to explain its ability to affect adults and children, the observed familial clustering, and its male predominance in both adults and children.

Case series and limited studies on natural history suggest that EoE can develop in children and in adults and persists in both groups.[27,28] Because the disease is chronic in children, some adults with EoE likely had the onset of the disease in childhood. However, studies of adults suggest that the disease can also arise after childhood.[2,28] While a subset of adults recall symptoms during childhood, others describe compatible clinical features beginning much later in life. Furthermore the disease has been reported in patients who first presented in their 70s.[2]

Thus, a theory explaining the development of EoE must consider mechanisms leading to food sensitization or loss of tolerance in adults. The much larger body of evidence related to the pathogenesis of food allergy in children may not be directly applicable. For example, an immature gastrointestinal immune response has been suggested as a cause of sensitization to foods in infants, but is unlikely to have a prominent role in adults.[29]

Multiple reports have described familial clustering of EoE across generations.[30–32] The degree to which this can be attributed to genetic predisposition or shared environmental risk factors is unknown. A study comparing familial with sporadic cases found no significant differences in the disease based upon genome-wide microarray analysis, suggesting that the pathogenesis of the sporadic form is similar to that of the familial form.[33]

Virtually every study on EoE has described a striking male predominance (approximately three to one), the magnitude of which has not been described in other forms of allergic disorders in adults.[34] Why boys and men should be relatively susceptible to the disease is unknown. Interestingly, a male predominance (about two to one) is also seen in Barrett's esophagus. Whether the two conditions are pathogenically linked is unclear, although an association has been suggested.[35,36]

ENVIRONMENTAL THEORIES

Multiple theories have been proposed to explain the increase in allergic disorders in recent decades. None of these theories have been studied directly in patients with EoE.

Hygiene Hypothesis

The hygiene hypothesis explains the rising incidence of allergic and immune disorders as a result of improvements in hygiene during the 20th century. An initial report described an inverse association between family size and the development of atopic disorders.[37] Several lines of epidemiologic and laboratory evidence provide support for the hygiene hypothesis in a variety of allergic and inflammatory disorders, although discordant data have been published and many unsettled questions remain.[38–40] For example, the relatively low disease burden of allergic disorders in developing nations is compatible with the theory that microbiological exposures can protect against the development of allergic disorders. On the other hand, this observation may at least in part be due to underreporting of allergic conditions and to genetic or epigenetic factors in the protected populations.

The hygiene hypothesis has not been extensively studied in the development of food allergies and the data that do exist are not highly compelling. For example, limited evidence has demonstrated an association between cesarean delivery and an increased risk of food allergy, implying that the lack of early colonization with colonic microflora during vaginal delivery increases the risk of developing food sensitivity.[41] However, such an association is potentially confounded by a number of factors, such as the effects of maternal age, number and ages of siblings, and a baseline risk for development of allergic disorders.

No studies have established a convincing link between general or specific changes in microbiological exposures that are compatible with the timetable for the inception of EoE described above. It is also difficult to identify general or specific changes in microbiological exposures that correlate well with the increasing incidence of EoE in recent decades.

Epidermal Barrier Function

A provocative theory in the pathogenesis of atopic dermatitis and asthma suggests that an underlying cause is genetically determined epithelial barrier dysfunction. One theory of asthma suggests that the epithelium is impaired through defective tight junction formation, thereby facilitating penetration of potentially toxic or damaging environmental insults.[42]

Similarly, accumulating evidence has suggested that abnormal epithelial barrier function may be fundamental to the development of atopic sensitization, eczema, and possibly to asthma in patients with eczema.[43,44] The abnormal function appears to be at least in part related to variations in the profilaggrin gene.[43] Filaggrin is a major component of the granular layer of the epidermis. In addition to atopic dermatitis, abnormalities of the profilaggrin system have been associated with ichthyosis vulgaris and possibly other skin conditions. Loss-of-function mutations in the profilaggrin gene have been detected in about 10% of the general population.[45]

The role of epithelial barrier function (including variations in the filaggrin gene) is currently being studied in EoE. However, abnormal barrier function itself cannot explain the rising incidence of EoE or other allergic conditions. The genetic susceptibility to abnormal epithelial barrier function preceded this trend. Thus, some form of environmental cause is needed to explain its deleterious consequences.

Helicobacter pylori

A decrease in disease burden related to *Helicobacter pylori* in recent decades coincided with the increase in allergic disorders, suggesting that *H pylori* may protect against the development of allergy.[46,47] Proponents of *H pylori* therapy also point toward a "dose-response" effect, whereby relatively virulent strains of *H pylori* (cytotoxin-associated gene A+) have the strongest protective effect against the development of asthma.[47,48]

On the other hand, some studies have found an association with the presence of *H pylori* and the development of food allergies and the resolution of atopic dermatitis after *H pylori* eradication.[49–51] In addition, the decline in the prevalence in *H pylori* infection in developed nations is believed to have preceded the increase in the incidence of allergy and atopic disorders. No study has directly evaluated whether *H pylori* infection has a role in the development of EoE.

Dietary Fat Hypothesis

The dietary fat hypothesis suggests that a relative increase in consumption of omega-6 fatty acids and a decrease in omega-3 fatty acids (mainly from fish oil) are responsible for the development of allergies.[52–54] There are only limited, inconclusive data evaluating this hypothesis in food allergy and none in EoE.

Vitamin D Hypothesis

A decrease in exposure to vitamin D (either because of maternal diet during pregnancy, early childhood diet, lack of exposure to sunlight, or variations in the vitamin D receptor) has been implicated in the development of allergic disorders, but data are mixed.[46,55–58] By contrast, an increase in exposure to vitamin D has also been linked to the development of allergies.[59–61] Vitamin D status has not been studied directly in EoE.

Acid Suppression

Acid-suppressive medications have been associated with development of IgE antibodies to foods in humans and in experimental models.[62–65] A decrease in gastric acidification may cause the persistence of labile food proteins, potentially leading to sensitization.[64]

No study has directly demonstrated the development of EoE in adults or children following exposure to acid-suppressive medications. It is likely (at least in children) that exposure to these drugs would follow the development of EoE rather than precede it because children with EoE would be unlikely to have previously used these drugs for other conditions.

Furthermore, clinical observations in patients with EoE taking proton-pump inhibitors do not suggest that they worsen food sensitivity or cause sensitivity to new foods, although there have been no formal studies. Indeed, there are case series of patients with severe esophageal eosinophilia that resolved upon treatment with a proton-pump inhibitor.[66] The question of whether such patients represent a variant of gastroesophageal reflux disease or a proton-pump inhibitor–responsive form of EoE remains unanswered. In the latter situation, it is interesting to speculate whether alteration in food proteins due to a relative lack of gastric digestion may have favorably altered immune reactivity against the implicated food proteins.

Changes in Food Composition and Other Environmental Exposures

Esophageal eosinophilia and symptoms resolve with an elemental or elimination diet in children with EoE, making a compelling case for a central role of food allergies in its pathogenesis.[27] Most theories related to food allergy have focused on mechanisms leading to sensitization or loss of tolerance to relevant food proteins.

By contrast, the question of whether there may have been clinically important changes in the characteristics of the implicated foods over time, making them more likely to cause allergy, has not been extensively evaluated. Some studies have found that foods grown under modern conditions (with the assistance of synthetic fertilizers and pesticides) differ in their composition of certain polyphenols and antioxidants than foods grown under organic conditions.[67–70] Whether these changes could influence the immunogenicity of the foods is unknown. However, some reports have found an association between a decrease in maternal antioxidant intake and childhood wheezing and eczema.[55,71–73]

Growth of foods under modern conditions may also stimulate plants to produce "pathogenesis-related proteins" or other allergens that protect the plants from pathogens but have the potential to contribute to sensitization in humans.[74] Interestingly, use of synthetic pesticides in the United States began in the 1930s and became widespread after World War II, a time-frame compatible with the onset of EoE.

Few studies have directly evaluated the impact of these effects on the clinical expression of allergy. At least one cohort study found a significantly lower risk of eczema in children who had consumed predominantly organic dairy products during the first 2 years of life.[75] No association was found for organic meats, fruits, vegetables, or eggs.

In addition, populations in developed nations have experienced dramatic changes in the ways that foods are processed and packaged and have been exposed to an enormous variety of new foods, food additives, pesticide residues, and other synthetic materials that are ultimately ingested or come into contact with the skin or respiratory epithelium. Several potential mechanisms in which these changes could lead to the development of allergy in susceptible individuals exist, but none has yet been extensively studied in food sensitivity. For example, these changes might have influenced the ecology of the gut flora; altered epithelial barrier function in the gut, skin, or respiratory mucosa; or influenced food protein characteristics, thus predisposing to sensitization.

An association of certain synthetic compounds and agricultural products, such as fungicides, with the development of contact dermatitis through direct skin contact or by exposure of the respiratory epithelium has been demonstrated repeatedly.[76–84] Certain fungicides also behave as haptens, small molecules that are capable of eliciting an immune response when conjugated with carrier molecules.[85] Furthermore, because these agents may be present on specific foods, sensitization to them may be confused with sensitization to the food. No studies have determined whether exposure to these agents contributes to the development of food sensitivities in patients with EoE or other forms of food-allergic disorders. Lack of standardization of methods and the long list of potential candidates are undoubtedly important obstacles to studying these potential associations.

Dual-Allergen Hypothesis

The dual-allergen hypothesis is based upon the observation that allergic sensitization to food may develop following low-dose cutaneous exposure while early oral exposure to food protein induces tolerance. Thus, according to this hypothesis, food allergy will develop if food proteins penetrate the skin, leading to sensitization before oral toler-ance develops.[86] Cutaneous exposure is hypothesized to occur when food proteins present on tabletops and the household environment contact the skin.

What has changed in the last half century to cause the implicated foods to lead to cutaneous sensitization by this mechanism is unexplained. It is interesting to specu-late whether environmental synthetic materials facilitate cutaneous sensitization either by serving as haptens for food proteins or by impairing epidermal barrier function in individuals who are already susceptible (such as those with loss-of-function mutations in the filaggrin gene). No studies have directly examined whether such an association exists.

Respiratory Allergens

Experimental evidence in EoE has linked the development of esophageal eosinophilia with sensitization to aeroallergens in the bronchial mucosa. Esophageal eosinophilia developed in mice exposed to respiratory allergens while exposure of the mice to oral or intragastric allergens did not promote eosinophilic esophagitis.[87]

The extent to which these observations are applicable to humans with EoE remains unclear. Limited data suggest there may be seasonal variation in the incidence of EoE with fewer cases in winter months, possibly implicating pollen or other aeroaller-gens.[88–90] However, no direct evidence has linked respiratory exposure to relevant food proteins or their mimics to the development of EoE in humans.

Changes in Gut Ecology

The gut microbiota influences intestinal permeability and the generation of proinflam-matory cytokines involved in the development of sensitization to luminal contents.[91] The composition of the gut microflora is influenced by multiple factors but particularly diet and use of antibiotics.[92] There is large variability in the composition of the flora among people, although it remains relatively constant in individuals.[93,94] Alterations in microbial flora in patients with inflammatory bowel diseases and in animal models of inflammatory bowel diseases have been repeatedly described and are also impli-cated in the pathogenesis of allergic diseases.[95] Multiple clinical trials have evaluated the role of probiotics in treatment of these conditions, but results have been mixed.[96]

The question of whether specific types of microflora are associated with the devel-opment of EoE has not yet been studied. There is no evidence that the composition of the fecal microbiota in the population has changed in recent decades to account for the development of allergic conditions, but the subject has not been well studied.

SUMMARY

The ultimate cause of EoE remains unknown even as the immune mechanisms in-volved are becoming clarified. The disease is unequivocally related to food allergies, but the steps involved that lead to sensitization to the implicated foods and account for the epidemiologic and clinical features described above remain a mystery. Solving the mystery is important not only to understand EoE but also to shed light upon the causes of other allergic conditions.

ACKNOWLEDGMENTS

I am grateful to Dr. Anna Feldweg for her insights during preparation of this manuscript.

REFERENCES

1. Bousvaros A, Antonioli DA, Winter HS. Ringed esophagus: an association with esophagitis. Am J Gastroenterol 1992;87(9):1187–90.
2. Croese J, Fairley SK, Masson JW, et al. Clinical and endoscopic features of eosinophilic esophagitis in adults. Gastrointest Endosc 2003;58:516.
3. Potter JW, Saeian K, Staff D, et al. Eosinophilic esophagitis in adults: an emerging problem with unique esophageal features. Gastrointest Endosc 2004;59:355.
4. Zimmerman SL, Levine MS, Rubesin SE, et al. Idiopathic eosinophilic esophagitis in adults: the ringed esophagus. Radiology 2005;236:159.
5. Katzka DA, Levine MS, Ginsberg GG, et al. Congenital esophageal stenosis in adults. Am J Gastroenterol 2000;95:32.
6. Langdon DE. Corrugated ringed and too small esophagi. Am J Gastroenterol 1999;94:542.
7. McKinley MJ, Eisner TD, Fisher ML, et al. Multiple rings of the esophagus associated with gastroesophageal reflux [case report]. Am J Gastroenterol 1996;91: 574.
8. Morrow JB, Vargo JJ, Goldblum JR, et al. The ringed esophagus: histological features of GERD. Am J Gastroenterol 2001;96:984.
9. Landres RT, Kuster GG, Strum WB. Eosinophilic esophagitis in a patient with vigorous achalasia. Gastroenterology 1978;74:1298.
10. Shiflett DW, Gilliam JH, Wu WC, et al. Multiple esophageal webs. Gastroenterology 1979;77:556.
11. Schatzki R, Gary JE. Dysphagia due to a diaphragm-like localized narrowing in the lower esophagus (lower esophageal ring). Am J Roentgenol Radium Ther Nucl Med 1953;70:911.
12. Kelley ML Jr, Frazer JP. Symptomatic mid-esophageal webs. JAMA 1966;197: 143.
13. Shamma'a MH, Benedict EB. Esopahgeal webs: a report of 58 cases and attempt at classification. N Engl J Med 1958;259:378.
14. Aceves SS, Newbury RO, Dohil R, et al. Distinguishing eosinophilic esophagitis in pediatric patients: clinical, endoscopic, and histologic features of an emerging disorder. J Clin Gastroenterol 2007;41:252.
15. Chehade M, Sampson HA, Morotti RA, et al. Esophageal subepithelial fibrosis in children with eosinophilic esophagitis. J Pediatr Gastroenterol Nutr 2007;45:319.
16. Vanderheyden AD, Petras RE, DeYoung BR, et al. Emerging eosinophilic (allergic) esophagitis: increased incidence or increased recognition? Arch Pathol Lab Med 2007;131:777.
17. Chadwick I, Kaplan G. Rising incidence of eosinophilic esophagitis in the Calgary Health Region: a population-based study [abstract]. Gastroenterology 2008;134: A291.
18. Cherian S, Smith NM, Forbes DA. Rapidly increasing prevalence of eosinophilic oesophagitis in Western Australia. Arch Dis Child 2006;91:1000.
19. Dellon ES, Woosley JT. Increasing incidence of eosinophilic esophagitis: persistent trend after accounting for procedure indication and biopsy rate [abstract]. Gastroenterology 2008;134:289.
20. Noel RJ, Putnam PE, Rothenberg ME. Eosinophilic esophagitis. N Engl J Med 2004;351:940.
21. Prasad GA, Smryk TC, Scleck C. Secular trends in the epidemiology and outcomes of eosinophilic esophagitis in Olmsted County, Minnesota (1976–2007) [abstract]. Gastroenterology 2008;134:A289.

22. Straumann A, Simon HU. Eosinophilic esophagitis: escalating epidemiology? J Allergy Clin Immunol 2005;115:418.
23. Furuta GT, Liacouras CA, Collins MH, et al. Eosinophilic esophagitis in children and adults: a systematic review and consensus recommendations for diagnosis and treatment. Gastroenterology 2007;133:1342.
24. Dellon ES, Aderoju A, Woosley JT, et al. Variability in diagnostic criteria for eosinophilic esophagitis: a systematic review. Am J Gastroenterol 2007;102:2300.
25. Kapel RC, Miller JK, Torres C, et al. Eosinophilic esophagitis: a prevalent disease in the United States that affects all age groups. Gastroenterology 2008;134:1316.
26. Karmam U, Gonsalves N, Hirano I. Differences in demographic and clinical characteristics of eosinophilic eophagitis in urban and rural US populations [abstract]. Gastroenterology 2008;134:A289.
27. Liacouras CA, Spergel JM, Ruchelli E, et al. Eosinophilic esophagitis: a 10-year experience in 381 children. Clin Gastroenterol Hepatol 2005;3:1198.
28. Straumann A, Spichtin HP, Grize L, et al. Natural history of primary eosinophilic esophagitis: a follow-up of 30 adult patients for up to 11.5 years. Gastroenterology 2003;125:1660.
29. Shah U, Walker WA. Pathophysiology of intestinal food allergy. Adv Pediatr 2002; 49:299.
30. Meyer GW. Eosinophilic esophagitis in a father and a daughter. Gastrointest Endosc 2005;61:932.
31. Patel SM, Falchuk KR. Three brothers with dysphagia caused by eosinophilic esophagitis. Gastrointest Endosc 2005;61:165.
32. Zink DA, Amin M, Gebara S, et al. Familial dysphagia and eosinophilia. Gastrointest Endosc 2007;65:330.
33. Collins MH, Blanchard C, Abonia JP, et al. Clinical, pathologic, and molecular characterization of familial eosinophilic esophagitis compared with sporadic cases. Clin Gastroenterol Hepatol 2008;6:621.
34. Jensen-Jarolim E, Untersmayr E. Gender-medicine aspects in allergology. Allergy 2008;63:610.
35. Francalanci P, De Angelis P, Minnei F, et al. Eosinophilic esophagitis and Barrett's esophagus: an occasional association or an overlap disease? Esophageal 'double trouble' in two children. Digestion 2008;77:16.
36. Wolfsen HC, Hemminger LL, Achem SR. Eosinophilic esophagitis and Barrett's esophagus with dysplasia. Clin Gastroenterol Hepatol 2007;5:A18.
37. Strachan DP. Hay fever, hygiene, and household size. BMJ 1989;299:1259.
38. Bach JF. Six questions about the hygiene hypothesis. Cell Immunol 2005;233:158.
39. Garn H, Renz H. Epidemiological and immunological evidence for the hygiene hypothesis. Immunobiology 2007;212:441.
40. Vercelli D. Mechanisms of the hygiene hypothesis—molecular and otherwise. Curr Opin Immunol 2006;18:733.
41. Bager P, Wohlfahrt J, Westergaard T. Caesarean delivery and risk of atopy and allergic disease: meta-analyses. Clin Exp Allergy 2008;38:634.
42. Holgate ST. The airway epithelium is central to the pathogenesis of asthma. Allergol Int 2008;57:1.
43. Baurecht H, Irvine AD, Novak N, et al. Toward a major risk factor for atopic eczema: meta-analysis of filaggrin polymorphism data. J Allergy Clin Immunol 2007;120:1406.
44. Henderson J, Northstone K, Lee SP, et al. The burden of disease associated with filaggrin mutations: a population-based, longitudinal birth cohort study. J Allergy Clin Immunol 2008;121:872.

45. McGrath JA, Uitto J. The filaggrin story: novel insights into skin-barrier function and disease. Trends Mol Med 2008;14:20.
46. Blaser MJ, Chen Y, Reibman J. Does Helicobacter pylori protect against asthma and allergy? Gut 2008;57:561.
47. Shiotani A, Miyanishi T, Kamada T, et al. Helicobacter pylori infection and allergic diseases: epidemiological study in Japanese university students. J Gastroenterol Hepatol 2007.
48. Chen Y, Blaser MJ. Inverse associations of Helicobacter pylori with asthma and allergy. Arch Intern Med 2007;167:821.
49. Corrado G, Luzzi I, Pacchiarotti C, et al. Helicobacter pylori seropositivity in children with atopic dermatitis as sole manifestation of food allergy. Pediatr Allergy Immunol 2000;11:101.
50. Galadari IH, Sheriff MO. The role of Helicobacter pylori in urticaria and atopic dermatitis. Skinmed 2006;5:172.
51. Murakami K, Fujioka T, Nishizono A, et al. Atopic dermatitis successfully treated by eradication of Helicobacter pylori. J Gastroenterol 1996;31(Suppl 9):77.
52. Almqvist C, Garden F, Xuan W, et al. Omega-3 and omega-6 fatty acid exposure from early life does not affect atopy and asthma at age 5 years. J Allergy Clin Immunol 2007;119:1438.
53. Hwang I, Cha A, Lee H, et al. N-3 polyunsaturated fatty acids and atopy in Korean preschoolers. Lipids 2007;42:345.
54. Miyake Y, Sasaki S, Tanaka K, et al. Fish and fat intake and prevalence of allergic rhinitis in Japanese females: the Osaka Maternal and Child Health Study. J Am Coll Nutr 2007;26:279.
55. Camargo CA Jr, Rifas-Shiman SL, Litonjua AA, et al. Maternal intake of vitamin D during pregnancy and risk of recurrent wheeze in children at 3 y of age. Am J Clin Nutr 2007;85:788.
56. Poon AH, Laprise C, Lemire M, et al. Association of vitamin D receptor genetic variants with susceptibility to asthma and atopy. Am J Respir Crit Care Med 2004;170:967.
57. Raby BA, Lazarus R, Silverman EK, et al. Association of vitamin D receptor gene polymorphisms with childhood and adult asthma. Am J Respir Crit Care Med 2004;170:1057.
58. Weiss ST, Litonjua AA. Maternal diet vs lack of exposure to sunlight as the cause of the epidemic of asthma, allergies and other autoimmune diseases. Thorax 2007;62:746.
59. Hypponen E, Sovio U, Wjst M, et al. Infant vitamin D supplementation and allergic conditions in adulthood: northern Finland birth cohort 1966. Ann N Y Acad Sci 2004;1037:84.
60. Milner JD, Stein DM, McCarter R, et al. Early infant multivitamin supplementation is associated with increased risk for food allergy and asthma. Pediatrics 2004; 114:27.
61. Wjst M. Another explanation for the low allergy rate in the rural Alpine foothills. Clin Mol Allergy 2005;3:7.
62. Scholl I, Untersmayr E, Bakos N, et al. Antiulcer drugs promote oral sensitization and hypersensitivity to hazelnut allergens in BALB/c mice and humans. Am J Clin Nutr 2005;81:154.
63. Untersmayr E, Bakos N, Scholl I, et al. Anti-ulcer drugs promote IgE formation toward dietary antigens in adult patients. FASEB J 2005;19:656.
64. Untersmayr E, Jensen-Jarolim E. The role of protein digestibility and antacids on food allergy outcomes. J Allergy Clin Immunol 2008;121:1301.

65. Untersmayr E, Scholl I, Swoboda I, et al. Antacid medication inhibits digestion of dietary proteins and causes food allergy: a fish allergy model in BALB/c mice. J Allergy Clin Immunol 2003;112:616.
66. Ngo P, Furuta GT, Antonioli DA, et al. Eosinophils in the esophagus—peptic or allergic eosinophilic esophagitis? Case series of three patients with esophageal eosinophilia. Am J Gastroenterol 2006;101:1666.
67. Carbonaro M, Mattera M, Nicoli S, et al. Modulation of antioxidant compounds in organic vs conventional fruit (peach, Prunus persica L., and pear, Pyrus communis L.). J Agric Food Chem 2002;50:5458.
68. Chassy AW, Bui L, Renaud EN, et al. Three-year comparison of the content of antioxidant microconstituents and several quality characteristics in organic and conventionally managed tomatoes and bell peppers. J Agric Food Chem 2006; 54:8244.
69. Lombardi-Boccia G, Lucarini M, Lanzi S, et al. Nutrients and antioxidant molecules in yellow plums (Prunus domestica L.) from conventional and organic productions: a comparative study. J Agric Food Chem 2004;52:90.
70. Williams CM. Nutritional quality of organic food: shades of grey or shades of green? Proc Nutr Soc 2002;61:19.
71. Devereux G, Turner SW, Craig LC, et al. Low maternal vitamin E intake during pregnancy is associated with asthma in 5-year-old children. Am J Respir Crit Care Med 2006;174:499.
72. Litonjua AA, Rifas-Shiman SL, Ly NP, et al. Maternal antioxidant intake in pregnancy and wheezing illnesses in children at 2 y of age. Am J Clin Nutr 2006; 84:903.
73. Martindale S, McNeill G, Devereux G, et al. Antioxidant intake in pregnancy in relation to wheeze and eczema in the first two years of life. Am J Respir Crit Care Med 2005;171:121.
74. Ronchetti R, Kaczmarski MG, Haluszka J, et al. Food allergies, cross-reactions and agroalimentary biotechnologies. Adv Med Sci 2007;52:98.
75. Kummeling I, Thijs C, Huber M, et al. Consumption of organic foods and risk of atopic disease during the first 2 years of life in the Netherlands. Br J Nutr 2008;99:598.
76. Campbell FA, Forsyth A. Dithiocarbamate-induced allergic contact dermatitis. Contact Dermatitis 2003;49:305.
77. Horiuchi N, Oguchi S, Nagami H, et al. Pesticide-related dermatitis in Saku district, Japan, 1975-2000. Int J Occup Environ Health 2008;14:25.
78. Lensen G, Jungbauer F, Goncalo M, et al. Airborne irritant contact dermatitis and conjunctivitis after occupational exposure to chlorothalonil in textiles. Contact Dermatitis 2007;57:181.
79. Lerbaek A, Menne T, Knudsen B. Cross-reactivity between thiurams. Contact Dermatitis 2006;54:165.
80. Nakamura M, Miyachi Y. Airborne photocontact dermatitis due to the insecticide phoxim. Contact Dermatitis 2003;49:105.
81. Nguyen SH, Dang TP, MacPherson C, et al. Prevalence of patch test results from 1970 to 2002 in a multi-centre population in North America (NACDG). Contact Dermatitis 2008;58:101.
82. Penagos H, Ruepert C, Partanen T, et al. Pesticide patch test series for the assessment of allergic contact dermatitis among banana plantation workers in Panama. Dermatitis 2004;15:137.
83. Verma G, Sharma NL, Shanker V, et al. Pesticide contact dermatitis in fruit and vegetable farmers of Himachal Pradesh (India). Contact Dermatitis 2007;57:316.

84. Yu KJ, Chen HH, Chang YC, et al. Ulcerative irritant contact dermatitis from lindane. Contact Dermatitis 2005;52:118.
85. Gunther S, Hempel D, Dunkel M, et al. SuperHapten: a comprehensive database for small immunogenic compounds. Nucleic Acids Res 2007;35:D906.
86. Lack G. Epidemiologic risks for food allergy. J Allergy Clin Immunol 2008;121: 1331.
87. Mishra A, Hogan SP, Brandt EB, et al. An etiological role for aeroallergens and eosinophils in experimental esophagitis. J Clin Invest 2001;107:83.
88. Fogg MI, Ruchelli E, Spergel JM. Pollen and eosinophilic esophagitis. J Allergy Clin Immunol 2003;112:796.
89. Prasad GA, Smryk TC, Schleck C, et al. Seasonal variation in the incidence of eosinophilic eosphagitis over 30 years: a population based study [abstract]. Gastroenterology 2008;134:W1033.
90. Wang FY, Gupta SK, Fitzgerald JF. Is there a seasonal variation in the incidence or intensity of allergic eosinophilic esophagitis in newly diagnosed children? J Clin Gastroenterol 2007;41:451.
91. Sartor RB. Therapeutic manipulation of the enteric microflora in inflammatory bowel diseases: antibiotics, probiotics, and prebiotics. Gastroenterology 2004; 126:1620.
92. O'Keefe SJ. Nutrition and colonic health: the critical role of the microbiota. Curr Opin Gastroenterol 2008;24:51.
93. Eckburg PB, Bik EM, Bernstein CN, et al. Diversity of the human intestinal microbial flora. Science 2005;308:1635.
94. Matsuki T, Watanabe K, Fujimoto J, et al. Use of 16S rRNA gene-targeted group-specific primers for real-time PCR analysis of predominant bacteria in human feces. Appl Environ Microbiol 2004;70:7220.
95. Noverr MC, Huffnagle GB. The 'microflora hypothesis' of allergic diseases. Clin Exp Allergy 2005;35:1511.
96. Osborn DA, Sinn JK. Probiotics in infants for prevention of allergic disease and food hypersensitivity. Cochrane Database Syst Rev 2007;4:CD006475.

Evaluation of the Patient with Suspected Eosinophilic Gastrointestinal Disease

David M. Fleischer, MD[a], Dan Atkins, MD[b,c,d,e],*

KEYWORDS

- Eosinophilic gastrointestinal disease
- Eosinophilic gastrointestinal disorders
- Eosinophilic gastritis • Eosinophilic gastroenteritis
- Eosinophilic enteritis • Eosinophilic colitis

Over the past decade, eosinophilic esophagitis (EoE) morphed from a rarely recognized entity into a frequently entertained diagnostic consideration in patients of all ages presenting with any of a variety of gastrointestinal complaints.[1] This miniepidemic has spawned interest in the appropriate evaluation and management of eosinophilic gastrointestinal diseases (EGIDs), of which EoE is the most common. Diagnostic consideration of EGIDs is prompted by identification of abnormal eosinophilic infiltration on morphologic evaluation of gastrointestinal tissues obtained by biopsy or resection from patients with gastrointestinal complaints. To solidify the diagnosis, other potential causes of gastrointestinal eosinophilia must be excluded. EGIDs have been classified in regard to the site involved (esophageal, gastric, small intestinal, colonic, or multiple) and tissue localization of the eosinophil accumulation (mucosal, muscular, serosal, diffuse, or transmural).[1-3]

In categorizing the larger group of all disorders associated with gastrointestinal eosinophilia, EGIDs are referred to as primary eosinophil-associated disorders to

[a] Department of Pediatrics, Division of Pediatric Allergy and Immunology, National Jewish Health, University of Colorado Health Sciences Center, 1400 Jackson Street, J321, Denver, CO 80206, USA
[b] Department of Pediatrics, Division of Pediatric Allergy and Immunology, National Jewish Health, University of Colorado Health Sciences Center, 1400 Jackson Street, J301, Denver, CO 80206, USA
[c] Pediatric Day Program, National Jewish Health, 1400 Jackson Street, Denver, CO 80206, USA
[d] Division of Ambulatory Pediatrics, National Jewish Health, 1400 Jackson Street, Denver, CO 80206, USA
[e] Department of Pediatrics, University of Colorado Health Sciences Center, 13123 East 16th Avenue, Aurora, CO 80045, USA
* Corresponding author. Department of Pediatrics, Division of Pediatric Allergy and Immunology, National Jewish Health, 1400 Jackson Street, J301, Denver, CO 80206.
E-mail address: atkinsd@njc.org (D. Atkins).

Immunol Allergy Clin N Am 29 (2009) 53–63
doi:10.1016/j.iac.2008.09.002
0889-8561/08/$ – see front matter © 2009 Elsevier Inc. All rights reserved.

immunology.theclinics.com

distinguish them from secondary eosinophil-associated disorders, where eosinophil accumulation is attributed to an identified cause. Thus, EGIDs, or primary eosinophil-associated gastrointestinal disorders, include EoE, eosinophilic gastritis, eosinophilic gastroenteritis, eosinophilic enteritis, and eosinophilic colitis or proctitis.[4] Demonstration of atopy in approximately 75% of these patients and recognition of familial involvement in more than 10% has prompted further categorization of EGIDs into atopic, nonatopic, and familial varieties.[1] Secondary eosinophil-associated gastrointestinal disorders include those disorders where eosinophil accumulation can be attributed to a distinct cause. These disorders are further categorized as (1) those due to eosinophilic disorders, usually hypereosinophilic syndrome; and (2) those due to noneosinophilic disorders, such as inflammatory bowel diseases, infectious diseases, connective tissue disorders, vasculitides, neoplasia, and iatrogenic causes. As EoE is covered elsewhere in this issue, this article focuses upon the approach to the evaluation and management of the remaining EGIDs.

HISTORY

As with any medical condition, the initial step in diagnosing EGID is a thorough history accurately delineating all symptoms, the timing of their onset, duration, progression, aggravating or alleviating factors, and response or lack thereof to previous treatment. Some EGIDs are age-limited, as exemplified by allergic proctocolitis of infancy, whereas others, such as eosinophilic gastroenteritis, occur at any age, although the peak incidence is between ages 20 to 50 years.[2,5,6] Curiously, serosal disease is much more common in women over 40 years of age (accounting for over 75% of these patients), whereas males outnumber females in other EGIDs.[7] Although the majority of reported cases involve Caucasians, isolated case reports from various locations throughout the world suggest no ethnic group is immune.[8]

Signs and symptoms vary depending upon the location and layer of gastrointestinal tissue involved. Classification of EGIDs by layer of gastrointestinal involvement was first proposed by Klein[2] in 1970. Mucosal involvement is by far the most common and is accompanied by one or more of the following symptoms: decreased appetite, early satiety, nausea, vomiting, gastric dysmotility, abdominal pain, malabsorption, diarrhea, anemia, failure to thrive, occult blood in the stool, and protein-losing enteropathy. Involvement of the muscular layer usually presents with colicky abdominal pain and symptoms of gastric outlet or intestinal obstruction. Serosal involvement, the least common, is accompanied by abdominal distention and eosinophilic ascites. Combinations of these symptoms occur with involvement of more than one tissue layer.

A personal history of allergic disease, such as eczema, asthma, allergic rhinitis, or animal dander sensitivity, heightens suspicion because the majority of patients with EGIDs are atopic, although the absence of other allergic disease does not preclude the diagnosis. Suspected foods and symptoms attributed to the ingestion of these foods should be listed, as questioning often reveals evidence of food allergy. Although comorbid food-induced anaphylaxis is relatively uncommon in these patients, it should not be overlooked. A dietary history is required to document regularly ingested foods, checking for the ingestion of those that increase the risk of parasite exposure, and to evaluate the nutritional adequacy of the diet.

Medication or environmental exposures predisposing to conditions associated with gastrointestinal eosinophilia should be identified and investigated. Where a person lives is an important variable as geographic location exerts a significant influence, with 35-fold higher numbers of colonic eosinophils associated with warmer climates, presumably because of differences in exposure to microbes and aeroallergens and because of regional differences in dietary allergen exposures.[9] Note that seasonal variations in symptoms may correlate with exposures to pollens or other allergens to which the patient is sensitized.[10] Make a complete record of medication history, including allergen immunotherapy and the use of over-the-counter medications, such as nonsteroidal anti-inflammatory drugs, vitamin supplements, and herbal remedies. Environmental exposures, including occupational and recreational exposures, should be elicited. Such exposures could include those related to foreign travel, camping, ingestion of well or stream water, farm work, and contact with animals.

Questioning about the presence of similar gastrointestinal symptoms in other family members is worthwhile because of the recognized familial tendency of these disorders. Allergic disease is often present in immediate family members. The presence of malignancy, immunodeficiency, inflammatory bowel disease, collagen vascular diseases, or other eosinophilic disorders in other family members should be ascertained.

An often-overlooked aspect of the history is questioning to determine the emotional well-being of the patient and other family members. Feeding difficulties and failure to thrive are often associated with EGIDs in infants and young children, and the frequent delay in obtaining an accurate diagnosis is often stressful for parents and patients alike. Detection of developmental delays in young children stemming from malnutrition or other causes is vital. Coping with elimination diets and chronic illness can be emotionally draining. By recognizing illness-related anxiety or depression and intervening early, and by providing education and psychologic support, the clinician can significantly improve the patient's quality of life.

PHYSICAL EXAMINATION

Although there are no physical findings diagnostic of EGID, a thorough physical examination is indicated to assess nutritional status and to identify physical findings suggestive of other diseases that might explain gastrointestinal symptoms. Longitudinal tracking of weight and other growth parameters, particularly in children, is necessary to monitor the impact of disease and dietary aberrations. Checking for physical findings of allergic rhinoconjunctivitis, asthma, or eczema is encouraged and, if present, noting whether these conditions are flared or well controlled provides useful information as total IgE levels and peripheral eosinophil counts often rise in patients with poorly controlled allergic disease. A careful examination of the abdomen to identify areas and degrees of tenderness, the presence of abdominal distention, organomegaly, ascites, or increased stool is an important aspect of the evaluation.

DIFFERENTIAL DIAGNOSIS

The differential diagnosis of EGIDs includes a host of conditions, referred to as secondary eosinophil-associated gastrointestinal disorders, that cause abdominal symptoms in combination with gastrointestinal eosinophilia.[1] Entities to be considered include systemic eosinophilic disorders with gastrointestinal involvement, such as hypereosinophilic syndromes, and other causes, including infections, inflammatory bowel diseases, celiac disease, food allergies, connective tissue disorders, vasculitis, neoplasia, responses to immunologic injury, and iatrogenic causes, such as reactions to medications. Parasitic infestations involving helminths, hookworms, pinworms, and a variety of other parasites have been associated with gastrointestinal tissue eosinophilia.[11–13] Clearing of gastric eosinophilia upon eradication of Helicobacter pylori has been reported, but further documentation of this association is warranted.[14] Increased numbers of activated eosinophils as evidenced by degranulation are noted in the inflamed gastrointestinal tissues of patients with Crohn's disease and ulcerative colitis where eosinophils are not the predominant cell type.[15] Interestingly, higher numbers of eosinophils in the mucosa of patients with ulcerative colitis have been reported as a favorable prognostic finding.[16] The hypercellular gastrointestinal lamina propria encountered in celiac disease contains increased eosinophil numbers, along with elevated numbers of lymphocytes, plasma cells, mast cells, and basophils.[4] The identification and removal of offending foods from the diet of food-allergic patients can lead to resolution of gastrointestinal eosinophilia, as is often seen in infants with allergic proctocolitis.[5] Varying levels of gastrointestinal eosinophilia have been observed in scleroderma, systemic lupus erythematosus, and dermatomyositis, in addition to vasculitides, such as Churg-Straus syndrome and periarteritis nodosa.[17] Graft-versus-host disease in bone marrow transplant patients is often associated with increased eosinophil numbers in the colon and rectum.[4] The use of oral tacrolimus for suppression of rejection in patients with solid organ transplants is associated with gastrointestinal eosinophilia accompanying food allergies in approximately 10% of the recipients.[18,19] A host of other medications have been implicated as causing gastrointestinal eosinophilia that usually resolves with discontinuation of the drug. Examples include nonsteroidal anti-inflammatory drugs, interferon, enalapril, carbamazepine, and co-trimoxazole.[20]

Hypereosinophilic syndromes must also be considered in patients presenting with gastrointestinal tissue eosinophilia and elevated peripheral eosinophil counts. The hypereosinophilic syndromes are recognized by the presence of more than 1500 circulating eosinophils per cubic millimeter for longer than 6 months without any identified cause, in association with organ damage not attributable to a cause other than eosinophilic infiltration. The presence of multiple organ involvement in these patients and the association of endomyocardial disease with prolonged eosinophilia prompt continued surveillance for extragastrointestinal involvement in patients presenting with EGIDs. These syndromes have been the topic of recent reviews and a previous issue of the *Immunology and Allergy Clinics*.[21] The diagnostic evaluation for hypereosinophilic syndromes is briefly detailed in **Box 1**.

DIAGNOSIS OF EOSINOPHILIC GASTROINTESTINAL DISEASE

Diagnosis of EGID requires a high index of suspicion, as the symptoms and presentations are nonspecific, often sharing features with more commonly encountered gastrointestinal disorders, such as infection, inflammatory bowel diseases, and iatrogenic and functional gastrointestinal disorders.[7] There are no confirmatory laboratory tests, and the morphologic evaluation of biopsies or surgical specimens is required to confirm the diagnosis. Because of the patchy nature of these disorders and, with the exception of EoE, the lack of uniformly accepted diagnostic criteria, the diagnosis can be overlooked or remain in question if multiple biopsies are not taken. When biopsy specimens are evaluated and eosinophilic infiltration is identified, other causes of eosinophil infiltration must be excluded before the diagnosis is confirmed. As a result, it is all too common for patients with these disorders to be symptomatic for extended periods before an accurate diagnosis is made.[22,23]

Laboratory Evaluation

Unfortunately, no laboratory tests are diagnostic of EGIDs. Laboratory tests that may be useful in distinguishing EGIDs from other diseases associated with tissue eosinophilia are listed in **Box 1**. Peripheral blood eosinophilia is noted in about two thirds of patients with eosinophilic gastroenteritis[24] and may be found in patients with

---

Box 1
Diagnostic evaluation of EGID

General

- Histologic evaluation of multiple biopsy specimens
- Immunohistological analysis of biopsy specimens for eosinophil or mast cell granule proteins: eosinophil cationic protein, eosinophil-derived neurotoxin, eosinophil peroxidase, and major basic protein for eosinophils; tryptase for mast cells
- Serum, urinary, and fecal markers: eosinophil cationic protein, eosinophil-derived neurotoxin, eosinophil protein X
- Complete blood count with differential
- Immunophenotyping of eosinophils and T cells: IL-5 receptor alpha-chain and chemokine receptor-3 for eosinophils; CD3 for T cells
- Total IgE and food-specific IgE (by ImmunoCAP, Phadia) levels
- Skin-prick testing and atopy patch testing
- Erythrocyte sedimentation rate/c-reactive protein
- Infection evaluation: *Helicobacter pylori*; helminths, hookworms, pinworms, and other parasites
- Autoantibody evaluation: tissue transglutaminase for celiac disease, antineutrophil cytoplasmic antibodies for vasculitides and inflammatory bowel disease; *Saccharomyces cerevisiae* IgG and IgA antibodies for inflammatory bowel disease

Additional testing in the presence of hypereosinophilia

- Bone marrow examination with cytogenetics and special staining
- ECG and echocardiogram
- Pulmonary function testing
- CT of chest, abdomen, and pelvis
- Tissue biopsies as indicated by other involved sites
- Measurement of serum vitamin B12 and tryptase
- Evaluation for *FIPL1-PDGFRA* mutation
- T and B cell receptor rearrangement studies

---

eosinophilic colitis. Higher levels of fecal eosinophilic cationic protein and serum eosinophilic cationic protein, eosinophil-derived neurotoxin, and eosinophil protein X have been found in patients with eosinophilic gastroenteritis, compared with those having ulcerative colitis or Crohn's disease.[25] Higher levels of urinary eosinophil-derived neurotoxin, serum eosinophil-derived neurotoxin, and eosinophilic cationic protein have been measured in patients with eosinophilic colitis.[26] Clinical studies have also shown that there is increased secretion of IL-4 and IL-5 by peripheral blood T cells in patients with eosinophilic gastroenteritis.[27] In patients with the mucosal form of eosinophilic gastroenteritis, who have malabsorption or protein-losing enteropathy, there may be increased fecal fat excretion, prolonged prothrombin time, reduced serum iron concentration, hypoalbuminemia, and hypogammaglobulinemia. Patients who have the serosal form of eosinophilic gastroenteritis usually have marked eosinophilia in the ascitic fluid.[2]

Evaluation of Allergic Disease

The majority of patients with eosinophilic gastroenteritis have increased total IgE levels and a history of other atopic diseases, including asthma, eczema, or allergic rhinitis. Most also have positive food-specific IgE levels and positive skin tests to food allergens.[1] The use of the atopy patch test in the food allergy workup of EGIDs has been shown to be beneficial in some studies as well.[28,29] However, the role of food allergy as an inciting agent in other forms of EGIDs besides EoE has not been as clearly defined. In contrast to EoE and eosinophilic gastroenteritis, eosinophilic colitis is more commonly a non-IgE–associated EGID, and thus skin tests to foods and food-specific IgE levels are more often negative.[30] Nonetheless, a thorough allergy history and food sensitization evaluations are warranted regardless of the type of EGID. Although it has primarily been reported in EoE, certain patients may also have seasonal variation of EGIDs due to exposure to seasonal environmental allergens, such as pollens,[31,32] so environmental allergen testing is recommended as well.

Radiological Evaluation

Radiological examinations generally do not provide much assistance in the diagnosis of EGIDs because they lack significant sensitivity or specificity. However, barium studies may suggest the diagnosis by revealing gastric antral stenosis with mucosal irregularity, gastric pseudopolyposis, or thickening in the small bowel due to edema.[33] Ultrasonography may show diffuse, nonspecific bowel wall infiltration with persistence of a multilayer echo pattern, and it can be useful in detecting ascites in the serosal form of eosinophilic gastroenteritis.[34,35] CT findings of EGID depend on the layer of involved tissue, but generally consist of nodular and irregular fold thickening in the stomach, bowel wall thickening, and luminal narrowing without obstruction. CT findings may also be useful for the evaluation of the degree and extent of eosinophilic infiltration and help guide transmural biopsy by endoscopy.[36,37]

Endoscopic Evaluation

While the esophageal tissue should not contain any eosinophils under normal conditions, eosinophils can be present at baseline throughout the remainder of the intestine. However, no standards for the normal number of baseline eosinophils have been established beyond the esophagus. Thus, there are no standards for the numbers of eosinophils diagnostic for EGIDs other than EoE. Nonetheless, there are certain endoscopic and pathologic findings that help support the diagnosis.

Endoscopic findings may be nonspecific and include erythema, friability, ulcerations, erosions, nodules, and loss of vascularity. Patients with eosinophilic gastritis may have micronodules or polyposis consisting of aggregates of lymphocytes and eosinophils.[1] Gross endoscopic findings may be normal as well because normal-appearing mucosa can harbor eosinophilic infiltration. Therefore, multiple biopsies should be taken from both normal- and abnormal-appearing tissue given the patchy involvement of EGIDs.

Pathologic Evaluation

On pathologic examination, the presence of infiltrating eosinophils within the intestinal crypts and gastric glands is supportive of eosinophilic gastroenteritis.[30] Histologic analysis of the tissue often reveals extracellular deposition of eosinophil remnants, including major basic protein and eosinophilic cationic protein.[1] Mast cells have also been detected in intestinal biopsies of eosinophilic gastroenteritis patients in numbers higher than those for normal control patients.[38] The diagnosis of the muscular form of eosinophilic gastroenteritis may require laparoscopic full-thickness biopsies because the lack of mucosal involvement often makes endoscopic biopsies nondiagnostic. In colonic biopsy specimens of patients with eosinophilic colitis, there may be diffuse eosinophilic infiltration in the lamina propria or focal aggregates of eosinophils in the lamina propria, crypt epithelium, and muscularis mucosa with preservation of the underlying mucosal architecture. Extracellular deposition of major basic protein and eosinophilic cationic protein, accumulation of mast cells, and, occasionally, submucosal multinucleated giant cells have also been noted in colonic tissue biopsies.[39,40]

TREATMENT

EGIDs other than EoE are relatively uncommon, so data on the treatment are limited to case reports and retrospective case series rather than prospective, randomized therapeutic clinical studies. For eosinophilic gastritis and eosinophilic gastroenteritis, referral to an allergist for skin testing to foods and environmental allergens, serum food-specific IgE testing by ImmunoCAP, and atopy patch testing is warranted. However, the role of food allergy in these EGIDs is not as well defined as it is in EoE. Nevertheless, if specific food sensitivities can be identified, patients have responded to targeted elimination diets.[38,41] If elimination diets are used, patients should be educated about the complexity of strict avoidance and should be evaluated by a nutritionist to ensure that no gaps in essential nutrients occur. Complete resolution of symptoms and disease has also been documented with the use of amino acid–based elemental formulas, although it is difficult for most patients to maintain such a strict diet.[42] If no food sensitization is discovered, or if a targeted elimination diet is not feasible or has failed to alleviate symptoms, then treatment with systemic corticosteroids, such as prednisone or methylprednisolone, or with topical corticosteroids, such as enteric coated budesonide, or with both systemic and topical corticosteroids is reasonable.[43–46] Various other treatment approaches have been used with varying degrees of success, including mast cell stabilizers (oral cromoglycate),[47,48] leukotriene antagonists (montelukast),[49–52] antihistamines (ketotifen),[53–55] suplatast tosilate,[56] humanized anti–IL-5 antibody,[57,58] and anti-IgE antibody (omalizumab).[59] If environmental allergens are identified, they should also be treated with antihistamines and intranasal corticosteroids.

For eosinophilic colitis, the treatment varies and depends on the clinical subtype. In eosinophilic colitis of infancy, it may be as simple as eliminating cow's milk or soy proteins, as these are the most frequent cause of this disease, which usually resolves by ages 1 to 3 years.[39] In milk-induced allergic proctocolitis, elimination of cow's milk protein results in resolution of bloody diarrhea with subsequent tolerance to milk, usually by age 1 year. However, treatment of eosinophilic colitis in older individuals is more problematic because IgE-mediated triggers are rarely identified. This means elimination diets are rarely effective. Therefore, treatment of eosinophilic colitis has primarily involved attempts at medical management with various drugs, including mast cell stabilizers (cromoglycate), leukotriene antagonists (montelukast), and antihistamines, although these are rarely efficacious. Anti-inflammatory drugs, such as topical or systemic corticosteroids and aminosalicylates, are more commonly used and appear to be more effective, although controlled clinical trials have not been performed.[1]

NATURAL HISTORY

Little is known about the natural history of eosinophilic gastritis, gastroenteritis, enteritis, and colitis as it has not yet been evaluated in longitudinal clinical studies, likely as a result of the difficulty in establishing a robust cohort of patients with these disorders for long-term follow-up. However, from currently available data and recent experience with EoE, it is likely that these diseases have similar courses, with complete resolution in some patients and recurrent or persistent disease in others.[60] When these diseases present in infancy and specific sensitization to foods can be identified, the prognosis appears favorable with possible remission in later childhood.[1] It is possible for different segments of the gastrointestinal tract to be affected over time and, because these diseases can be predecessors to other disease processes, such as hypereosinophilic syndromes, routine endoscopic and cardiopulmonary evaluations are recommended.

SUMMARY

EGIDs can affect any segment of the gastrointestinal tract, singly or in combination, and are named accordingly: EoE, gastritis, gastroenteritis, enteritis, and colitis. The diagnosis of EGID is primarily dependent on the clinical history and histopathology of multiple biopsy specimens after ruling out other causes of intestinal eosinophilia. The diagnosis of EGID other than EoE is complicated by the lack of uniformly accepted diagnostic criteria. Treatment involves evaluation for food sensitivity, elimination diets, and the use of antiallergy and anti-inflammatory medications with varying degrees of success. Little is known about the natural history of EGIDs, underscoring the need for long-term follow-up studies of patients with these disorders.

REFERENCES

1. Rothenberg ME. Eosinophilic gastrointestinal disorders. J Allergy Clin Immunol 2004;113:11–28.
2. Klein NC, Hargrove RL, Sleisenger MH, et al. Eosinophilic gastroenteritis. Medicine 1970;49(4):299–319.
3. Mueller S. Classification of eosinophilic gastrointestinal diseases. Best Pract Res Clin Gastroenterol 2008;22:425–40.
4. Zuo L, Rothenberg ME. Gastrointestinal eosinophilia. Immunol Allergy Clin North Am 2007;27:443–55.
5. Lake AM. Food-induced eosinophilic proctocolitis. J Pediatr Gastroenterol Nutr 2000;30:S58–60.
6. Kahn S, Orenstein SR. Eosinophilic gastroenteritis: epidemiology, diagnosis and management. Paediatr Drugs 2002;4:563–70.
7. Straumann A. Idiopathic eosinophilic gastrointestinal diseases in adults. Best Pract Res Clin Gastroenterol 2008;22:481–96.
8. Kahn S, Orenstein SR. Eosinophilic gastroenteritis. Gastroenterol Clin North Am 2008;37:333–48.
9. Pascal RR, Gramlich KM, Gansler TS. Geographic variations in eosinophil concentration in normal colonic mucosa. Mod Pathol 1997;10:363–5.
10. Polydorides AD, Banner BF, Jannaway PJ, et al. Evaluation of site-specific and seasonal variation in colonic mucosal eosinophils. Hum Pathol 2008;39:832–6.
11. Chira O, Badea R, Dumitrascu D, et al. Eosinophilic ascites in a patient with toxocara canis infection. A case report. Rom J Gastroenterol 2005;14:397–400.
12. Tsibouris P, Galeas T, Moussia M, et al. Two cases of eosinophilic gastroenteritis and malabsorption due to Enterobius vermicularis. Dig Dis Sci 2005;50:2389–92.
13. Kocabay G, Gul E, Cagatay A, et al. Is eosinophilic gastroenteritis a primary disease or a secondary developing entity due to parasitosis? South Med J 2006;99: 901.

14. Papadopoulos AA, Tzathas C, Polymeros D, et al. Symptomatic eosinophilic gastritis cured with Helicobacter pylori eradication. Gut 2005;54:1822.
15. Carvalho AT, Elia CC, de Souza HS, et al. Immunohistochemical study of intestinal eosinophils in inflammatory bowel disease. J Clin Gastroenterol 2003;36:120–5.
16. Heatley RV, James PD. Eosinophils in the rectal mucosa. A simple method of predicting the outcome of ulcerative proctocolitis? Gut 1979;20:787–91.
17. Barbie DA, Mangi AA, Lauwers GY. Eosinophilic gastroenteritis associated with systemic lupus erythematosus. J Clin Gastroenterol 2004;38:883–6.
18. Lykavieris P, Frauger E, Habes D, et al. Angioedema in pediatric liver transplant recipients under tacrolimus immunosuppression. Transplantation 2003;75:152–65.
19. Atkins FM. Systemic FK506 and post transplant food allergy in children. J Pediatr Gastroenterol Nutr 2003;37(4):525–6.
20. Talley NJ. Gut eosinophilia in food allergy and systemic and autoimmune diseases. Gastroenterol Clin North Am 2006;37:307–32.
21. Klion AD, Alam R. Hypereosinophilic syndromes. Immunol Allergy Clin N Am 2007;27(3):333–570.
22. Attwood SE, Smyrk TC, Demeester TR, et al. Esophageal eosinophilia with dysphagia. A distinct clinicopathologic syndrome. Dig Dis Sci 1993;38:109–16.
23. Straumann A, Spictin HP, Bernoulli R, et al. Idiopathic eosinophilic esophagitis: a frequently overlooked disease with typical clinical aspects and discrete endoscopic findings. Schweiz Med Wochenschr 1994;124:1419–29.
24. Straumann A, Simon HU. The physiological and pathophysiological roles of eosinophils in the gastrointestinal tract. Allergy 2004;59:15–25.
25. Bischoff SC, Mayer J, Nguyen QT, et al. Immunohistological assessment of intestinal eosinophilic activation in patients with eosinophilic gastroenteritis and inflammatory bowel disease. Am J Gastroenterol 1999;94:3521–9.
26. Inamura H, Tomita M, Okano A, et al. Serial blood and urine levels of EDN and ECP in eosinophilic colitis. Allergy 2003;58:959–60.
27. Jaffe JS, James SP, Mullins GE, et al. Evidence for an abnormal profile of interleukin-4 (IL-4), IL-5, and gamma-interferon (gamma-IFN) in peripheral blood T cells from patients with allergic eosinophilic gastroenteritis. J Clin Immunol 1994;14:299–309.
28. Spergel JM, Brown-Whitehorn T, Beausoleil JL, et al. Predictive values for skin prick test and atopy patch test for eosinophilic esophagitis. J Allergy Clin Immunol 2007;119:509–11.
29. Spergel JM, Andrews T, Brown-Whitehorn TF, et al. Treatment of eosinophilic esophagitis with specific food elimination diet directed by a combination of skin prick and patch tests. Ann Allergy Asthma Immunol 2005;95:336–43.
30. Conus S, Simon HU. General laboratory diagnostics of eosinophilic GI diseases. Best Pract Res Clin Gastroenterol 2008;22:441–53.
31. Fogg MI, Ruchelli E, Spergel JM. Pollen and eosinophilic esophagitis. J Allergy Clin Immunol 2003;112:796–7.
32. Spergel JM. Eosinophilic esophagitis and pollen. Clin Exp Allergy 2005;35:1421–2.
33. MacCarty RL, Talley NJ. Barium studies in diffuse eosinophilic gastroenteritis. Gastrointest Radiol 1990;15:183–7.
34. Stevof C, Rao S, Parsons W, et al. EUS and histopathologic correlates in eosinophilic esophagitis. Gastrointest Endosc 2001;54:373–7.
35. Maroy B. Nonmucosal eosinophilic gastroenteritis: sonographic appearance at presentation and during follow-up of response to prednisone therapy. J Clin Ultrasound 1998;26:483–6.

36. Horton KM, Corl FM, Fishman EK. CT of non-neoplastic diseases of the small bowel: spectrum of disease. J Comput Assist Tomogr 1999;23:417–28.
37. Zheng X, Cheng J, Pan K, et al. Eosinophilic enteritis: CT features. Abdom Imaging 2008;33:191–5.
38. Chehade M, Magid MS, Mofidi S, et al. Allergic eosinophilic gastroenteritis with protein-losing enteropathy: intestinal pathology, clinical course, and long-term follow-up. J Pediatr Gastroenterol Nutr 2006;42:516–21.
39. Guajardo JR, Rothenberg ME. Eosinophilic esophagitis, gastroenteritis, gastroenterocolitis, and colitis. In: Metcalfe DD, Sampson HA, Simon RA, editors. Food allergy: adverse reactions to foods and additives. 3rd edition. Malden (MA): Blackwell Publishing; 2003. p. 217–26.
40. Ohtsuka Y, Shimizu T, Shoji H, et al. Neonatal transient eosinophilic colitis causes lower gastrointestinal bleeding in early infancy. J Pediatr Gastroenterol Nutr 2007; 44:501–5.
41. Chen MJ, Chu CH, Lin SC, et al. Eosinophilic gastroenteritis: clinical experience with 15 patients. World J Gastroenterol 2003;9:2813–6.
42. Justinich C, Katz A, Gurbindo C, et al. Elemental diet improves steroid-dependent eosinophilic gastroenteritis and reverses growth failure. J Pediatr Gastroenterol Nutr 1996;23:81–5.
43. Tan AC, Kruimal JW, Naber TH. Eosinophilic gastroenteritis treated with non-enteric-coated budesonide tablets. Eur J Gastroenterol Hepatol 2001;13:425–7.
44. Siewert E, Lammert F, Koppitz P, et al. Eosinophilic gastroenteritis with severe protein-losing enteropathy: successful treatment with budesonide. Dig Liver Dis 2006;38:55–9.
45. Elsing C, Placke J, Gross-Weege W. Budesonide for the treatment of obstructive eosinophilic jejunitis. Z Gastroenterol 2007;45:187–9.
46. Lombardi C, Salmi A, Savio A, et al. Localized eosinophilic ileitis with mastocytosis successfully treated with oral budesonide. Allergy 2007;62:1343–5.
47. Van Dellen RG, Lewis JC. Oral administration of cromolyn in a patient with protein-losing enteropathy, food allergy, and eosinophilic gastroenteritis. Mayo Clin Proc 1994;69:441–4.
48. Perez-Millan A, Martin-Lorente JL, Lopez-Morante A, et al. Subserosal eosinophilic gastroenteritis treated efficaciously with sodium cromoglycate. Dig Dis Sci 1997;42:342–4.
49. Neustrom MR, Friesen C. Treatment of eosinophilic gastroenteritis with montelukast. J Allergy Clin Immunol 1999;104:506.
50. Schwartz DA, Pardi DS, Murray JA. Use of montelukast as steroid-sparing agent for recurrent eosinophilic gastroenteritis. Dig Dis Sci 2001;46:1787–90.
51. Quack I, Sellin L, Buchner NJ, et al. Eosinophilic gastroenteritis in a young girl—long term remission under montelukast. BMC Gastroenterol 2005;5:24.
52. Urek MC, Kujundzic M, Banic M, et al. Leukotriene receptor antagonists as potential steroid sparing agents in a patient with serosal eosinophilic gastroenteritis. Gut 2006;55:1363–4.
53. Melamed I, Feanny SJ, Sherman PM, et al. Benefit of ketotifen in patients with eosinophilic gastroenteritis. Am J Med 1991;90:310–4.
54. Katsinelos P, Pilpilidis I, Xiarchos P, et al. Oral administration of ketotifen in a patient with eosinophilic colitis and severe osteoporosis. Am J Gastroenterol 2002;97:1072.
55. Bolukbas FF, Bolukbas C, Uzunkoy A, et al. A dramatic response to ketotifen in a case of eosinophilic gastroenteritis mimicking abdominal emergency. Dig Dis Sci 2004;49:1782–5.

56. Shirai T, Hashimoto D, Suzuki K, et al. Successful treatment of eosinophilic gastroenteritis with suplatast tosilate. J Allergy Clin Immunol 2001;107:924–5.
57. Prussin C, James SP, Huber MM, et al. Pilot study of anti-IL-5 in eosinophilic gastroenteritis [Abstract]. J Allergy Clin Immunol 2003;111:S275.
58. Kim YJ, Prussin C, Martin B, et al. Rebound eosinophilia after treatment of hypereosinophilic syndrome and eosinophilic gastroenteritis with monoclonal anti-IL-5 antibody SCH55700. J Allergy Clin Immunol 2004;114:1449–55.
59. Foroughi S, Foster B, Kim NY, et al. Anti-IgE treatment of eosinophilic-associated gastrointestinal disorders. J Allergy Clin Immunol 2007;120:594–601.
60. Lee CM, Changchien CS, Chen PC, et al. Eosinophilic gastroenteritis: 10 years experience. Am J Gastroenterol 1993;88:70–4.

Clinical Presentation of Feeding Dysfunction in Children with Eosinophilic Gastrointestinal Disease

Angela M. Haas, MA, CCC-SLP[a],*, Nancy Creskoff Maune, OTR[b]

KEYWORDS

- Esophageal disease • Feeding • Food refusal
- Dysphagia • Children

CLINICAL PRESENTATION OF FEEDING DYSFUNCTION IN CHILDREN WITH EOSINOPHILIC GASTROINTESTINAL DISEASE

Feeding issues may affect many aspects of a child's health, development, growth, nutrition and overall well-being. No other activity of daily living consumes more time, attention, and energy in the life of a family than feeding and eating.[1] Food refusal, dysphagia, and reduced volume and variety of intake are common complaints associated with eosinophilic gastrointestinal disorders (EGIDs) in children.[2,3] Oftentimes, before a diagnosis of EGID is made, a feeding specialist is the first contact for children with eating difficulties. Accurate diagnosis of eosinophilic gastrointestinal disease is frequently missed as many of its features are similar to other gastrointestinal diseases.[4] Gastroenterologists, allergists, feeding specialists, dietitians, psychologists, and social workers are now collaborating to provide integrated comprehensive care for optimal diagnosis and treatment of children with EGIDs. In the general population, feeding difficulties are present in 25% of typically developing children and in 75% to 80% of children with developmental disabilities[4–6] Although prevalence numbers for feeding issues in children with EGIDs are unknown, it is anticipated that the prevalence will fall closer to that of children with developmental disabilities.

---

[a] Audiology, Speech Pathology, and Learning Services, Feeding and Swallowing Program, The Children's Hospital Denver, B030, 13123 E. 16th Avenue, Aurora, CO 80045, USA
[b] Department of Occupational Therapy, Feeding and Swallowing Program, The Children's Hospital Denver, B335, 13123 E. 16th Avenue, Aurora, CO 80045, USA
* Corresponding author.
E-mail address: haas.angela@tchden.org (A.M. Haas).

Immunol Allergy Clin N Am 29 (2009) 65–75
doi:10.1016/j.iac.2008.09.014   immunology.theclinics.com

There is a developmental continuum for the acquisition of feeding skills, which includes motor skills, sensory systems, behavioral/emotional components, and communication.[7,8] As clinicians' experience in working with children with EGIDs has evolved, it has been recognized that feeding difficulties are a prevalent feature, which disrupt the progress along the typical developmental feeding continuum. This disruption manifests itself in a variety of ways depending on the age of the child, the symptoms of the disease, and the unique family or social situation. Knowledge of the normal acquisition of feeding skills is critical to interpret the impact of the disease and plan appropriate intervention (**Table 1**).

PREVALENT SYMPTOMS ASSOCIATED WITH FEEDING DYSFUNCTION

Frequently cited symptoms of eosinophilic gastrointestinal disease are: vomiting, pain, and dysphagia.[2,3] Interestingly, symptoms promoting referral and evaluation have been grouped by age: food refusal in infants and toddlers; abdominal pain and vomiting in preschool and school-aged children; and dysphagia in older children.[9] Additional characteristics are emerging, including: oral motor, oral sensory, behavioral and developmental variances.

Dysphagia

Swallow function is typically described as having three distinct phases: oral, pharyngeal, and esophageal.[8,10,11] The type of swallow dysfunction most commonly associated with esophageal disease is intermittent esophageal dysphagia, characterized by food impaction or the sensation of food "getting stuck."[12] This difficulty is in contrast to pharyngeal dysphagia, which is related to aspiration, laryngeal penetration, or compromised airway protection. Pharyngeal dysphagia is not commonly associated or reported with this population. Treatment for food impaction and esophageal dilation are interventions related to esophageal narrowing or strictures. An emerging characteristic of children with eosinophilic esophageal disease is avoidance of solid foods or higher textured foods, presumably a result of altered ability to pass the food comfortably through the esophagus. Oral phase dysphagia, characterized by oral motor dysfunction, is less likely than oral motor immaturity in this population. Oral and pharyngeal dysphagia may be present in children who have concomitant neurologic and/or neuromotor disease, such as cerebral palsy.

Gagging and Vomiting

A variety of reasons may cause a child to gag and vomit. It is important to differentiate between gagging and choking, as caregivers often use these terms interchangeably. The gag response is a protective reflex, reflecting the sensation that a bolus is too big to be swallowed.[8] Gagging can also be due to nausea or related to other gastrointestinal disorders, such as gastroesophageal reflux. For a child who has a history of frequent vomiting, gagging may be more easily elicited and may more readily trigger vomiting. Gagging may occur secondary to altered oral motor and/or oral sensory skills. It may also be a learned response, as a strategy to avoid eating. Determining the cause of gagging and vomiting is critical to planning appropriate feeding treatment.

Learned Behaviors and Food Refusal

Eating is a learned behavior with a predictable developmental sequence in the healthy, thriving child. When this sequence is interrupted by illness, discomfort, or environmental stressors, the result can be altered patterns of mealtime behavior for the child and the caregiver. Children can learn how to eat as well as learn how not to eat with operant and classical conditioning influencing both processes. A child who repeatedly experiences a cycle of hunger, successful eating, satiety, and comfort is reinforced to continue eating. This experience is rewarding and satisfying to the caregiver as well. A child who repeatedly experiences hunger, followed by pain or discomfort with eating is reinforced to avoid eating. This experience can be frustrating, confusing, and unsatisfying to the caregiver, often resulting in altered feeding practices in an effort to feed their child.[1,13,14] Children with eosinophilic gastrointestinal disease may reduce the volume of food they eat, reduce the variety of food in their diet, or engage in maladaptive behaviors at mealtimes, all in an effort to reduce pain or discomfort.

Oral Motor

The sequence for the development of mature oral motor skills occurs between birth and 24 months of age.[7] There are critical windows in the developmental continuum related to the sensory and motor aspects of learning to eat, when the child's maturation and opportunities to learn a new skill coincide. If the opportunities to learn are not there at the same time, or the child does not experience feeding during a particular portion of the developmental sequence, it becomes more difficult for the child to learn the skill at a later date.[15] Children who have eosinophilic gastrointestinal disease may not have had well-aligned "maturation" and "opportunities to learn" in terms of feeding and eating. The influence of the disease on this process can be dramatic in that oral motor skill development may be interrupted due to conditioned food refusal as a result of discomfort or pain. In this case, a child may not progress his diet to include foods that require advanced oral motor skills, resulting in an immature skill set. Treatment itself may require a child to be on a liquid elemental diet or significantly restrict the range of foods or textures, with a similar impact on skill development. Thus far, it has been our experience that these children tend to present with issues of oral motor immaturity rather than oral motor dysfunction. A child may also have true oral motor dysfunction related to altered tone, strength, or coordination with coexisting diagnoses such as cerebral palsy or Down syndrome.

Oral Sensory

Oral sensory development is not as easy to observe and measure as oral motor development, and it is much more reliant on a child's behavior to assess. As part of successful feeding, a child must have appropriate perception of tactile input and the ability to adaptively respond.[8] The motor system is reliant on the sensory system to supply accurate information regarding food properties for the most efficient motor response. Oral sensory dysfunction may present as food refusal, gagging in response to a particular taste or texture, or inability to manage certain foods. These difficulties may be related to lack of experience and exposure, which may be self-imposed or as a result of treatment. Frequent discomfort related to food and eating may lead to reduced motivation for oral exploration and play in younger children, which may negatively impact oral sensory development. Children may present with food aversion, oral aversion, or global sensory processing disorders, all of which have distinct characteristics. Food aversion, or specific refusal to bring food items to the mouth, is the most common oral sensory disturbance the authors have encountered in children with eosinophilic gastrointestinal disease.

Developmental Differences

In addition to the above characteristics, feeding can also be impacted by the behaviors associated with chronic discomfort. The authors have observed children with the

Table 1
Developmental acquisition of feeding skills

Age	Food Type	Positioning	Oral Patterns	Self-Feeding
1 month	Liquid from bottle or breast	Semi-reclined or side, lying with neck slightly flexed	Sucking pattern, loses some liquid; sequences two or more sucks before pausing to breathe or swallow.	Brings hands to mouth
4–6 months	Liquids, baby cereals, puréed foods	Supported semi-sitting or sitting positions	Sucking pattern. No longer loses liquid during sucking, although may lose some when initiating or terminating the suck or as the nipple is removed. By 4 months, sequences 20 or more sucks from breast or bottle. Uses a sucking pattern with puréed foods with tongue protrusion past the lips. Some food is pushed out of the mouth. At 6 months, jaw quiets and remains in a stable, open position until the spoon enters the mouth. The tongue quiets to accept the spoon.	At 4 months, infant pats bottle and holds both hands on the bottle. Infant holds bottle independently 6 months. Cup may be introduced at 6 months.
9 months	Liquids, puréed foods, ground or junior foods, mashed table foods, soft cookies and crackers	Sitting, usually in a highchair with a tray table for spoon feeding and finger feeding	No longer loses any liquid during sucking initiation or when the nipple is removed from the mouth. Child may use wide jaw excursions with cup drinking, and loss of liquid is common. Upper lip is active in food removal from the spoon. Uses vertical jaw movements when chewing solids. Begins to transfer food from the center of the mouth to the side. Child uses vertical and diagonal rotary jaw movements for chewing.	Capable of independent finger feeding. Holds and bangs spoon. Drinks from cup held by caregiver.

Age	Foods	Positioning	Oral motor skills	Self-feeding
12 months	Liquids and coarsely chopped table foods including easily chewed meats.	Sitting unsupported in a highchair or a similar seat (eg, clip-on chair, booster chair)	Sucking pattern. Takes liquid primarily from a cup. Tongue may protrude slightly for stability. Uses a controlled, sustained bite on a soft cookie. Minimal loss of food from mouth with spoon-feeding. Lips are active to clear utensil of food and contain food while chewing.	Child holds cup and drinks with some spilling. Brings filled spoon to mouth with spilling
18 months	Liquids and coarsely chopped table foods including most meats and some raw vegetables	Sitting unsupported at the family table or at a small child's chair and table	Jaw stabilization is obtained by biting down on the edge of the cup. Upper lip is closed on the edge of the cup, providing a good seal for drinking. Child uses a controlled, sustained bite on a hard cookie. Can chew with the lips closed and does so intermittently. Diagonal rotary jaw movements are smooth and well coordinated.	Child scoops food onto spoon and brings it to the mouth.
24 months	Liquids, wide variety of table foods except for some raw fruits, vegetables, nuts	Sitting at table	Jaw stabilization is emerging. Jaw movement in chewing is variable and includes diagonal rotary and circular rotary movements. Tongue is used in a free, sweeping motion to and clean food from the upper and lower lips. Child swallows solid foods including those with a combination of textures with easy lip closure as needed.	Child brings spoon or fork to mouth with the hand palm-up, uses well. Typically, child is fully weaned from the bottle or breast (may occur earlier) and drinks entirely from the cup.

> **Box 1**
> **Feeding problems associated with eosinophilic gastrointestinal disease in children**
>
> - Compromised nutritional status
> - Dysphagia or discomfort with the esophageal phase of swallowing
> - Food refusal
> - Decreased variety and volume of oral intake
> - Gagging, coughing, and vomiting
> - Delayed attainment of mature eating patterns
> - Delayed attainment of self-feeding skills
> - Chronic discomfort associated with food and mealtimes
> - Behavioral or learned feeding problems
> - In the tube-fed child, altered feeding development and mealtime dynamics

following: decreased initiation, low energy, decreased motivation, flat affect, altered pragmatics (social/language skills), and emotional lability. Following appropriate treatment for their disease, many of these behaviors improve without the need for additional interventions. These children can be mislabeled as having developmental differences, when it is actually the chronic disease process that appears to be responsible (**Box 1**).

ASSESSMENT

Understanding the role of eosinophilic gastrointestinal disease is a critical first step in the assessment of a child's feeding difficulties. Collaboration with a team of treating professionals in gastroenterology, allergy, and nutrition is often necessary to determine the baseline status of the patient. This baseline information, combined with a patient's previous history provides the feeding specialist with a foundation to begin the analysis of the feeding behaviors of the child and the caregiver, and to form hypotheses regarding developmental function, experiences and learning. Assessment must include an observation of a meal that replicates the mealtime in the home as closely as possible, and the meal should include accepted and challenging food items. A child's oral motor patterns, oral sensory responses, mealtime behaviors and child/caregiver mealtime dynamics are carefully observed. Assessment should also include the impact of overall development, muscle tone, postural alignment and stability, breathing, global sensory processing, and communication on feeding and the mealtime experience.

CASE STUDIES

The following case studies illustrate the role of the feeding specialist in the management of children with eosinophilic gastrointestinal disease at varied ages.

Case #1: 18-Month-Old Boy

Background
This young boy had a long-standing history of vomiting since early infancy. At 6 months of age, he received the diagnosis of gastroesophageal reflux. He was treated with several medications, but he continued to struggle with vomiting, low volume of intake,

refusal to eat, and poor growth. Due to additional issues of persistent eczema and skin rashes, he was referred to an allergist. Allergy testing revealed multiple food allergies at age 12 months, and an endoscopy led to the diagnosis of eosinophilic esophagitis. He was started on a strict elimination diet, continued on a high dose of proton pump inhibitor treatment, and a course of topical steroid treatment. All nutrition was provided via elemental formula, with a goal of 32 ounces a day set by the dietitian. In an effort to meet that intake goal, his parents did not adhere to a mealtime schedule, but they tended to leave bottles and cups around the house for him to take sips throughout the day. His parents reported the greatest volume of intake when he was in his crib and while he was watching TV, but he had never been able to meet the intake goal of 32 ounces. He was often playing in the next room during family mealtimes because he was not able to eat any food, and his parents thought he might become upset or frustrated watching them eat.

Treatment plan
Initially, consultation with a feeding specialist emphasized building a foundation for learning about mealtimes and provided parent education regarding developing a mealtime schedule, structure, and routine. Other goals of therapy were to increase his daily volume of formula and to establish a schedule that would help him develop hunger to meet this goal. He was encouraged to sit in a highchair for family meals and he was provided with opportunities to interact with the "tools" of mealtimes such as a spoon, bowl, and cup. He was offered ice chips in his bowl to practice self-feeding skills. Follow-up visits with the feeding specialist focused on oral motor and oral sensory skill development, using toys and nonfood items. Other ideas to support his learning about eating included reading books about foods or eating and pretend play with plastic foods in a play kitchen.

Progress
His parents were able to create a mealtime schedule for him that was age-appropriate, with five to six planned opportunities for him to drink his formula. He sat at the table or in a highchair to drink, and no longer "grazed" all day. His daily formula intake increased, and he was able to meet the goal set by the dietitian. He appeared to be comfortable sitting with his parents for family meals and he enjoyed practicing with his spoon, bowl and cup. At age 18 months, his treatment plan was updated and food trials were initiated. He initially refused to eat the food; feeding therapy was resumed to provide intervention strategies of promoting food interaction, modeling, positive reinforcement, and teaching the mechanics of eating. Over the course of 8 months of weekly treatment he was able to progress from touching and smelling food, to licking, biting and finally eating the food in small quantities.

Case #2: 4-Year-Old Girl

Background
This child received a diagnosis of eosinophilic esophagitis at 3 years of age, with a long history of gagging, vomiting, and poor weight gain. In addition to medications, she was treated with a diet of specialized formula and dietary exclusions based on her food allergies. She presented with many maladaptive behaviors at mealtimes, such as refusal to stay seated at the table, throwing food, accepting only a few foods, and gagging with the introduction of any new foods. She did not like the new formula and refused to drink it. Her parents reported feeling very frustrated and concerned; they felt they had tried "everything," including force-feeding, to no avail.

Treatment plan
This little girl was initially seen for one-on-one feeding therapy with primary goals of helping her transition to the new formula and reducing the high stress and anxiety around mealtimes. A thorough assessment revealed that her oral motor skills were immature and that her inability to manage many of the foods she was offered resulted in gagging and then strong refusal behaviors. Parent education was provided on recommended food textures and emphasized offering purees, soft solids, and meltable solids (solids that soften or "melt" with saliva). A technique of liquid fading was introduced to help gradually move her from her preferred formula to her new formula. A small amount of new formula was added to her preferred formula with a gradual increase of new formula over time. A consistent, predictable routine for meals was developed in therapy sessions and carried over in the home. As positive reinforcement and social modeling were found to be very effective for this child, she was seen in a group feeding therapy program with four other children with feeding issues.

Progress
Over a 4-week period, she was able to successfully transition to her new specialized formula. In the 8-month course of one-on-one therapy and group feeding therapy, she was able to stay seated at the table for mealtimes, had decreased her behaviors of throwing, gagging and refusal, and added six new foods to her accepted diet. She continued to have overall low volume of oral intake and she continued to have slow growth. A decision to place a gastrostomy tube was made to optimize her nutrition and growth, while continuing to support her progress with oral eating. She continued her participation in the feeding group program with goals of expanding her repertoire and increasing her intake by mouth. This program was also a valuable experience for her parents as they were able to meet with other caregivers of children with feeding difficulties, network, and share resources.

Case #3: 9-Year-Old Boy

Background
This child presented with the primary complaint of abdominal pain, constipation, and esophageal dysphagia, particularly with solid foods. He had been diagnosed with attention deficit disorder with hyperactivity, obsessive–compulsive disorder, and sensory processing dysfunction. His parents described him as anxious, with a flat affect and a long-standing history of picky eating and food refusal. This child was home-schooled due to frequent abdominal discomfort resulting in absences from school. Mealtime in the home was described as a "battle." He also avoided social situations where food or eating was the activity (ie, school cafeteria, birthday parties). Endoscopy confirmed the diagnosis of eosinophilic esophagitis, and allergy testing revealed multiple foods allergies. This child was placed on a diet of an elemental formula for 6 months, with no other foods allowed. He was also treated with a proton pump inhibitor, topical steroids, and laxative (in addition to medication for ADHD). He was able to meet caloric needs with an elemental formula, however, only by drinking the formula in small volumes throughout the entire day and into the evening. He was subsequently retested for food allergies with several foods now safely allowed. Upon introduction, these foods were generally refused, despite the child reporting that he was motivated to eat again.

Treatment
Intensive, daily feeding treatment was established for 2 weeks with a feeding specialist working in concert with this child's treating allergist, gastroenterologist, and dietician.

Caregiver teaching was provided to establish a mealtime schedule of predictable mealtimes and snacks at regular intervals throughout the day to limit grazing on formula. Direct therapy sessions were held to introduce strategies to approach, interact with and eventually eat newly re-introduced foods, as well as model and provide caregiver education to use these strategies in the home. Elemental formula was reduced by 40%. Foods were presented before formula, with all formula presented during a meal or snack time while sitting at the table. Ongoing consultation with a dietician occurred to make adjustments to his elemental formula needs as oral intake increased.

Progress
The intensive treatment schedule was weaned from daily to three times weekly, twice weekly, and then once weekly before discharge after 4 months. This child benefited from ongoing outpatient therapy to develop rapport and trust around mealtimes and eating. This relationship also contributed to an atmosphere that allowed him to use the treatment strategies effectively. Significantly improved affect and decreased anxiety were noted by all team members. Establishing a mealtime schedule and reducing formula intake supported natural hunger/satiety cues that led to improved motivation to eat newly re-introduced foods. Ongoing caregiver education was provided which resulted in significantly fewer mealtime battles. Elemental formula need was reduced by 80% overall at the time of discharge. Occupational therapy with a focus on global sensory processing was also initiated. Follow-up at 8 months revealed that elemental formula could be discontinued, and this child was able to return to school. Occupational therapy had been reduced to twice monthly.

GASTROSTOMY (FEEDING) TUBES

In many cases, a feeding tube may be a consideration.[16] It can provide relief from the stress and anxiety which often surrounds insufficient intake, help diffuse difficult mealtime dynamics, and discourage the temptation to force feed. Feeding tubes can provide energy and nutrition for health and development, and in the majority of cases, do not need to be in place of oral feeding but can be a supplement to insure growth. Children can remain oral feeders and develop oral motor skills, appropriate mealtime behaviors, and opportunities for positive learning about eating with those foods that are identified as safe. It is important that a feeding tube not be presented or viewed as a failure on the part of the child or caregiver but rather a temporary tool to consider for a child who needs additional support during the treatment process.

GENERAL TREATMENT STRATEGIES

Feeding treatment can take many forms, from intensive one-on-one daily sessions to weekly group treatment sessions with peer models. Early diagnosis and timely intervention can minimize or avoid maladaptive feeding practices. When feeding treatment is recommended, commitment to the treatment regime from a child's caregivers is critical for a successful outcome. Parent education must be provided regarding mealtime schedules and routines, reinforcement (physiologic and behavioral), and systematic interaction with food at mealtimes. Anticipatory guidance is recommended to support the developmental progression of feeding when a child is on an exclusive elemental diet. Success is also dependent upon the status of any coexisting diagnoses, which all require consideration for their potential impact on feeding and need for additional treatment.[17] It is important to appreciate that feeding difficulties can require a great deal of energy, effort, and time to change in the course of treatment.

SUMMARY

Eating is a dynamic learning experience. Eosinophilic gastrointestinal disease and its symptoms can derail the development of oral feeding and alter family dynamics at mealtimes. Despite effective medical treatment, the residual effects on feeding can persist and need to be addressed. Specific strategies may be required to help children move toward the goals of increased intake, increased variety in diet, developing appropriate oral motor and oral sensory skills, and addressing mealtime behaviors and environment. A multidisciplinary team approach affords the opportunity to provide comprehensive care for this unique population. Collaboration regarding the medical, nutritional, and developmental plan of care optimizes outcomes for the well-being of children and families affected by this disease.

REFERENCES

1. Satter E. Child of mine: feeding with love and good sense. Palo Alto (CA): Bull Publishing Co; 1991. p. 406–27.
2. Furuta GT, Liacouras CA, Collins MH, et al. Eosinophillic esophagitis in children and adults: a systematic review and consensus recommendations for diagnosis and treatment. Gastroenterol 2007;133:1342–63.
3. Spergel JM. Eosinophilic esophagitis in adults and children: evidence for a food allergy component in many patients. Curr Opin Allergy Clin Immunol 2007;7: 274–8.
4. Aceves SS, Furuta GT, Spechler SJ. Integrated approach to treatment of children and adults with eosinophilic esophagitis. Gastrointest Endosc Clin N Am 2008;18: 195–217.
5. Kerwin ME, Ahearn WH, Eicher PS, et al. The costs of eating: a behavioral economic analysis of food refusal. J Appl Behav Anal 1995;28:245–60.
6. Eicher PM. Feeding. In: Batshaw ML, editor. Children with disabilities. 4th edition. Baltimore (MD): Paul H. Brookes Publishing Co; 1997. p. 621–41.
7. Morris SE, Klein MD. Pre-feeding skills: a comprehension resource for feeding development. 2nd edition. Tucson (AZ): Therapy Skill Builders; 1987. p. 59–94.
8. Wolf L, Glass RP. Feeding and swallowing disorders in infancy: assessment and management. Tucson (AZ): Therapy Skill Builders; 1992.
9. Putnam P. Eosinophilic esophagitis in children: clinical manifestations. Gastrointest Endosc Clin N Am 2008;18:11–23.
10. Logemann JA. Evaluation and treatment of swallowing disorders. 2nd edition. San Diego (CA): College Hill Press; 1997.
11. Stevenson D, Allaire JH. The development of normal feeding and swallowing. Pediatr Clin North Am 1991;38(6):1439–53.
12. Nurko S, Rosen R. Esophageal dismotility in patients who have eosinophillic esophagitis. Gastrointest Endosc Clin N Am 2008;18:73–89.
13. Kedesdy JL, Budd KS. Childhood feeding disorders: biobehavioral assessment and intervention. Baltimore (MD): Paul H. Brookes Publishing Co; 1998.
14. Iwata B, Riordan M, Wohl MK, et al. Pediatric feeding disorders: behavioral analysis and treatment. In: Accardo PJ, editor. Failure to thrive in infancy and early childhood. Baltimore (MD): University Park Press; 1982. p. 297–329.
15. Illingworth RS, Lister J. The critical or sensitive period, with special reference to certain feeding problems in infants and children. J Pediatr 1964; 65:839–48.

16. Young C. Nutrition. In: Arvedson JC, Brodsky L, editors. Pediatric swallowing and feeding: assessment and management. Thousand Oaks (CA): Singular Publishing; 1985. p. 157–208.
17. Pentiuk SP, Miller CK, Kaul A. Eosinophillic esophagitis in infants and toddlers. Dysphagia 2007;22:44–7.

Nutritional Management of Children who have Food Allergies and Eosinophilic Esophagitis

Catherine M. Santangelo, RD[a], Emily McCloud, MS, RD[b],*

KEYWORDS

- Eosinophilic esophagitis • Food allergies
- Nutritional management

Over the past decade, eosinophilic esophagitis (EoE) has become increasingly prevalent in the United States.[1] The diagnosis of EoE requires the presence of symptoms such as food impaction and dysphagia in adults, and feeding intolerance, failure to thrive, or gastroesophageal reflux disease (GERD) symptoms in children, accompanied by esophageal biopsies with more than 15 eosinophils per high-power field, and the exclusion of other disorders with similar clinical or endoscopic features, such as GERD.[1,2]

One of the effective treatment approaches is dietary management, which aims to eliminate exposure to food allergens. Approaches to dietary management include the use of elemental diets, elimination diets, and tailored elimination diets, each of which poses potential nutrition risks. Therefore, a complete nutrition assessment by a registered dietitian (RD) with expertise in the management of food allergies is recommended for all patients diagnosed with EoE.[2]

Obtaining a complete diet history is critical to a RD's evaluation of a patient who has EoE. Care must be taken to determine current dietary exclusions, preferences, amounts consumed, eating behaviors, and meal preparation.[2] Three-day foods records are frequently analyzed to assess a child's macro- and micronutrient intake.

[a] Division of Gastroenterology/Nutrition, The Children's Hospital, 1260 South York Street, Denver, CO 80210, USA
[b] National Jewish Health, 1400 Jackson Street, A02D, Denver, CO 80206, USA
* Corresponding author.
E-mail address: mccloude@njc.org (E. McCloud).

Immunol Allergy Clin N Am 29 (2009) 77–84
doi:10.1016/j.iac.2008.09.009
0889-8561/08/$ – see front matter © 2009 Elsevier Inc. All rights reserved.
immunology.theclinics.com

The data obtained often dictate the degree of nutrition intervention that may be necessary.

Assessment of growth and nutrition is fundamental for children who have EoE. Nutritional assessment includes a review of the child's Center for Disease Control growth charts and anthropometric measurements, and an evaluation of current dietary intake by way of 3-day food records, 24-hour diet recalls, and food frequency questionnaires. Growth charts are used to establish baseline data, including weight/age, height/age, and weight-for-height percentiles. Growth velocity (the increase in height per unit of time), weight gain, and weight-for-height-ratios monitor children's growth and determine the possibility of nutritional deficiency.[3]

Another key component of the RD's assessment of a child who has EoE is determining the child's nutrient needs. Nutritional requirements are established for both macro- and micronutrients. Macronutrients refer to carbohydrate, protein, and fat. Children require sufficient total calories to promote adequate weight gain and growth. For pediatric populations, nutritional requirements are determined based on recommended dietary allowances and, since 1998, dietary reference intakes (DRIs).[4,5] Estimated nutritional requirements for children who have EoE are generally the same as those of healthy children. In children presenting with poor weight gain and growth, additional calories and protein would likely be recommended.[2,3]

In pediatric populations, carbohydrate intake should comprise 45% to 55% of total calories consumed.[3] Preferred carbohydrate sources include whole grains, fresh fruit, vegetables, and legumes. However, alternative grain sources may need to be used and legumes might be restricted based on individual allergy testing.

Protein should comprise 15% to 20% of the diet. Children who have EoE often have a difficult time meeting their protein needs with high-quality protein, such as iron-rich meat and eggs, secondary to feeding difficulties, eating aversions, and diet restrictions. Therefore, care must be taken to assure children consume either dietary sources of high-quality protein, which supply all eight essential amino acids, or complementary proteins to meet protein requirements.[2,3] Use of a protein hydrolysate or an amino acid–based formula may be necessary if dietary intakes of high-quality protein are insufficient.

Fat should comprise 30% to 35% of the diet. Dietary fat provides a concentrated source of calories and helps children meet total calorie requirements while on restricted diets. Furthermore, adequate dietary fat is important to prevent essential fatty acid deficiency. Essential fatty acids are linoleic (C18:2n-6) and alpha-linolenic (C18:3n3) acids.[1] Butter is commonly eliminated for children who follow a milk-free diet and it must be replaced by an alternative source of fat (often vegetable oils). A wide variety of fat in children's diets helps assure that appropriate amounts of saturated, monounsaturated, and polyunsaturated fats are consumed.[2,3]

The adequacy of micronutrient intake of vitamins, minerals, and trace elements is dependent on the variety of foods in the diet. The DRIs for vitamins, minerals, and trace elements can be used as guidelines for children who have food allergies. Salman and colleagues[6] recently reviewed nutritional intakes of children who had food allergies; several key nutrients, including calcium, iron, vitamin D, vitamin E, and zinc, provided less than 67% of the DRIs. Christie and colleagues[7] also found that children who had more than one food allergy consumed less than 67% of the DRI for calcium, vitamin D, and vitamin E. Dietary intakes of less than 67% of the DRI strongly suggest that consumption of these nutrients warrants improvement. An important finding of the aforementioned study was that children significantly improved their intakes of calcium, vitamin D, and vitamin E when they received nutrition counseling.

Overall, the macro-micronutrient intake in children on elimination diets may be inadequate. A study by Henriksen and colleagues[8] found that children on milk-free diets had overall lower energy (calorie), fat, protein, calcium, riboflavin, and niacin intakes than children consuming milk. Inadequate nutrition in children may have long-lasting implications, such as poor growth, delayed development, and failure to thrive, again emphasizing the importance of using a RD's expertise to assess a child's nutrient intake when he/she is on an elimination diet.

DIET THERAPY

Fifty to eighty percent of children who have EoE are atopic, as defined by the coexistence of other atopic diseases (atopic dermatitis, allergic rhinitis, or asthma) and the presence of allergic sensitization based on prick skin testing or measurement of serum allergen–specific IgE.[9] Although no studies have clearly defined a universal, food-specific elimination diet, many patients indeed improve on several different allergen-free diets. Three different dietary approaches to treating EoE are amino acid–based elemental diets, six-food elimination diets, and tailored elimination diets based on prick skin testing.

Elemental Diets

Several studies demonstrate the use of elemental diets as an effective treatment modality in patients who have EoE. Elemental diets provide relief from clinical symptoms and normalize esophageal histology. The elemental or amino acid–based dietary approach was first described by Kelly and colleagues,[10] when 10 children who did not respond to standard antireflux treatments completed a minimum 6-week trial on an elemental formula (Neocate or Neocate 1+). Eighty percent of the children's symptoms resolved and 20% showed improvement while following this diet therapy.[10] The results of this initial study were confirmed by Markowitz and colleagues,[11] when 51 children who had EoE out of 346 children who had chronic GERD treated with an elemental diet demonstrated significant improvement in vomiting, abdominal pain, or dysphagia. Forty-nine of the 51 children's symptoms improved in an average of 8.5 days. In a study by Liacourus and colleagues,[9] 95% of the 172 children, using an amino-acid based formula, demonstrated significant improvement in symptoms and esophageal eosinophilia.

Elemental diets have been considered the "gold standard" in determining whether food allergens play a role in EoE. Elemental diets require removal of all solid foods and use a nutritionally complete formula to meet recommended nutrient needs. The protein provided by an elemental formula is composed of 100% nonallergenic free amino acids. Products used most commonly in the pediatric population include Neocate, Neocate Junior, Neocate One Plus, E028 Splash (Nutricia North America, Rockville, Maryland, www.Neocate.com), EleCare (Ross Products Division, Abbott Laboratories, Columbus, Ohio), and Nutramigen AA (Mead Johnson & Company, Evansville, Indiana). Extensively hydrolyzed formulas such as Nutramigen (Mead Johnson & Company) or Alimentum (Ross Products Division, Abbott Laboratories) contain small amounts of hydrolyzed milk protein and are not suitable for a complete elemental diet.

The dramatic resolution of symptoms when using elemental diets makes this an alluring approach to disease management. However, when determining the best dietary approach for a child, it is important to consider potential obstacles that may preclude the use of this form of nutritional management. The predominant barrier to the use of an elemental diet is patient compliance. Although formula manufacturers have made significant strides to improve the taste of their products by providing both flavored and unflavored formula, the use of amino acids instead of complete protein in the formula alters palatability. As a result, children are often unable to drink the required amount of formula or may refuse the formula altogether. Therefore, implementing an elemental diet frequently requires the use of a nasogastric or gastrostomy tube. Families and patients are often unaccustomed to these feeding modalities and may find them intrusive to children's active lifestyles; thus, these factors need to be addressed when considering the possibility of using elemental diets. Another factor to consider when recommending an elemental diet is the formula's cost. Although some insurance companies provide payment for formulas, long-term use may pose a financial burden to families.

Young children with limited food experience are more receptive to an elemental diet and transition more easily to this treatment. Older patients, who have had full exposure to a wide variety of foods, experience more difficulties adhering to these recommendations. In order to increase acceptance of the elemental formulas, approved flavorings can be used to alter their taste. These include, but are not limited to, adding sugar-based flavor packets provided by the formula manufacturer, mixing the formula with an approved 100% juice, and flavoring the formula with Kool-aid and sugar. An allergist should be involved to approve any flavorings.

Six-Food Elimination Diet

In response to the limitations of elemental diets, Kagawalla and colleagues[12] treated children by removing the six most common causative foods (milk, soy, eggs, wheat, peanuts/tree nuts, and seafood) from their diets. Thirty-five children were treated with a six-food elimination diet while continuing to eat other table foods. These children were compared with 25 children who had EoE who received an elemental diet only. After 6 weeks of diet therapy, 74% of the children following the six-food elimination diet and 88% of the children following elemental diets showed significant histologic improvement.[12] These results support the use of a six-food elimination diet as an effective treatment that improves symptoms and decreases inflammation for most children who have EoE.[12]

An advantage of implementing a six-food elimination diet is that it allows children to continue ingesting solid foods, which tends to be less disruptive to the child's lifestyle and therefore may increase compliance with dietary therapy. Another advantage to the six-food elimination diet is that it empirically removes potential allergens and does not require extensive skin testing. Additionally, this diet limits the number of food allergens to be reintroduced into a child's diet after resolution of symptoms and histology. Although allergen-free foods can increase monthly food costs, it can be more affordable than an elemental formula.

A disadvantage to a six-food elimination diet is that it may unnecessarily remove foods and simultaneously increase nutrient risk. Without allergy testing, it is difficult to determine if all food allergens have been eliminated and, as a result, symptoms or pain may remain in a child treated with the six-food elimination diet.

Tailored Elimination Diets

Another dietary treatment of EoE is the removal of specific foods from the diet based on food allergy testing. In an initial study investigating potential food antigens in EoE, Spergel and colleagues[13] identified milk, egg, peanut, shellfish, peas, beef, fish, rye, tomato, and wheat as the most commonly identified allergic foods through prick skin testing. These foods differed slightly from those identified through atopy patch testing, which included wheat, corn, beef, milk, soy, rye, egg, chicken, oats, and potato.[13] In this study, children were instructed to eliminate positive foods from their diet for 6 weeks. Seven children were instructed to follow elemental diets based on multiple positive skin tests. Following the 6-week diet therapy, biopsies were performed in 24 children. Biopsy results were normal in 13 children and significantly improved in 11 children, demonstrating that causative foods could be identified and eliminated through selective allergy testing.[13] In select individuals, the reintroduction of eliminated foods led to the return of symptoms.[13] In a follow-up study, Spergel and colleagues[14] completed comprehensive food allergy evaluations using prick skin testing and atopy patch testing to identify and remove causative foods from children's' diets. At the 6-week clinical follow-up, 112 out of 146 children (76%) had resolution of inflammation and were considered "responders" to diet therapy.

In tailored elimination diets, children undergo extensive skin testing using commercial and fresh food extracts. These tests are done to eliminate all positive foods and to build a nutritionally complete diet using only foods with negative prick skin testing. Some children undergo minimal skin testing based on history, whereas others experience extensive testing. Prick skin testing typically includes the top eight allergens (milk, eggs, wheat, soy, peanuts, tree-nuts, fish, and shellfish), common sources of both complete and incomplete protein (beef, pork, lamb, chicken, turkey, kidney bean, black bean), complex carbohydrates (rice, corn, oats, rye, barley, buckwheat, quinoa, white potato, sweet potato), and any fruits or vegetables identified through a complete diet history. Children eliminating multiple foods from their diets may require supplementation with an elemental formula to meet their total calorie or protein needs.

Children are often more responsive and open to making dietary changes based on the results of testing. Children appear more compliant to this dietary approach because it enhances their quality of life. Although the flexibility of a tailored eliminated diet is beneficial, the removal of additional problematic foods can increase a child's risk for nutrient deficiency. Additionally, the ability of allergy testing to identify inciting foods correctly is still questionable.

Even when children are able to meet their nutrient needs through an elimination diet or an elemental formula, it is sometimes necessary to provide additional supplements to meet their micronutrient needs. Many over-the-counter supplements contain allergens. Therefore, careful label reading and selection of supplements is recommended. Complete hypoallergenic children's multivitamins often recommended include Kirkman Children's Multivitamins (www.kirkmanlabs.com), Nano VM (www.solacenutrition.com), and Freeda Vitamin Vitalets (www.freedavitamins.com).

IMPLEMENTING DIET THERAPY

A critical aspect of implementing diet therapy involves having a RD assess nutrient intake, provide education on practical aspects of food avoidance, and ensure the nutritional adequacy of restricted diets. Inadequate calorie intake is common in children avoiding multiple foods. The foods that pose the greatest nutritional risk when removed from a child's diet include dairy, wheat, and egg. Inadequate protein intake often occurs in elimination diets as common sources of protein (milk, eggs, soy, meat/poultry, fish, shellfish, legumes, peanuts, and tree nuts) are avoided. Adequate fat is required for energy, growth, brain development, and transport of fat-soluble vitamins. Common fat sources, such as dairy, eggs, meat, and nuts, are often avoided, and foods often used in elimination diets, such as fruits, vegetables, and rice, are low in fat. Vitamin and mineral deficiency can occur when avoiding multiple foods or entire food groups, or when the overall diet is nutritionally incomplete. Calcium and vitamin D deficiency can occur when children are not fed a formula or a milk alternative. Additionally, many medications children take may decrease absorption of these nutrients. For instance, children have increased needs for calcium, vitamins A, C, and D, and potassium when taking corticosteroids. A RD skilled in food allergy counseling can provide specific recommendations for meeting nutrient needs while avoiding the allergens.

Successful Allergen Avoidance

To implement an elimination diet successfully, RDs can educate families about how to identify specific allergens and confidently replace excluded nutrients through alternative food sources. The Food Allergen Labeling and Consumer Protection Act (FALCPA) of 2004 (effective in January 2006) provides mandatory guidelines for the labeling of foods containing the six most common allergens (milk, eggs, soy, wheat, peanuts/tree nuts, and fish or shellfish).[15] This law requires all imported and domestic food packages in the United States to clearly state the presence of "major food allergens."[15] If a product contains any of these allergens, it must be listed in clear common terms, which can be accomplished in one of two ways. Manufacturers are in compliance if the allergen is clearly listed in ingredient statements or if the allergen is listed in a "contains" statement on the food product. Many families quickly glance at food products looking only for the "contains" statement without reading the ingredient list and accidentally purchase foods that should be avoided. Therefore, diet education should specifically address label reading.

Cross contamination is another concern at home and when dining out. Common causes of cross contamination include delicatessen slicers, cutting boards, grills, pans, serving trays, bulk bins, salad bars, and shared utensils. Foods are often manufactured in facilities with other allergens and it is important for consumers to contact manufacturers to determine which methods are used to minimize cross contamination.

RDs can emphasize which foods are allowable, in addition to teaching families how to follow strict elimination diets. They can educate families about the nutritional risks posed by allergen avoidance and provide dietary guidance to help children meet their nutrient needs with alternative food sources.

Milk is a significant source of protein, fat, vitamin A, vitamin D, riboflavin (B2), pantothenic acid, vitamin B12 (cobalamin), calcium, and phosphorus. Soy milk and rice milk are typically fortified to be equivalent to cow's milk in regards to calcium and vitamin D. These milk alternatives are also frequently fortified with B12, riboflavin, vitamin A, and phosphorus. Therefore, replacing cow's milk with either soy milk or rice milk helps meet micronutrient needs. Soy milk provides more fat, protein, and calories per serving and is preferable if allowed in the diet. Rice milk contains minimal protein and fat; therefore, it is imperative to assure these needs are met through alternative sources, such as meat, legumes, milk-free margarine, and oils.

Wheat is a staple grain in the United States and avoidance of this food significantly impacts a child's macronutrient intake. Wheat is a good source of thiamin (vitamin B1), riboflavin, niacin, chromium, and iron (when product is enriched). Alternative grain sources include rice, corn, oats, rye, barley, buckwheat, quinoa, amaranth, millet, and tapioca. Over the last decade, more commercially prepared products made with alternative grains have become available to consumers. RDs can direct families to these alternative products and also provide recipes using alternative ingredients.

Eggs are common sources of protein, vitamin B12, riboflavin (B2), pantothenic acid, biotin, choline, and selenium. Eggs are used in many complex carbohydrates such as bread, muffins, pancakes, waffles, and many other baked goods. When eggs are eliminated from the diet, baked goods may also be eliminated, which can significantly reduce a child's total energy intake. RDs can educate families on egg alternatives that can be used in baked goods and breads to provide safe, egg-free options. Egg substitutes sold in the grocery store contain egg whites, a significant source of egg protein, and must be avoided in the egg-free diet.

Soy is a good source of protein, thiamin, riboflavin, pyridoxine (vitamin B6), folic acid, calcium, phosphorus, magnesium, iron, and zinc. Although soy does not traditionally appear in large quantities in many children's diets, its avoidance in combination with other allergens can increase nutritional risk. Including an alternative grain beverage like rice or oat milk can help meet micronutrient needs, but it is essential for a soy-free diet to also provide alternative sources of protein and fat. Highly refined soybean oil and soy lecithin are allowable ingredients because they typically contain nondetectable levels of protein. The inclusion of highly refined soybean oil and soy lecithin allows children to enjoy a wider variety of manufactured foods. However, soybean oil that is cold pressed, expeller pressed, extracted, or extruded should be avoided because these are less-refined oils and could potentially contain protein.

Peanuts, tree nuts, fish, and shellfish provide protein, vitamin E, niacin, magnesium, manganese, chromium, iron, zinc, and essential fatty acids. Removal of these foods alone does not pose nutritional risk; however, in combination with additional food avoidance, the elimination of these alternative sources of nutrients can increase risk for nutrient deficiency. When avoiding these foods, it is important to recommend alternative sources of zinc (beef, pork, chicken, turkey, beans, leafy greens, whole grains, and multivitamins) and essential fatty acids (safflower oil, corn oil, sunflower oil, sunflower seeds, soybean oil, flaxseed oil, and canola oil).

In addition to micro-macronutrient concerns, food elimination diets can have significant psychosocial impacts on the child and his/her family. Food elimination diets require children and their families to learn how to avoid the forbidden foods. They are required to invest tremendous amounts of time and energy in learning to read food labels, understanding how to alter recipes, and educating other family members or caregivers.[16]

Food plays an integral part in our lives and social gatherings; thus, constant food avoidance can interfere with a child's socialization. Children may be teased at school and have a difficult time feeling accepted. The effort involved in avoiding potential allergens can dissuade families from attending parties or dining out with friends. Providing guidance on how to prepare and plan ahead can alleviate a great deal of stress for children and their families. Therefore, it is important to empower children and their families to participate actively in the management of their food allergies so informed decisions can be made without constant deliberation and stress.

In conclusion, three different dietary approaches may be considered for the management of EoE. When determining the best diet therapy for a child, it is important to consider the benefits and deterrents of the treatment. The elemental diet removes all solid foods and meets nutrient needs through an amino acid–based formula. This diet removes all potential food allergens, but compliance may prove challenging because of formula taste and cost. The six-food elimination diet empirically removes the top six allergens without allergy testing. However, this diet may remove foods incorrectly, increasing nutrition risk while symptoms remain. Tailored elimination diets remove foods based on positive allergy testing. This diet may prove more flexible; however, whether current allergy tests can identify all problematic foods correctly remains questionable. Regardless of the diet therapy selected, involvement of a RD is essential to assess a child's nutrient needs and to provide appropriate diet education.

REFERENCES

1. Furuta GT, Liacouras CA, Collins MH, et al. Rothenberg ME and members of the FIGERS subcommittees. Eosinophilic esophagitis in children and adults: a systematic review and consensus recommendations for diagnosis and treatment. Gastroenterology 2007;133:1342–63.
2. Spergel JM, Shuker M. Nutritional management of eosinophilic esophagitis. Gastrointest Endosc Clin N Am 2008;18:179–94.
3. Mofidi S. Nutritional management of pediatric food hypersensitivity. Pediatrics 2003;111:1645–53.
4. Food and nutrition board NRC. Recommended dietary allowances. 10th edition. Washington, DC: National Academy Press; 1989.
5. Food and nutrition board IoM. Dietary reference intakes–applications in dietary assessment. A report of the subcommittee on interpretation and uses of dietary reference intakes and the standing committee on the scientific evaluation of dietary reference intakes. Washington, DC: National Academy Press; 2000.
6. Salman S, Christie L, Burks A, et al. Dietary intakes of children with food allergies: comparison of the food guide pyramid and the recommended dietary allowances. J Allergy Clin Immunol 2002;109:S214.
7. Christie L, Hine RJ, Parker JG, et al. Food allergies in children affect nutrient intake and growth. J Am Diet Assoc 2002;102:1648–51.
8. Henriksen C, Eggesbo M, Halvorsen R, et al. Nutrient intake among two-year-old children on cow's milk-restricted diets. Acta Paediatr 2000;89(3):272–8.
9. Liacouras CA, Spergel JM, Ruchelli E, et al. Eosinophilic esophagitis: a 10-year experience in 381 children. Clin Gastroenterol Hepatol 2005;3:1198–206.
10. Kelly K, Lazenby A, Rowe PC, et al. Eosinophilic esophagitis attributed to gastroesophageal reflux: improvement with amino acid-base formula. Gastroenterology 1995;109(5):1503–12.
11. Markowitz JE, Spergel JM, Ruchelli E, et al. Elemental diet is an effective treatment for eosinophilic esophagitis in children and adolescents. Am J Gastroenterol 2003;98(4):777–82.
12. Kagawalla AF, Sentongo TA, Ritz S, et al. Effect of six-food elimination diet on clinical and histologic outcomes in eosinophilic esophagitis. Clin Gastroenterol Hepatol 2006;4(9):1097–102.
13. Spergel JM, Beasusoleil JL, Mascarenhas M, et al. The use of skin prick tests and patch tests to identify causative foods in eosinophilic esophagitis. J Allergy Clin Immunol 2002;109:363–8.
14. Spergel JM, Andrews T, Brown-Whitehorn TF, et al. Treatment of eosinophilic esophagitis with specific food elimination diet directed by a combination of skin prick and patch tests. Ann Allergy Asthma Immunol 2005;95:336–43.
15. United States, Food and Drug Administration. Questions and answers regarding food allergens including the Food Allergen Consumer Protection Act of 2004, 4th edition. Available at: http://www.cfsan.fda.gov/~dms/alrguid4.html. Accessed June 24, 2008.
16. Munoz-Furlong A. Daily coping strategies for patients and their families. Pediatrics 2003;111:1654–61.

Association of Eosinophilic Gastrointestinal Disorders with Other Atopic Disorders

Soma Jyonouchi, MD, Terri A. Brown-Whitehorn, MD,
Jonathan M. Spergel, MD, PhD*

KEYWORDS

- Eosinophilic esophagitis • Atopy • Asthma
- Food allergy • Atopic dermatitis

Atopy involves an exaggerated immune response to common environmental allergens. Atopy can be defined in various ways: elevated total IgE; physician diagnosis of asthma, allergic rhinitis (AR), or atopic dermatitis (AD); or a positive allergy test (skin prick test or specific IgE to an allergen). In general, allergic/atopic diseases are associated with an expansion of T helper (Th) 2 cell population and secretion of cytokines (interleukin [IL]-4, IL-5, and IL-13) that favor IgE synthesis and eosinophilia. The most common atopic diseases are asthma, AR, food allergy, and AD.

Atopic diseases have common features: inflammation (often eosinophilic), hyperresponsiveness to stimuli, remodeling of tissues, and Th2 cellular production. Asthma is a chronic, inflammatory lung disease characterized by reversible airway obstruction and increased airway hyperresponsiveness. Thickening of airway tissue observed in asthma includes subepithelial fibrosis, increased matrix deposited in the submucosa, and increased smooth muscle (hyperplasia and hypertrophy). The symptoms of hyperresponsiveness are experienced as cough or wheeze with exercise, cold air, or other stimuli. The airway inflammation in asthma consists of Th2 cells and eosinophils and, in severe disease, neutrophils are found in bronchoalveolar lavage and lung biopsies.[1] AR involves eosinophilic inflammation of the nasal membranes triggered by an IgE-mediated response to environmental proteins.[2] Similar to asthma, AR has nasal hyperresponsiveness seen as sneezing in response to stimulation by allergens. AD is

Division of Allergy and Immunology, The Children's Hospital of Philadelphia, University of Pennsylvania School of Medicine, 34th Street and Civic Center Boulevard, Philadelphia, PA 19104, USA
* Corresponding author.
E-mail address: Spergel@email.chop.edu (J.M. Spergel).

Immunol Allergy Clin N Am 29 (2009) 85–97
doi:10.1016/j.iac.2008.09.008
immunology.theclinics.com

a disease of chronic skin inflammation with eosinophilic inflammation and Th2 cells in early lesions on skin biopsies. In chronic lesions, a mixed picture of Th1 cells and spongiosis is observed. In asthma, remodeling occurs with chronic lesions, homologous to the thickened skin, lichenification, in the AD. AD can be triggered by IgE-mediated sensitivity to food or aeroallergens and non–IgE-mediated reactions. The third common component, hyperresponsiveness, is seen as itching to normal stimuli such as dry skin (xerosis).[3] Another form of atopy is food allergies. Food allergies can be classified into two broad categories: IgE-mediated and non–IgE-mediated. Classic IgE-mediated food allergies involve mast cell degranulation following exposure to food proteins, causing urticaria, rhinorrhea, emesis, diarrhea, wheezing, angioedema, and anaphylaxis. Non–IgE-mediated food allergies include cell-mediated disease processes, such as food protein–induced enterocolitis, dermatitis herpetiformis, and eosinophilic esophagitis (EoE).[4] In asthma, AR, AD, and food allergies, the acute hypersensitivity reaction is mediated by mast cell degranulation following cross linking of IgE and its receptor. The subsequent release of preformed mediators results in swelling from increased blood flow and increased vascular permeability. However, a late-phase reaction can also occur, characterized by infiltration of tissues by neutrophils, eosinophils, macrophages, and Th2 cells that help to sustain inflammation.

Similar to eosinophilic inflammation seen in atopy, the presence of increased eosinophils in the gastrointestinal tract, without other known cause, is seen in a group of conditions known as eosinophilic gastrointestinal disorders (EGIDs). The most common of these disorders, namely EoE, is hypothesized to be caused by IgE- and cell-mediated reactions (non–IgE-mediated) to foods and other triggers. The mixed picture is similar to that of AD.

This article discusses the similarities between EoE and other atopic disorders. The authors first review the existing murine and human data that suggest a link between asthma, AR, AD, and food allergy themselves, followed by the link between EoE and these allergic conditions. This article also discusses atopic conditions in patients who have eosinophilic gastroenteritis (EG), a disease that occurs with much less frequency than EoE.

SIMILARITIES BETWEEN EOSINOPHILIC GASTROINTESTINAL DISORDERS AND ATOPIC DISORDERS

Rise in Atopic Diseases and Eosinophilic Gastrointestinal Disorders

Over the past few decades, the reported prevalence of allergic diseases has increased dramatically. In industrialized countries, approximately 25% to 30% of the population suffers from AD, food allergy, or AR.[5] Data from the Centers for Disease Control and Prevention National Health Information survey confirm a rise in all atopic diseases. The reported prevalence of asthma in 1990 was only 3%. According to 2007 data, the prevalence has increased to 7.7%.[6] A similar rise in AD prevalence was also noted between 1998 (7.3% of children under 17) and 2006 (10% of children under 17).[7] Mirroring this rise in allergic disorders has been an increase in the diagnosis of EGIDs, in particular EoE. Perth, Australia, has seen an 18-fold rise in the prevalence of EoE over 10 years.[8] At the authors' institution in Philadelphia, they saw a 35-fold increase between 1994 and 2003.[9]

Common Pathology: Eosinophilic and T Helper 2 Inflammation

EGIDs are a spectrum of disease that includes EoE, EG, and eosinophilic colitis. EGIDs are characterized by eosinophilic inflammation of the gastrointestinal tract in the absence of other secondary causes of eosinophilia.[10] The normal esophagus is void of eosinophils and their presence signifies either gastroesophageal reflux or EoE in most cases. Unlike the esophagus, the stomach, small intestine, and colon normally contain eosinophils, which aid in parasitic defense and do not cause tissue damage. However, an increase in tissue eosinophilia may signify EG, eosinophilic colitis, a parasitic disease, drug allergy, or inflammatory bowel disease. This eosinophilic inflammation in EGIDs mirrors the eosinophilic inflammation seen in asthma and AR.

Similar to thickening of the basement membrane in the lung in asthma and lichenification of the skin in AD, thickening of the esophagus in EoE is observed. In EoE, the membrane has an increased in basal layer. Aceves and colleagues[11] have seen increased collagen and fibrosis on esophageal biopsies in EoE. They have also observed a mechanism for this thickening on EoE that is similar to that of asthma, with increases in vascular cell adhesion molecule (VCAM)-1, profibrotic molecule, transforming growth factor-beta (TGF-β) and transcription factor, Smad2/3 in esophageal biopsies, which is similar to changes observed in asthma.[12,13] In murine models, IL-13 has been shown to play a critical role.

One frequently cited explanation of allergic disease involves the Th1 versus Th2 paradigm. Following antigen presentation by a dendritic cell, the naïve T cell becomes polarized to either a Th1 or Th2 cell. The Th1 subclass produces interferon-gamma (which helps clear viruses and intracellular pathogens) and down-regulates Th2 cells and the production of IgE. Th2 cells produce IL-4, IL-5, and IL-13 and down-regulate Th1 cells. Th2 cells promote isotype switching to IgE and the production of eosinophils, which confers protection against parasitic worms but also creates a favorable environment for the development of atopy.[3]

Th2 cells and their cytokines have been seen in EoE and other atopic diseases (asthma, AD, and AR). Simon and colleagues[14–16] have demonstrated high expression of the Th2 cytokines, IL-5 and IL-13, in patients who have acute AD. Assessment of bronchoalveolar lavage fluid from patients who have asthma has shown elevated levels of IL-4 and IL-5 cytokines.[1] Similarly, in nasal lavage samples from patients who have AR, high levels of IL-4, IL-5, and IL-13 can be detected.[17] Straumann and colleagues[18] have demonstrated that EoE is also associated with a Th2 allergic phenotype. In patients who have EoE, esophageal biopsy specimens were found to have greater numbers of T cells and mast cells and increased expression of IL-5. In mouse models of EoE, IL-5 knockout mice are resistant to developing disease.[19] Chemokines are small 8- to 10-kilodalton molecules that attract cells to specific locations. These homing signals (chemokine and their receptors) for Th2 cells and eosinophils are also increased in EoE and atopic disease, and include thymus and activation-regulated chemokine (TARC) and CXC chemokine receptor 3 (CXCR3) in asthma;[20,21] decreased TARC levels after immunotherapy in AR;[22] cutaneous T-cell-attracting chemokine (CTACK) and TARC in the peripheral blood in AD;[23] and eotaxin-3 in EoE,[24] which indicates further pathogenetic links between atopic disease and EoE.

A common end point in asthma, AD, and EoE is remodeling. Some patients who have asthma develop airway remodeling and a permanent decline in lung function thought to be due to subepithelial fibrosis and angiogenesis.[25] For AD, the remodeling is seen in chronic lesions as lichenification and thickening of the skin.[26] In patients who have untreated EoE, the development of strictures is a concern. Aceves and colleagues[11] have demonstrated basement membrane thickening and increased vascular activation in untreated patients who have EoE, which is similar to changes seen in airway remodeling with elevated TGF-β and VCAM-1 expression. Adults who have EoE have more strictures and food impaction than children, suggesting a natural course of disease.[27]

Similarities in Murine Models of Atopy and Eosinophilic Gastrointestinal Disorders

In addition to the prevalence and biopsy similarities, murine models predict a similar mechanism of disease pathogenesis. Spergel and colleagues[28] originally created a mouse model linking AD and asthma. Mice were first exposed to ovalbumin allergen by the epicutaneous route (an allergen patch was applied to a shaved area on the back), which induced AD-like changes to the skin. Following sensitization, a single aerosolized exposure to the same allergen induced airway hyperresponsiveness to methacholine and eosinophilia on bronchoalveolar lavage.

In a murine model of EoE, Akei and colleagues[29] used the same epicutaneous sensitization as Spergel with *Aspergillus fumigatus* or ovalbumin. These mice did not develop EoE after skin sensitization alone, although they did develop AD-like skin changes. However, following the single intranasal challenge to allergen, the development of marked EoE was observed. The investigators concluded that epicutaneous sensitization to allergen primes the esophagus for inhaled allergen-induced EoE in their model, similar to asthma.[9] The importance of Th2 cytokines and signaling in this model was further demonstrated with the use of specific knockout mice. IL-5 knockout mice were completely resistant to developing EoE using this protocol. IL-13, IL-4, and STAT 6 knockout mice developed milder forms of EoE.[29] Other similarities between the murine models were that CD4+ T cells were necessary for the development of AD[30] and Th2 cytokines were necessary for the development of airway sensitization,[11] as described in the EoE model.

The model created by Akei and colleagues[29] provides evidence for a link between AD and EoE, and Mishra and colleagues[31] created a murine model that suggests a link between asthma and EoE. This model was adapted from a protocol used to create airway inflammation. Anesthetized mice were exposed to 100 μg of *Aspergillus fumigatus* intranasally. A total of nine treatments were given over the course of 3 weeks. These mice developed esophageal eosinophilia and epithelial cell hyperplasia. Although mice exposed to intranasal allergen developed EoE, the same allergen delivered by oral or intragastric route failed to elicit eosinophilia. Furthermore, the eosinophilia was isolated to the esophagus, with no eosinophils seen in the stomach or small intestine.

Association of Atopic Diseases to Each Other: Linkage Between Asthma and Allergic Rhinitis

Human data also mimic the murine models of disease, demonstrating a connection between different atopic conditions. In the United Airway model, (linkage of asthma–AR), AR and asthma are linked by an anatomic and immunologic connection between the upper and lower airways. A European population-based survey showed a threefold asthma increase in subjects who suffered from AR.[32] The treatment of AR with nasal corticosteroids is associated with a reduced risk for asthma-related ER visits and hospitalizations and decreased airway hyperreactivity.[33,34] Conversely, inhaled steroid use has been shown to decrease eosinophilia in the nose and AR symptoms, despite the lack of direct medication contact.[35]

Braunstahl and colleagues[36,37] have helped elucidate the pathophysiology of the connection between the upper and lower airways. In one study, human subjects who had AR who underwent nasal allergen provocation developed tissue eosinophilia and up-regulation of adhesion molecules in the nasal and bronchial epithelium.[37] In a related experiment, atopic subjects who underwent a bronchial allergen challenge were shown to develop inflammatory cell infiltrate and increased expression of IL-5 in the nasal mucosa.[36]

Atopic March: The Link Between Atopic Dermatitis and Asthma

A similar link exists between AD and asthma, known as the atopic march. Typically, AD marks the first manifestation, followed by the emergence of food allergy, asthma, and AR. AD may improve or even disappear over time.[38] The evidence is from longitudinal, genetic, and mechanistic studies. Gustafsson and colleagues[39] conducted a longitudinal study of 94 children who had AD aged 4 months to 3 years. After 7 years, one third of the patients had resolution of AD. However, 43% had developed asthma and 45% had developed AR. In another study, involving 2270 children who had AD, aged 2 years to 17 years, 33% of the patients had either asthma or AR and 38% had both asthma and AR.[40] In the general population, 8.5% of children have asthma and 25% have AR,[6,41] which suggests that AD is an important risk factor in the development of other allergic diseases.

The proposed mechanism for this relationship is based on the supposition that the skin acts as the site of primary sensitization.[38] Sensitized T cells then would migrate to the nose and lungs, causing asthma and AR. Recent genetic studies suggest patients who have "leaky skin," as evidenced by filaggrin mutations,[42] have an increased risk for asthma and AD. The allergen penetrates the leaky skin, causing sensitization and airway disease, like the murine model.[28]

Sensitization to Allergens and Atopy

Sensitization to food allergens has also been shown to be predictive of future asthma. In a birth cohort of 100 infants in England, patients who had skin prick test sensitivity to egg and cow's milk were more likely to develop asthma later in life (odds ratio 10.7; 95% CI 2.1–55.1).[43] Likewise, sensitization to inhalant allergens, in particular *Alternaria* mold and dust mites, is associated with asthma.[44]

COMMON CLINICAL FEATURES OF EOSINOPHILIC GASTROINTESTINAL DISORDER AND ATOPIC DISEASES

Like other allergic conditions, EoE is a chronic disease that leads to either persistent symptoms or, at times, intermittent "flares." Infants and young children often present with persistent vomiting, failure to thrive, or abdominal pain, whereas adolescents and adults present with abdominal pain, dysphagia, or food impaction. Those who have dysphagia will often modify their behavior and learn to eat slowly and cautiously, similar to asthmatics, who modify their behavior by limiting physical activity. The flaring observed in EGIDs is similar to the exacerbations seen in asthma and AD with baseline underlying inflammation. Another common feature in atopic disease is hyperresponsiveness to stimuli, seen as coughing and wheezing to methacholine in asthma, and itching in AD. It appears that patients who have EGIDs have an increased sensitivity to acid reflux or gastrointestinal symptoms, but this has not been not confirmed in a rigorous manner.

The treatment approach for EoE is similar to that for other forms of atopy. The key to therapy is avoidance of known allergens or triggers. In EoE, food is often the culprit and thus, removal is recommended. Removal of the allergen leads to normalization of esophageal biopsies, indicating the role of food allergens in EoE.[9,45] In asthma, removal of the aeroallergen (animal dander or dust mites) leads to reduction of symptoms and airway inflammation.[46,47] If dietary management of EoE fails or is not tolerated by the patient, topical "swallowed" forms of corticosteroids are used to control the underlying inflammation and symptoms. Similarly, topical steroids are the cornerstone of the authors' approach to treating asthma, AD, and AR.[48,49]

Link Between Eosinophilic Esophagitis and Atopic Diseases

The authors and others have reported that most children and adults who have EoE have concomitant atopy (**Table 1**). In contrast, 20% of adults in the general United States population have AR and 6.7% of adults have asthma (the prevalence of asthma in children in the United States is 8.5%)[50] and approximately 17% of children in the United States are affected by AD.[51] At the authors' institution, a 14-year follow-up of more than 600 pediatric patients who had EoE showed that two thirds had evidence of other allergic disease,[52] approximately threefold greater than the general population. Data from Cincinnati also indicated a high prevalence of environmental (79%) and food allergies (75%) in children who had EoE.[53] In addition, genetic links between allergy and EoE are likely. Of 381 patients who had EoE, 164 were found to have AR, or AD in a first-degree relative.[9] Guajardo and colleagues[54] reported an even higher prevalence of AR (77%) and asthma (51%) in immediate family members.

Adults who have EoE appear to show similar atopic features as children. For instance, Roy-Ghanta and colleagues[55] recently evaluated 23 adult patients who had EoE and found that most showed evidence of sensitization to environmental aeroallergens (78%) and the presence of specific IgE to food allergens (82%). Simon and colleagues[56] have described a similar pattern of increased atopy in 31 adult patients who had EoE. Of these adult patients who had EoE, 68% experienced asthma, AD, or AR. The prevalence of atopic diseases in EoE in children and adults is summarized in **Table 2**.

The prevalence of atopic diseases in EoE varies; some studies have reported it to be as low as 50%, whereas others report it to be as high as 80%. The differences could be due to the particular region where the study was done or the physician diagnosing the disorder. Studies done by an allergist-immunologist have a higher prevalence of atopic diseases than a similar study done by a gastroenterologist. This difference could be a selection bias or it may reflect the fact that an allergist-immunologist can make the diagnosis sooner because he/she sees those diseases more frequently.

Link Between Eosinophilic Esophagitis and Food Allergens

The strongest evidence for food allergy as a cause of EoE comes from the clinical response of patients who are placed on restricted or elemental diets. In 1996, Kelly and

Table 1
Studies showing the development of other atopic diseases in patients who have atopic dermatitis, allergic rhinitis, or egg allergy

Study	Number in Study	AD → Asthma[a]	AD → AR[a]	AR → Asthma[a]	EA → Asthma (OR)
Kapoor et al[40]	2270	33%	33%	—	—
Ricci et al[69]	252	34%	57%	—	—
Gustafsson et al[39]	96	43%	45%	—	—
Greisner et al[70]	306	—	—	21%	—
Wright et al[71]	129	—	—	32%	—
Sibbald et al[72]	—	—	—	—	—
Kotaniemi-Syrjanen et al[73]	82	—	—	—	2.85
Rhodes et al[43]	63	—	—	—	10.70

Abbreviations: EA, egg allergy; OR, odds ratio.
[a] Percentage is the prevalence of the second atopic disease developing in the initial population.

Table 2							
Studies showing the frequency of atopic disease in patients who have eosinophilic esophagitis							
Author/Year [Ref]	No. EoE Patients	Age (y)	Asthma	AR	AD	FA (Anaphylaxis)	
Spergel et al. 2008[52]	620	9.1 ± 3.1	50%	61%	21%	5.7%	
Assa'ad et al. 2007[58]	89	6.2 ± 4.8	39%	30%	19%	9.0%	
Sugnanam et al. 2007[59]	45	3 mo to 16 y	66%	93%	55%	24.0%	
Guajardo et al. 2002[54]	39	8 ± 12	38%	64%	26%	23.0%	
Roy-Ghanta et al. 2008[55]	23	18 to 57	26%	78%	4%	—	

Abbreviation: FA, food allergy.

colleagues[45] examined 10 children who had persistent GERD and esophageal eosinophilia refractory to pharmacotherapy; in fact, 6 of the 10 patients had already received Nissen fundoplication as a treatment of medically resistant GERD. Following a 6-week trial of elemental formula, a significant decrease in esophageal eosinophils and clinical symptoms was observed in all of the patients, with 8 patients demonstrating complete resolution.[45]

At the authors' institution, with their last published report of the 160 patients who had EoE treated with an elemental diet, 97% achieved symptom resolution and esophageal biopsy normalization. The use of specific elimination diets of foods identified by skin prick testing and patch testing led to improvement in 75% of cases.[9] In the authors' current practice, which includes more than 700 children who have EoE, they have found that 98% responded to elimination or elemental diet (Jyonouchi, Brown, and Spergel, unpublished data, August 2008).

Additional support for food allergy as a participant in EoE is provided by Kagalwalla and colleagues,[57] who demonstrated improvement of EoE in patients after implementation of an empiric six-food elimination diet. Instead of extensive skin testing, these investigators eliminated, for a 6-week period, the six most common food allergens (milk, soy, egg, wheat, nuts, and seafood) from the diets of 35 patients who had EoE and compared them with a control group of children who had EoE who were provided with an elemental diet alone. They found significant improvement in esophageal eosinophils (<10 per high-power field) for the six-food elimination group (74% of patients), as compared with an 88% response in children treated with an elemental diet.

Most patients who have EoE have evidence of IgE-mediated sensitization to food based on in vitro–specific IgE or skin prick testing. However, the reported incidence of actual food-induced anaphylaxis has been variable. In the cohort reported by Assa'ad and colleagues[58] and in the authors' patient population, the incidence has been 9% and 8.1%, respectively. Rates of food anaphylaxis were significantly higher in the data reported by Sugnanam[59] and Guajardo[54] (24% and 23%). The difference of 8.1% and 23% both from Cincinnati Children's Hospital is probable due to two reasons (time period studied and method of studies).[55,58] The higher number was found in a Web-based study versus lower number in the chart review.

Evidence indicates that the mechanism underlying the immunologic reaction to foods in EoE is not only IgE mediated but also cell mediated. In his cohort, Kelly and colleagues[45] demonstrated that the introduction of skin test–negative foods into the diet could induce clinical disease. Further support comes from the finding that flares of symptoms following reintroduction of offending foods occurred within 30 minutes for some patients, but took up to 8 hours for others. In the authors' experience, some patients remain asymptomatic for days to months with food reintroduction, and esophageal inflammation is found on repeat biopsy. To help address this issue, they have used patch testing as a tool for identifying delayed, cell-mediated allergic reactions in EoE/EG. In pediatric patients, they have found this testing method, along with skin prick testing, to be effective in guiding management. The combination of skin prick and patch testing had a negative predictive value of 88% to 100% for 20 foods (except milk), whereas the positive predictive value was greater than 74% for the most common foods causing EoE.[60]

The link between foods and EoE is not as clear in adult patients because limited data exist regarding the use and efficacy of elemental and elimination diets. In one study, Simon and colleagues[61] evaluated the effect of wheat and rye removal from the diet in six adults, who had skin tests (sensitization) to these foods. These patients were also sensitized to grass pollen, which can account as wheat/rye cross react with grass pollen. First, the patients underwent double-blind placebo-controlled food challenges to wheat and rye. The food challenges failed to provoke any EoE symptoms. In addition, a 6-week trial of wheat and rye removal from the diet failed to produce any histologic improvement in biopsy. However, a series of case reports published in abstracts indicates that diet can also be helpful in adults. Gonsalves reported a 50% response rate in adults on a six-food elimination diet and near 100% resolution on an elemental diet.[62]

ROLE OF AEROALLERGENS AND EOSINOPHILIC ESOPHAGITIS

Some evidence suggests that aeroallergens may play a causative role in the development of EoE in humans. A seasonal variation in cases of newly diagnosed EoE has been described, with fewer cases being diagnosed in the winter when the air contains less pollen.[63] Magnusson and colleagues[64] have demonstrated increased duodenal eosinophils and mast cells during pollen season in non-EoE patients allergic to birch pollen. Similarly, esophageal biopsies from patients who have AR during pollen season have shown elevated numbers of eosinophils compared with controls. However, the number of eosinophils observed was lower than values typically seen in patients who have EoE (5.5 $\pm$ 7.3 eosinophils per high-power field in the proximal esophagus and 3.2 $\pm$ 3.7 eosinophils per high-power field in the distal esophagus).[65]

In a study of adult patients, the symptoms of AR and asthma significantly preceded the onset of dysphagia and EoE diagnosis. This finding raises the possibility that sensitization to aeroallergens similar to the murine model created by Mishra could also cause EoE in humans.[31] Fogg and colleagues[66] described a 21-year-old female patient who had asthma, AR, and EoE, who suffered seasonal flares of esophageal inflammation. The patient was skin test and patch test negative to foods and her diet remained stable during the observation period. Esophageal biopsies taken during the spring or summer pollen months revealed moderate-to-severe EoE. However, biopsies performed during the winter months showed little or no esophageal inflammation. The one case reported by Fogg also noted worsening symptoms during pollen seasons.

In the authors' EoE population, they have confirmed seasonal/pollen variation in 55 patients, with worsening symptoms and esophageal eosinophilia during pollen seasons. Food allergies were still the primary cause of disease in these patients. However, during pollen season in the spring or fall, an exacerbation of disease (confirmed by biopsy) was documented. Full disease control was achieved only during non–pollen seasons and on proper dietary therapy.[52]

Although direct deposition of pollens onto the esophageal mucosa is one potential mechanism for inflammation, experimental evidence points toward other potential pathways. Greiff and colleagues[35] have previously demonstrated that eotaxin, which plays a key role in eosinophil migration into the esophagus, is secreted by the nasal mucosa of patients who have AR. Eotaxin release by nasal mucosa on exposure to aeroallergens provides a possible explanation as to why AR can lead to flares of EoE in some patients. Intranasal steroid therapy has been shown to decrease nasal secretion of eotaxin in patients who have AR and in the authors' patients they recommend its use regularly.

EOSINOPHILIC GASTROENTERITIS AND ATOPY

EG remains a rare disease and the exact incidence is difficult to estimate. Eosinophilic infiltration is seen throughout the gastrointestinal tract and must be differentiated from inflammatory bowel disease, Crohn's disease, or other gastrointestinal pathology. Clinical symptoms include abdominal pain, nausea, diarrhea, and vomiting. EG can be classified according to the depth of eosinophilic infiltration into the gut wall: mucosal, submucosal, muscularis, and serosa. As with EoE, an increased prevalence of atopic conditions has been reported in patients who have EG. Results from a Web-based registry of patients who had EG (n = 57) showed a high incidence of AR (63%), drug allergies (53%), asthma (39%), and eczema (40%).[54]

Insights into the pathogenesis of EG come from the diabetic biobreeding lymphopenic (lyp) rat model. The Lyp gene encodes a guanosine triphosphatase (GTPase) of the immunity-associated protein (GIMAP5), which may protect cells from apoptosis. Lyp/lyp mutation homozygous mice developed gastroenteritis strikingly similar to human EG.

Affected mice developed weight loss, listlessness, diarrhea, and gut ascites. Examination of the large and small intestines revealed increased eosinophils, mast cells, and basophils. Lyp/lyp T cells expressed high levels of IL-4, IL-5, and IL-13, which confirmed a Th2 phenotype. Mice also expressed high levels of serum IgE.[67]

The importance of IgE-mediated mechanisms in EG is supported by the work done by Foroughi and colleagues.[68] In their open-label study, nine patients who had EG were treated with omalizumab, a monoclonal anti-IgE antibody. Treatment was shown to decrease peripheral eosinophilia and lower eosinophil numbers in the gastric antrum and duodenum. The fact that only a partial decrease in the absolute eosinophil count was seen in most patients suggests that non-IgE–mediated mechanisms are also involved in the pathogenesis. Additionally, omalizumab led to a 63% reduction of symptoms at 8 weeks and a 70% reduction of symptoms at 16 weeks.

The role of food allergy in the pathogenesis of EG is supported by the success of elemental food diets. Chehade and colleagues[74] reported that children who had EG and protein-losing enteropathy who were placed on an elemental diet showed a significant decrease in symptoms. The efficacy of specific food elimination diets based on skin prick testing and patch testing for foods has not been well studied in this population of patients.

SUMMARY

The emergence of EGIDs has paralleled a rise in atopic diseases such as asthma, AR, AD, and food allergy. Significant similarities exist between EoE and other allergic diseases, including common cell types (mast cells and eosinophils), cytokines (IL-4, IL-5, and IL-13), and chemokines. Patients who have EoE and EG have a higher incidence of asthma, AR, AD, and food allergy. The underlying pathogenesis is still being pursued. Once understood, therapeutic interventions may be available not only to treat EoE or EG but also to prevent their development.

REFERENCES

1. Robinson D, Hamid Q, Ying S, et al. Predominant Th2-like bronchoalveolar T-lymphocytes population in atopic asthma. N Engl J Med 1992;326:298–304.
2. Spergel JM. Atopic march: link to upper airways. Curr Opin Allergy Clin Immunol 2005;5(1):17–21.
3. Bieber T. Atopic dermatitis. N Engl J Med 2008;358(14):1483–94.
4. Sampson HA. Food allergy. Part 1: immunopathogenesis and clinical disorders. J Allergy Clin Immunol 1999;103(5 Pt 1):717–28.
5. Kiyohara C, Tanaka K, Miyake Y. Genetic susceptibility to atopic dermatitis. Allergol Int 2008;57(1):39–56.
6. Brim SN, Rudd RA, Funk RH, et al. Asthma prevalence among US children in underrepresented minority populations: American Indian/Alaska Native, Chinese, Filipino, and Asian Indian. Pediatrics 2008;122(1):e217–22.
7. Laughter D, Istvan JA, Tofte SJ, et al. The prevalence of atopic dermatitis in Oregon schoolchildren. J Am Acad Dermatol 2000;43(4):649–55.
8. Cherian S, Smith NM, Forbes DA. Rapidly increasing prevalence of eosinophilic oesophagitis in Western Australia. Arch Dis Child 2006;91(12):1000–4.
9. Liacouras CA, Spergel JM, Ruchelli E, et al. Eosinophilic esophagitis: a 10-year experience in 381 children. Clin Gastroenterol Hepatol 2005;3(12):1198–206.
10. Rothenberg ME. Eosinophilic gastrointestinal disorders (EGID). J Allergy Clin Immunol 2004;113(1):11–28, quiz 29.
11. Aceves SS, Newbury RO, Dohil R, et al. Esophageal remodeling in pediatric eosinophilic esophagitis. J Allergy Clin Immunol 2007;119(1):206–12.
12. Cho J, Miller M, Baek K, et al. Immunostimulatory DNA inhibits transforming growth factor-beta expression and airway remodeling. Am J Respir Crit Care Med 2004;30:651–61.
13. McMillan S, Xanthou G, Lloyd C. Manipulation of allergen-induced airway remodeling by treatment with anti-TGF-beta antibody: effect on the Smad signaling pathway. J Immunol 2005;174:5774–80.
14. Grewe M, Walther S, Gyufko K, et al. Analysis of the cytokine pattern expressed in situ in inhalant allergen patch test reactions of atopic dermatitis patients. J Invest Dermatol 1995;105(3):407–10.
15. Thepen T, Langeveld-Wildschut EG, Bihari IC, et al. Biphasic response against aeroallergen in atopic dermatitis showing a switch from an initial Th2 response to a Th1 response in situ: an immunocytochemical study. J Allergy Clin Immunol 1996;97:828–37.
16. Simon D, Vassina E, Yousefi S, et al. Reduced dermal infiltration of cytokine-expressing inflammatory cells in atopic dermatitis after short-term topical tacrolimus treatment. J Allergy Clin Immunol 2004;114(4):887–95.
17. Erin EM, Zacharasiewicz AS, Nicholson GC, et al. Topical corticosteroid inhibits interleukin-4, -5 and -13 in nasal secretions following allergen challenge. Clin Exp Allergy 2005;35(12):1608–14.
18. Straumann A, Bauer M, Fischer B, et al. Idiopathic eosinophilic esophagitis is associated with a T(H)2-type allergic inflammatory response. J Allergy Clin Immunol 2001;108(6):954–61.
19. Mishra A, Hogan SP, Brandt EB, et al. IL-5 promotes eosinophil trafficking to the esophagus. J Immunol 2002;168(5):2464–9.
20. Thomas SY, Banerji A, Medoff BD, et al. Multiple chemokine receptors, including CCR6 and CXCR3, regulate antigen-induced T cell homing to the human asthmatic airway. J Immunol 2007;179(3):1901–12.

21. Ying S, O'Connor B, Ratoff J, et al. Thymic stromal lymphopoietin expression is increased in asthmatic airways and correlates with expression of Th2-attracting chemokines and disease severity. J Immunol 2005;174(12):8183–90.
22. Takeuchi H, Yamamoto Y, Kitano H, et al. Changes in thymus- and activation-regulated chemokine (TARC) associated with allergen immunotherapy in patients with perennial allergic rhinitis. J Investig Allergol Clin Immunol 2005;15(3):172–6.
23. Song TW, Sohn MH, Kim ES, et al. Increased serum thymus and activation-regulated chemokine and cutaneous T cell-attracting chemokine levels in children with atopic dermatitis. Clin Exp Allergy 2006;36(3):346–51.
24. Blanchard C, Wang N, Stringer KF, et al. Eotaxin-3 and a uniquely conserved gene-expression profile in eosinophilic esophagitis. J Clin Invest 2006;116(2):536–47.
25. Hoshino M, Nakamura Y, Sim J, et al. Bronchial subepithelial fibrosis and expression of matrix metalloproteinase-9 in asthmatic airway inflammation. J Allergy Clin Immunol 1998;102(5):783–8.
26. Leung DY. Atopic dermatitis: the skin as a window into the pathogenesis of chronic allergic diseases. J Allergy Clin Immunol 1995;96(3):302–18, quiz 319.
27. Furuta G, Liacouras C, Collins M, et al. Eosinophilic esophagitis in children and adults: a systematic review and consensus recommendations for diagnosis and treatment. Gastroenterology 2007;133(4):1342–63 [epub].
28. Spergel JM, Mizoguchi E, Brewer JP, et al. Epicutaneous sensitization with protein antigen induces localized allergic dermatitis and hyperresponsiveness to methacholine after single exposure to aerosolized antigen in mice. J Clin Invest 1998;101(8):1614–22.
29. Akei HS, Mishra A, Blanchard C, et al. Epicutaneous antigen exposure primes for experimental eosinophilic esophagitis in mice. Gastroenterology 2005;129(3):985–94.
30. Spergel JM, Mizoguchi E, Oettgen H, et al. Roles of TH1 and TH2 cytokines in a murine model of allergic dermatitis. J Clin Invest 1999;103(8):1103–11.
31. Mishra A, Hogan SP, Brandt EB, et al. An etiological role for aeroallergens and eosinophils in experimental esophagitis. J Clin Invest 2001;107(1):83–90.
32. Leynaert B, Neukirch C, Kony S, et al. Association between asthma and rhinitis according to atopic sensitization in a population-based study. J Allergy Clin Immunol 2004;113(1):86–93.
33. Corren J, Manning BE, Thompson SF, et al. Rhinitis therapy and the prevention of hospital care for asthma: a case-control study. J Allergy Clin Immunol 2004;113(3):415–9.
34. Watson WT, Becker AB, Simons FE. Treatment of allergic rhinitis with intranasal corticosteroids in patients with mild asthma: effect on lower airway responsiveness. J Allergy Clin Immunol 1993;91(1 Pt 1):97–101.
35. Greiff L, Petersen H, Mattsson E, et al. Mucosal output of eotaxin in allergic rhinitis and its attenuation by topical glucocorticosteroid treatment. Clin Exp Allergy 2001;31(8):1321–7.
36. Braunstahl GJ, Kleinjan A, Overbeek SE, et al. Segmental bronchial provocation induces nasal inflammation in allergic rhinitis patients. Am J Respir Crit Care Med 2000;161(6):2051–7.
37. Braunstahl GJ, Overbeek SE, Kleinjan A, et al. Nasal allergen provocation induces adhesion molecule expression and tissue eosinophilia in upper and lower airways. J Allergy Clin Immunol 2001;107(3):469–76.
38. Spergel JM, Paller AS. Atopic dermatitis and the atopic march. J Allergy Clin Immunol 2003;112(6 Suppl):S118–27.

39. Gustafsson D, Sjoberg O, Foucard T. Development of allergies and asthma in infants and young children with atopic dermatitis–a prospective follow-up to 7 years of age. Allergy 2000;55(3):240–5.
40. Kapoor R, Menon C, Hoffstad O, et al. The prevalence of atopic triad in children with physician-confirmed atopic dermatitis. J Am Acad Dermatol 2008;58(1): 68–73.
41. O'Connell EJ. The burden of atopy and asthma in children. Allergy 2004;59(Suppl 78):7–11.
42. Weidinger S, O'Sullivan M, Illig T, et al. Filaggrin mutations, atopic eczema, hay fever, and asthma in children. J Allergy Clin Immunol 2008;121(5):1203–9, e1201.
43. Rhodes HL, Sporik R, Thomas P, et al. Early life risk factors for adult asthma: a birth cohort study of subjects at risk. J Allergy Clin Immunol 2001;108(5):720–5.
44. Peat J, Tovey E, Mellis C, et al. Importance of house dust mite and Alternaria allergens in childhood asthma: an epidemiological study in two climatic regions of Australia. Clin Exp Allergy 1993;23:813–20.
45. Kelly KJ, Lazenby AJ, Rowe PC, et al. Eosinophilic esophagitis attributed to gastroesophageal reflux: improvement with an amino acid-based formula. Gastroenterology 1995;109(5):1503–12.
46. Simpson A, Custovic A, Pipis S, et al. Exhaled nitric oxide, sensitization, and exposure to allergens in patients with asthma who are not taking inhaled steroids. Am J Respir Crit Care Med 1999;160(1):45–9.
47. Johnson JR, Wiley RE, Fattouh R, et al. Continuous exposure to house dust mite elicits chronic airway inflammation and structural remodeling. Am J Respir Crit Care Med 2004;169(3):378–85.
48. Expert panel report 3 (EPR-3): guidelines for the diagnosis and management of asthma - summary report 2007. J Allergy Clin Immunol 2007;120(5 Suppl): S94–138.
49. Akdis CA, Akdis M, Bieber T, et al. Diagnosis and treatment of atopic dermatitis in children and adults: European Academy of Allergology and Clinical Immunology/ American Academy of Allergy, Asthma and Immunology/PRACTALL Consensus Report. Allergy 2006;61(8):969–87.
50. Pearce N, Ait-Khaled N, Beasley R, et al. Worldwide trends in the prevalence of asthma symptoms: phase III of the International Study of Asthma and Allergies in Childhood (ISAAC). Thorax 2007;62(9):758–66.
51. Peroni DG, Piacentini GL, Bodini A, et al. Prevalence and risk factors for atopic dermatitis in preschool children. Br J Dermatol 2008;158(3):539–43.
52. Spergel J, Brown-Whitehorn TF, Beausoleil J, et al. 14 years of eosinophilic esophagitis: clinical features and prognosis. J Pediatr Gastroenterol Nutr, in press.
53. Noel RJ, Putnam PE, Rothenberg ME. Eosinophilic esophagitis. N Engl J Med 2004;351(9):940–1.
54. Guajardo J, Plotnick L, Fende J, et al. Eosinophil-associated gastrointestinal disorders: a world-wide-web based registry. J Pediatr 2002;141(4):576–81.
55. Roy-Ghanta S, Larosa DF, Katzka DA. Atopic characteristics of adult patients with eosinophilic esophagitis. Clin Gastroenterol Hepatol 2008;6(5):531–5.
56. Simon D, Marti H, Heer P, et al. Eosinophilic esophagitis is frequently associated with IgE-mediated allergic airway diseases. J Allergy Clin Immunol 2005;115(5): 1090–2.
57. Kagalwalla AF, Sentongo TA, Ritz S, et al. Effect of six-food elimination diet on clinical and histologic outcomes in eosinophilic esophagitis. Clin Gastroenterol Hepatol 2006;4(9):1097–102.

58. Assa'ad AH, Putnam PE, Collins MH, et al. Pediatric patients with eosinophilic esophagitis: an 8-year follow-up. J Allergy Clin Immunol 2007;119(3):731–8.
59. Sugnanam KK, Collins JT, Smith PK, et al. Dichotomy of food and inhalant allergen sensitization in eosinophilic esophagitis. Allergy 2007;62(11):1257–60.
60. Spergel JM, Brown-Whitehorn T, Beausoleil JL, et al. Predictive values for skin prick test and atopy patch test for eosinophilic esophagitis. J Allergy Clin Immunol 2007;119(2):509–11.
61. Simon D, Straumann A, Wenk A, et al. Eosinophilic esophagitis in adults–no clinical relevance of wheat and rye sensitizations. Allergy 2006;61(12):1480–3.
62. Gonsalves. A prospective clinical trial of allergy testing and food elimination diet in adults with eosinophilic esophagitis (EE) [abstract]. Digestive Disease Week 2007.
63. Wang FY, Gupta SK, Fitzgerald JF. Is there a seasonal variation in the incidence or intensity of allergic eosinophilic esophagitis in newly diagnosed children? J Clin Gastroenterol 2007;41(5):451–3.
64. Magnusson J, Lin XP, Dahlman-Hoglund A, et al. Seasonal intestinal inflammation in patients with birch pollen allergy. J Allergy Clin Immunol 2003;112(1):45–50.
65. Onbasi K, Sin AZ, Doganavsargil B, et al. Eosinophil infiltration of the oesophageal mucosa in patients with pollen allergy during the season. Clin Exp Allergy 2005;35(11):1423–31.
66. Fogg MI, Ruchelli E, Spergel JM. Pollen and eosinophilic esophagitis. J Allergy Clin Immunol 2003;112(4):796–7.
67. Cousins L, Graham M, Tooze R, et al. Eosinophilic bowel disease controlled by the BB rat-derived lymphopenia/Gimap5 gene. Gastroenterology 2006;131(5):1475–85.
68. Foroughi S, Foster B, Kim N, et al. Anti-IgE treatment of eosinophil-associated gastrointestinal disorders. J Allergy Clin Immunol 2007;120(3):594–601.
69. Ricci G, Patrizi A, Baldi E, et al. Long-term follow-up of atopic dermatitis: retrospective analysis of related risk factors and association with concomitant allergic diseases. J Am Acad Dermatol 2006;55(5):765–71.
70. Greisner WA 3rd, Settipane RJ, Settipane GA. Co-existence of asthma and allergic rhinitis: a 23-year follow-up study of college students. Allergy Asthma Proc 1998;19(4):185–8.
71. Wright AL, Holberg CJ, Martinez FD, et al. Epidemiology of physician-diagnosed allergic rhinitis in childhood. Pediatrics 1994;94(6 Pt 1):895–901.
72. Sibbald B, Rink E. Epidemiology of seasonal and perennial rhinitis: clinical presentation and medical history. Thorax 1991;46(12):895–901.
73. Kotaniemi-Syrjanen A, Reijonen TM, Romppanen J, et al. Allergen-specific immunoglobulin E antibodies in wheezing infants: the risk for asthma in later childhood. Pediatrics 2003;111(3):e255–61.
74. Chehade M, Magid MS, Mofidi S, et al. Allergic eosinophilic gastroenteritis with protein-losing enteropathy: intestinal pathology, clinical course, and long-term follow-up. J Pediatr Gastroenterol Nutr 2006;42(5):516–21.

Psychological Impact of Eosinophilic Esophagitis on Children and Families

Mary D. Klinnert, PhD

KEYWORDS

- Eosinophilic esophagitis (EoE) • Children and adolescents
- Chronic illness • Psychological adjustment • Quality of life

Eosinophilic esophagitis (EoE) is a newly recognized disorder marked clinically by symptoms of upper gastrointestinal distress and by histologic findings of increased eosinophils in the esophagus.[1] Recent reports have documented that EoE occurs in children and adults, with initial diagnoses made in children as young as 6 months of age.[1] Most EoE symptoms among children are triggered by allergic hypersensitivity to foods.[2] For pediatric patients and their families, symptom experiences, diagnostic procedures, and recommended treatments related to the disease can have a tremendous impact on quality of life and on psychological and social adjustment. However, the manner in which parents and children respond to, and cope with, elements of the disease can significantly influence the impact of EoE on resulting quality of life. The goal of this article is to describe how the EoE disease experience affects the quality of life of children and their families, and to raise key questions regarding the unique physical and emotional challenges posed by this disease.

Because EoE in children has only recently been recognized and defined as a clinical syndrome, much about the natural history of the disease has yet to be discovered. Similarly, although some clinical studies have investigated treatment strategies for differing clinical presentations, much remains to be learned about optimal treatment. Systematic research is lacking regarding the psychological effects of EoE on children and the impact of the disease on children's quality of life and that of their families. However, some lessons can be learned by drawing on existing research regarding health-related quality of life (HRQL) for children who have similar chronic illnesses. By combining existing research findings with the clinical experience of a pediatric behavioral health team that has worked with children with EoE and their families, it is

This work was supported by the Department of Pediatrics, National Jewish Health.
Department of Pediatrics, National Jewish Health, 1400 Jackson Street, Denver, CO 80206, USA
E-mail address: klinnertm@njc.org

Immunol Allergy Clin N Am 29 (2009) 99–107
doi:10.1016/j.iac.2008.09.011
0889-8561/08/$ – see front matter © 2009 Elsevier Inc. All rights reserved.

possible to formulate a view of the impact of EoE on quality of life and the primary coping challenges faced by these children and their families.

Research regarding other pediatric chronic illnesses has shown that the disease experience depends on multiple factors. Studies of HRQL among children who have medical illnesses are concerned with the effects of the disease and associated medical treatments not only on physical status, but also on the psychological and social aspects of children's lives.[3] Chronic illness influences children's psychological adjustment, with short-term effects on emotional responses to symptoms and treatment, and long-term effects on overall adjustment.[4] Although the presence of a chronic illness has several general effects on children and families, other effects of pediatric chronic illnesses are related to the unique characteristics of the disease and the treatments.[4] Effects also depend on the developmental status of the affected child and on the life context being considered, such as the family environment within which children and adolescents experience their disease. Finally, chronic illness in children also has major effects on the children's caregivers.[5] Thus, it can be expected that the experience of having EoE will have effects on quality of life similar to those of other diseases, along with effects that are unique to EoE; that those effects will differ, depending on the characteristics of individual children and their families; and that caregivers will be greatly affected, in addition to the children and adolescents diagnosed with EoE.

QUALITY-OF-LIFE EFFECTS OF EOSINOPHILIC ESOPHAGITIS SYMPTOMS

In infants and young children, EoE most commonly presents as reflux or vomiting, early satiety, feeding aversion or intolerance, and failure to thrive.[1] Many of these symptoms are indistinguishable from those of gastroesophageal reflux disease (GERD); only the presence of increased numbers of eosinophils and the failure to respond to standard treatment of GERD indicate that the underlying disease is EoE.[1] As with GERD, symptoms in infants and young children are observed and reported by caregivers. When infants spit up or vomit, or they are fussy and irritable, their caregivers infer that they are experiencing discomfort or pain. Food aversion or intolerance are believed to stem from experiences of discomfort or pain with eating, leading to learned avoidance behavior in children too young to verbalize their pain. In fact, infants who have GERD during their first year of life were significantly more likely than healthy children to develop feeding problems within the following year,[6] and it is likely that infants who have EoE have a similar pattern. Because of infants' and toddlers' developmental status, their EoE symptoms, including reflux, food aversion, and failure to thrive, have a major impact on the quality of life of their caregivers. The impact on caregivers' quality of life will be discussed later, when the effects of EoE on families are addressed.

In children who are of school age and older, EoE symptom patterns are different from those of younger children, which, in part, may be because of the older children's ability to report internal sensations, but also because the disease may manifest differently with increased age.[1] Typical symptoms among older children and adolescents include heartburn, abdominal pain, early satiety, reflux, and vomiting. In addition, older children experience dysphasia (difficulty swallowing), choking, or esophageal food impaction. As with younger children, a large overlap with GERD symptoms occurs; however, those symptoms that are different from typical GERD symptoms and are most often associated with EoE, such as difficulty swallowing and food impaction, can be extremely distressing and may have significant effects on psychological functioning in older children and adolescents.

Research information is available regarding quality of life for children who have several gastrointestinal diseases, including GERD, and may be applicable to those children whose EoE symptoms mimic those of GERD. Using a generic instrument, children aged 5 to 18 reported on their quality of life in the domains of physical, emotional, social, and school functioning.[7] Their quality of life scores were comparable to those of children and adolescents who have diagnoses of inflammatory bowel disease and functional abdominal pain, and all were somewhat lower than scores for a healthy control group. Although these results confirm that children who have GERD symptoms experience a decrement in quality of life similar to that of other gastrointestinal conditions, they nevertheless provide limited insight into quality-of-life effects that are specific either for children who have GERD or for those who have EoE with GERD-like symptoms. To learn about the impact of symptoms on quality of life among children who have EoE, it is necessary to learn which children are experiencing specific EoE symptoms, the symptom frequency and severity, and the associated emotional distress and social and psychological impact.

Swallowing problems have been commonly reported among older children and adolescents who have EoE. The severity of swallowing problems varies a great deal, as does the children's related distress. For example, an 11-year-old boy said that having EoE seldom bothered him. About once a month he felt as if a ball were in his esophagus but he was able to eliminate the sensation by taking a sip of water. In contrast, another 12-year-old boy, in describing his "throat problem," had reported difficulties swallowing and choking on a daily basis. As a result, he never ate solid food at school, instead drinking only milk. His school friends were aware of his tendency to choke and looked out for him. At home, he ate small amounts of food continuously because he was often ravenously hungry. For the latter patient, the swallowing problems that characterized his EoE had a great impact on his day-to-day life in terms of his eating behavior and his nutritional intake; however, his emotional response to the symptoms appeared matter-of-fact. For other youngsters, the experience of choking on food on a regular basis is more than unpleasant; it is extremely frightening. It is not uncommon for children and adolescents who have these symptoms to develop strong anxiety reactions related to swallowing food. The experience of having a food impaction may be especially traumatic. For example, following an impaction and the emergency procedure required for removal of the food from his throat, an older adolescent began having panic attacks, and he required psychological treatment to help him eat without anxiety.

In sum, available information suggests that EoE symptoms affect children and adolescents' quality of life, and also possibly their psychological adjustment. However, no systematic information is available about the frequency with which various EoE symptoms are associated with meaningful effects within the key domains of child functioning across developmental stages. It appears that persistent symptoms in infancy may put children at high risk for feeding disorders, but the frequency and persistence of this outcome is unknown. It is unknown what level of swallowing difficulty or regular choking affects a child's or adolescent's nutritional status or social relationships. Similarly, no information is available regarding the emotional sequelae of an episode of food impaction, such as the frequency with which anxiety reactions occur. It would be helpful to discover the coping strategies that children and adolescents use when they experience symptoms, and their effectiveness in managing them. Thus, many questions remain regarding the relationship between the symptoms experienced by children who have EoE and the effects on quality of life and psychological adjustment.

QUALITY-OF-LIFE EFFECTS OF EOSINOPHILIC ESOPHAGITIS TREATMENTS

Children and adolescents who have EoE are impacted not only by the disease symptoms but also by the treatment of the disease. Recommended treatments of EoE in children usually involve medication or dietary manipulations.[1] Pharmacologic treatment may include reflux medications or swallowed topical corticosteroids. Because the removal of causative foods from the diet has been clearly demonstrated to be successful in the treatment of EoE, dietary elimination is a key component of most children's experience with EoE. Dietary interventions range from the elimination of several specific foods from the diet, to removal of about six of the most common allergenic foods, to allowing ingestion of only elemental formulas. The time course of dietary restrictions can range from a few days (eg, for trials of specific foods) to weeks, months, or even years. To provide sufficient calories with the elemental formulas, it is common to place a nasogastric tube for feeding for a limited time. When an elemental formula diet is deemed necessary over a longer period of time, a gastric tube (G-tube) may be placed directly into the stomach. Thus, treatment strategies vary in their bodily invasiveness and in the extent of required lifestyle changes.

The impact on children and adolescents of diagnostic procedures and treatments of EoE varies widely. In general, the ways in which children respond to procedures such as blood draws, skin testing, and endoscopies and to swallowed medications related to EoE appear to be similar to the ways in which children cope with procedures and treatments of other diseases.[8] The psychological impact depends on the individual child's age and stage of development, especially on the ability to understand what is involved in the procedure or treatment, and the reasons for it. Much also depends on the quality of emotional communications and coping assistance provided for the child by parents. Apart from parenting methods, children's temperamental styles are a key determinant of their response to procedures and treatments. A child who tends to be emotionally reactive, anxious, or inhibited responds differently from one who is flexible and easy-going, and a robust and strong-willed child will have yet a different response.

Although many of the EoE procedures and treatments, such as diagnostic tests and medication administration, might be considered routine, the illness-specific dietary restrictions that comprise a primary treatment strategy for children and adolescents who have EoE frequently pose a unique and difficult psychological challenge for children and their families. Extensive restrictions on children's diets may have the potential for a severe negative impact on all components of HRQL for children: their physical, emotional, social, and school functioning. Several aspects of dietary restrictions make this treatment particularly difficult. Eating habits and favorite foods are pervasive and deeply emotional aspects of children's lives. Family routines and social events alike revolve around meals and treats. Given the centrality of food in children and families' lives, dietary restrictions have a major impact on children who have EoE in much the same way as for children who have food allergies. However, for children who have EoE, a wide range of foods is often eliminated, in comparison with one or several foods for food allergic children. Also, the consequences of eating the offending foods are often not readily obvious to children who have EoE in the way that immediate reactions are to children who have food allergies so, unless they experience dramatic symptoms such as vomiting or food impactions, children who have EoE may fail to make the connection between their dietary restrictions and fluctuations in their disease. Given these factors, elimination diets that are central to the treatment of EoE may have a profound effect on children's quality of life.

Not every child responds negatively to implementation of an elimination diet. Clinical experience has shown that infants and very young children who require an elemental formula often do well. Their mothers point out that they have never known anything different, and they are enormously relieved when the symptoms remit and the child begins to thrive. The elimination of foods can be more difficult for toddlers who have begun eating solids, who are often selective in their food choices, and for whom withdrawal of a favorite food can lead to distress. For them, the experience of having new foods introduced and then removed from their diet, a process that occurs with food trials, can be particularly difficult, and reducing the emotional impact requires a great deal of parental and professional strategizing.

For preschool-aged children, the implementation of a restricted diet is often extremely difficult. At this age, children's understanding of their bodies is expanding, their emerging sense of self is facilitated by the discovery of favorite foods, and development of the ability to regulate emotions and behavior is intertwined with their expectation and mastery of routine. Although cognitive abilities are expanding, preschoolers are as yet unable to understand the rationale for the imposition of dietary restrictions. For example, a 4-year-old girl was accustomed to a wide range of food, but her frequent vomiting dictated the elimination of dairy and wheat from her diet. Her response was pervasive, with extreme anger at friends and family members, especially at her younger 2-year-old brother who was allowed to eat what he pleased. The brother, on the other hand, stopped eating what he was allowed and began restricting his diet to match that of his sister (illustrating one type of effect elimination diets can have on siblings!).

Despite their greater cognitive abilities, older children also can have much difficulty when food is partially or completely removed from their diet. Children may become anxious and depressed, or they may become oppositional. One child stole food from other family members, and her parents locked their kitchen cabinets to keep her from eating prohibited food. On the other hand, it is not unusual for teenagers, who typically have independent access to food, to angrily disregard the dietary prohibitions to be able to eat favorite foods such as pizza.

Some children who have EoE require gastrostomy tubes (G-tubes) to ensure that they receive adequate nutrition. Little information is available regarding the quality-of-life effects of tube feeding for patients whose lives are not in immediate danger. It may be that psychological adjustment in children who have EoE and have G-tubes is dependent on the same factors that affect children's adjustment to other treatments. These include the child's age at the time the G-tube is placed, the child's temperament and psychological adjustment before G-tube placement, and the family emotional context. For example, a 2-year-old vomited so frequently that he failed to gain weight over a 10-month period, and his cognitive and emotional development was compromised. His mother was vastly relieved when a G-tube was placed. Along with weight gain, this child evidenced brightened affect and accelerated cognitive and motor development. Unfortunately, the reinstatement of oral feeding can be extremely challenging for children, because of either recurring symptoms or learned patterns of food refusal.[9] Many questions remain regarding the short- and long-term emotional and social consequences of the use of G-tubes in the treatment of children who have EoE.

For children and adolescents who have EoE, quality of life is further impacted by additional medical disorders. Seventy percent of children diagnosed with EoE have one or more coexisting atopic disorders such as asthma, atopic dermatitis, allergic rhinitis, or food allergies.[1,10] Each of these disorders presents with symptoms that require attention and a treatment regimen, so that the coexistence of EoE with additional atopic disorders makes for a highly complex disease experience, impacting quality of life in multiple ways. The coexistence of EoE and food allergy can be a particularly challenging combination. Children who have EoE and immediate hypersensitivity food allergies are restricted from a wide array of foods, with varying levels of negative effects, including the possibility of anaphylaxis. An anxious 8-year-old boy who had both conditions explained: "Some food makes me sick if I eat it; some other food, if I eat it I could die." Clinical observations suggest that the combination of EoE and food allergies increases the likelihood of symptom confusion and high anxiety related to food exposure.

Children's characteristic temperamental style before onset of EoE is an additional influence on their response to the disease. From infancy onward, children exhibit distinct tendencies to respond to their environment in characteristic ways. Infants may show behavioral inhibition, or wariness, that often is manifested as shyness, or even anxiety, as they get older. Young children may respond to circumstances in an easygoing, flexible manner, or they may tend to be more emotionally reactive, sensitive, or inflexible, requiring much parental modulation to navigate their daily lives. With the onset of EoE, children's predisposing temperamental characteristics influence their experiences of and responses to their internal sensations such as those of hunger or pain, to diagnostic procedures such as skin testing or endoscopies, and to the changes in their routines necessitated by treatments such as elimination diets. As children get older, those who have tendencies to anxiety or depression have increased vulnerability when they are faced with elimination diets or invasive medical procedures. For one 9-year-old boy who had EoE triggered by hypersensitivity to almost all foods, and who also had food allergies, treatment consisted of eliminating all orally ingested foods and placing a G-tube to meet his nutritional needs. Unable to attend school or engage in activities with peers, this emotionally reactive and anxious child became profoundly depressed. His depression subsided somewhat when orally ingestible food was reintroduced into his diet, but his anxiety level remained high and he required further treatment to address his emotional response. In this manner, children and adolescents who are already vulnerable to stress because of their tendency toward anxiety or depression may develop serious psychological reactions when faced with deprivation or trauma; others may be able to take such events in stride.

To summarize, the treatments of EoE can have a significant impact on children's quality of life, although the effects depend on both child and family factors. Because of the centrality of food in children's lives, elimination diets have an especially great potential to profoundly impact children's adjustment. Research is needed if we are to better understand the psychological effects on children of elimination diets and to weigh them against the improvement in quality of life brought about by short-term symptom reduction and the prevention of long-term physical effects on the gastrointestinal system.

THE DISEASE EXPERIENCE FOR FAMILIES OF CHILDREN WHO HAVE EOSINOPHILIC ESOPHAGITIS

Chronic illness in children impacts not only the quality of life of the ill child but also that of the parents and siblings. Parents of chronically ill children report increased emotional strain and financial burdens, as well as effects on relationships within the family and social contacts outside the family.[5] In addition to providing information on children's quality of life, studies of similar diseases, such as GERD and food allergy, give insight into the effects on parents and siblings of children who have EoE.

In a study of caregivers of young children who had GERD, investigators conducted focus groups to identify issues affecting the parents' quality of life.[11] Parents talked about how routine childcare activities for children who have GERD required extra work and care, such as special feeding techniques involving small portions, frequent feedings, and preparation of special meals or formulas. They needed to spend additional time making meals because of their children's dietary needs, and they had extra housework because of soiled clothing or furnishings. The parents also talked about emotional concerns specific to their children's reflux and feeding problems. For example, they expressed fears that the child might choke on their vomit, especially when they put them to bed at night. Parents of children who had food refusal and failure to thrive, in particular, worried a great deal about their children's condition and prognosis. This finding is consistent with other studies that have documented high levels of parenting stress among parents of children who have feeding disorders.[12] Although feeding tubes can initially bring relief to parents concerned about their children's nutritional intake, one study showed that parents of children who had G-tubes had poorer quality of life in terms of social life, family life, sex life, and work.[13] The additional burden and high levels of emotional stress reported in these studies are consistent with clinical experience with parents of children who have EoE.

Because treatment of EoE typically involves dietary restrictions, many of the lifestyle changes required for families of children who have EoE are similar to those faced by families of children who have food allergies. However, although parents of food-allergic children often suffer from anxiety related to the possibility of life-threatening reactions, central worries for parents of children who have EoE concern avoiding precipitating foods while meeting their children's nutritional needs. A study of the impact of food allergies on families' lives investigated the effects on daily care giving and on family members' emotional lives.[14] As expected, meal preparation and family social activities were most strongly affected. However, caregiver stress received high impact ratings, and a sizable proportion of the caregivers reported large effects on sibling and spousal relationships. The diagnosis and management of EoE appear to be accompanied by significant increases in caregiver burden, parental anxiety and distress, and strain and tension within couples' relationships.

Caregiver anxiety and relationship strain are worsened by uncertainty related to children's chronic illness.[5] Because EoE is newly recognized, limited information is available about the natural history of the disease or about the short- and long-term effects of treatment, leaving parents in an even greater state of uncertainty than that experienced by parents of children who have well-characterized pediatric illnesses. The effect of the uncertainty surrounding EoE becomes apparent when compared with families' experiences with better known diseases such as diabetes, where diagnostic tests are available, risk factors and prognosis are known, treatment has been agreed on, educational and coping programs are advanced, and even psychological contributions and ramifications are known. In contrast, diagnostic criteria for EoE have only just been determined, and because the condition is less well known among general practitioners, parents have found themselves searching the Internet for an explanation for their children's symptoms. Parents report experiencing considerable stress during the process of trying to decipher their child's medical problem (eg, when reflux symptoms persisted despite routine treatment). Once a diagnosis was made, parents became aware that experts could disagree about optimal treatment, engendering further uncertainty and anxiety.

Despite limited information available about EoE, much variability exists in levels of distress and anxiety that parents experience in response to their children's disease. This variability may be related, in part, to differences among individuals in their tolerance for uncertainty. In general, high levels of uncertainty intolerance are related to anxiety, worry, and depression, and a need for cognitive closure.[15] For such parents, the current dearth of available information is intolerable, and they cope by searching for any available information, whether it portends positive or negative outcomes. For example, because little is known about the natural history of EoE, parents' natural inclination to prepare for their children's future motivates them to seek information from other parents whose children may have a much different disease profile. Having some information, even if it erroneously indicates a negative outcome, allows individuals who have little tolerance for uncertainty to experience anxiety-relieving cognitive closure. Strain in marital relationships may be exacerbated by parents' anxiety, especially when spouses' use of antithetical coping strategies leads to conflict. For one couple, conflict ensued when the mother sought information on the Internet regarding prognosis and treatment options, whereas her husband questioned the validity of the EoE diagnosis and the necessity of treatment beyond symptom management. An intervention aimed at increasing uncertainty tolerance and reducing anxiety may provide help for some anxious parents of children who have EoE to cope more effectively.

To summarize, EoE may have a profound effect on the quality of life and psychosocial adjustment of parents and siblings of the affected child. Much time and work is required to decipher and monitor symptoms, to meet dietary requirements, and to plan medical follow-up, resulting in tremendous emotional and financial stress. The emotional stress and resultant strain on family relationships is exacerbated by the limited information currently available about the natural history and treatment outcome of EoE in children and adolescents.

SUMMARY

Because EoE has only recently been recognized and described, systematic research regarding the natural history of the disease and the short- and long-term effects of treatment is in its infancy. Although no research has addressed the psychosocial impact of EoE, clinical experience indicates that disease symptoms and treatments can have profound effects on the quality of life of affected children and their families. The responses of children and adolescents are variable, and are dependent on developmental level, temperament, and pre-existing psychological adjustment. Although parents of chronically ill children typically experience increased burden and stress, it is possible that the uncertainties currently associated with EoE contribute to even higher levels of anxiety. Research studies are needed to investigate the impact of EoE symptoms and of current treatments on quality of life and psychological adjustment in children and their families, and to discover how best to help families cope in an optimal manner.

REFERENCES

1. Furuta G, Liacouras C, Collins M, et al. Eosinophilic esophagitis in children and adults: a systematic review and consensus recommendations for diagnosis and treatment. Gastroenterology 2007;133:1342–63.
2. Spergel J. Eosinophilic esophagitis in adults and children: evidence for a food allergy component in many patients. Curr Opin Allergy Clin Immunol 2007;7: 274–8.
3. Maity S, Thomas A. Quality of life in pediatric gastrointestinal and liver disease: a systematic review. J Pediatr Gastroenterol Nutr 2007;44:540–54.

4. Lavigne J, Faier-Routman J. Psychological adjustment to pediatric physical disorders. J Pediatr Psychol 1992;17:133–57.
5. Stein R, Riessman C. The development of an impact-on-family scale: preliminary findings. Med Care 1980;18:465–72.
6. Nelson S, Chen E, Synair G, et al. One-year follow-up of symptoms of gastro-esophageal reflux during infancy. Pediatrics 1998;102(6):1–4.
7. Youssef N, Langseder A, Verga B, et al. Chronic childhood constipation is associated with impaired quality of life: a case-controlled study. J Pediatr Gastroenterol Nutr 2005;41:56–60.
8. Lloyd M, Urquhart G, Heard A, et al. When a child says 'no': experience of nurses working with children having invasive procedures. Paediatr Nurs 2008;20(4): 29–34.
9. Byars K, Burklow K, Ferguson K, et al. A multicomponent behavioral program for oral aversion in children dependent on gastrostomy feedings. J Pediatr Gastroenterol Nutr 2003;34:473–80.
10. Assa'ad A, Putnam P, Collings M, et al. Pediatric patients with eosinophilic esophagitis: an 8-year follow-up. J Allergy Clin Immunol 2007;119:731–8.
11. Kim J, Keininger DL, Becker S, et al. Simultaneous development of the Pediatric GERD Caregiver Impact Questionnaire (PGCIQ) in American English and American Spanish. Health Qual Life Outcomes 2005;3: 1–12 [e-pub].
12. Greer A, Gulotta C, Masler E, et al. Caregiver stress and outcomes of children with pediatric feeding disorders treated in an intensive interdisciplinary program. J Pediatr Psychol 2008;33:612–20.
13. Wong C, Akobeng A, Miller V. Quality of life of parents of children on home parenteral nutrition. Gut 2000;46:294–5.
14. Bollinger M, Dahlquist L, Mudd K, et al. The impact of food allergy on the daily activities of children and their families. Ann Allergy Asthma Immunol 2006;96: 415–21.
15. Berenbaum H, Bredemeier K, Thompson R. Intolerance of uncertainty: exploring its dimensionality and associations with need for cognitive closure, psychopathology, and personality. J Anxiety Disord 2008;22:117–25.

Histopathology Associated with Eosinophilic Gastrointestinal Diseases

Margaret H. Collins, MD

KEYWORDS

- Pathology • Eosinophilic gastrointestinal disease
- Eosinophilic esophagitis • Eosinophilic gastritis
- Eosinophilic enteritis • Eosinophilic colitis

Eosinophils normally reside in the mucosa of most segments of the gastrointestinal tract (GIT) and normally perform protective functions.[1,2] Eosinophilic gastrointestinal disorders (EGIDs) are broadly defined as diseases that characteristically exhibit excessive numbers of eosinophils, in normal and abnormal locations, in one or more GIT segment. Eosinophilic esophagitis (EE), eosinophilic gastritis, eosinophilic enteritis, and eosinophilic colitis refer to eosinophilic inflammation in the esophagus, stomach, small bowel, and colon, respectively, and are all forms of localized EGIDs. If the inflammation involves more than one GIT segment, the specific segments affected should be designated in pathology reports. The term *eosinophilic gastroenteritis* (EG) signifies inflammation specifically involving the stomach and small intestine but has also been used more broadly as a synonym for EGIDs.[3,4]

In addition to involving one or more segments of the GIT, the eosinophilic inflammation in EGIDs may affect one or more layers of the wall of the affected segment.[3] The inflammation in EGIDs may occur in the mucosa, submucosa, muscularis propria, serosa, or in any combination of these layers. Although the mucosa is commonly involved, in approximately 10% of EGIDs cases, the mucosa does not exhibit changes diagnostic of EGIDs, possibly because of sampling error in a disease that may be patchy.[5] Because bowel biopsy samples obtained by endoscopy generally consist of mucosa only, endoscopy may not yield diagnostic tissue. The absence of mucosal eosinophilic inflammation, however, does not exclude the possibility that other layers

Division of Pathology and Laboratory Medicine, ML 1010 B4.180, Cincinnati Children's Hospital Medical Center, University of Cincinnati, 3333 Burnet Avenue, Cincinnati, OH 45229, USA
E-mail address: margaret.collins@cchmc.org

Immunol Allergy Clin N Am 29 (2009) 109–117
doi:10.1016/j.iac.2008.10.005
0889-8561/08/$ – see front matter © 2009 Elsevier Inc. All rights reserved.

of the underlying bowel wall are inflamed with eosinophils. In such cases, the diagnosis can be made by examination of a transmural biopsy or resected specimen.

NORMAL DISTRIBUTION OF EOSINOPHILS IN THE GASTROINTESTINAL TRACT

Few studies report the number of eosinophils present in normal GIT mucosa. Two reports of normal pediatric GIT mucosa have documented that eosinophils are normally found in mucosa in the stomach, small intestine, and colon [6,7] but are rarely present in esophageal epithelium.[7] One report of eosinophils in mucosal biopsy specimens of the descending and sigmoid colon of adults demonstrated that the mean number of eosinophils is greatest in samples obtained in the southern part of the United States compared with those from the northern United States.[8] A similar study has not been performed in children. In addition to varying according to geographic site in the United States, GIT mucosal eosinophil density may also show seasonal variation.[9]

Knowledge about the density of eosinophils in various parts of the GIT, in the various layers of the GIT wall, and at various ages is essential to accurately diagnose EGIDs. Some studies of EGIDs have based the diagnosis on finding greater than 20 eosinophils per high-power field (HPF) in mucosal biopsy specimens.[10–13] Although one study of normal biopsy specimens from adults reported a peak mucosal eosinophil count of 21/HPF in samples from descending and sigmoid colon,[8] another study of normal biopsy specimens from adults reported a peak eosinophil count of 68/HPF in the ascending colon and 50/HPF in the descending colon.[9] Studies of normal biopsy specimens from children have identified peak eosinophil counts exceeding 21/HPF in small intestine and colon,[6,7] including a peak eosinophil count in the right colon of 50 to 52/HPF. Quantitative eosinophil evaluations of normal biopsy tissue from infants are rarely reported. In one study, rectal biopsy tissue from infants to evaluate for Hirschsprung's disease contained an average of 1.3 eosinophils per HPF; a peak count was not provided.[14] In a different study of rectal biopsy tissue obtained to evaluate for Hirschsprung's disease in patients aged 3 days to 5 years, a mean number of 2 eosinophils per HPF was reported in samples lacking ganglion cells, and a mean of 5.3/HPF was reported in samples containing ganglion cells; a peak count of 18/HPF was reported in the ganglionated biopsy samples. In that study, mucosal eosinophil density did not differ significantly with patient age.[6] A somewhat higher peak count, 32/HPF, was found in normal rectal biopsy tissue from patients beyond infancy.[7]

Asymptomatic children do not undergo endoscopy; therefore, analyzing normal tissue remains difficult and problematic in pediatrics. Nonetheless, it is extremely important for pathologists and gastroenterologists to be aware that based on current evidence, normal mucosal eosinophil density varies among segments of the GIT, and for that reason, a single peak value cannot be applied to all segments of the GIT in children or in adults. Pathologists must avoid overdiagnosis of EGIDs by applying site-specific criteria for eosinophil density to mucosal biopsy specimens. Gastroenterologists must avoid contributing to overdiagnosis by submitting biopsy samples from each segment of the GIT separately, especially from the colon where the maximum mucosal eosinophil density in the right side normally exceeds that of the more distal colon.

RECOMMENDED HISTOPATHOLOGIC TERMINOLOGY

Studies of large numbers of normal biopsy specimens from multiple sites in the GIT, from multiple areas of the United States and the world, at multiple times of the year, and in multiple age groups are lacking, but pathologists are nonetheless required to render diagnoses based on mucosal biopsy. Some studies report mean mucosal eosinophil numbers with standard deviations and do not provide a peak, or maximum, number. Counting eosinophils in multiple or in every HPF of a biopsy sample yields more complete information and may be preferable for research, but a peak count of eosinophils in the most densely inflamed HPF is informative and more practical for daily surgical pathology sign-out.

Using the results of published studies or of unpublished intradepartmental studies to establish norms for peak eosinophil numbers in endoscopic biopsy samples, pathologists should consider the diagnosis of mucosal eosinophilia to signify mildly increased numbers of eosinophils without other pathologic changes (**Fig. 1**). Biopsy samples showing only mildly increased numbers of eosinophils may indicate diseases other than EGIDs. For example, small numbers of intraepithelial eosinophils in esophageal biopsy specimens are consistent with gastroesophageal reflux disease (GERD) but not with EE. Genome-wide analysis of esophageal biopsy tissue shows different transcriptomes for samples containing no or few eosinophils compared with those containing numerous eosinophils, consistent with EE;[15] these data may serve as a molecular basis to distinguish EE from GERD and from normal tissue. Similarly, mildly increased numbers of eosinophils without other histologic changes in other parts of the GIT may represent potentially normal variations including those associated with geographic region of the United States, season of the year, or an early nonspecific sign of inflammatory bowel disease.[5] Until more studies of normal GIT biopsy tissue in children and adults are reported, pathologists should acknowledge that eosinophil density that appears to be mildly increased but does not include other alterations may or may not indicate EGIDs. This approach avoids potential overdiagnosis that could lead to inappropriate or unnecessary therapy, including the use of steroids, which has more potential adverse effects in children than in adults. Because EGIDs may be patchy, when initial mucosal biopsy specimens are normal or only mildly inflamed and when clinical suspicion for EGIDs remains strong, repeat biopsies may be indicated and may provide more definitive results.

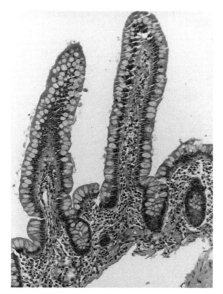

Fig. 1. Mucosal eosinophilia. In this section of ileum, numerous eosinophils are present in the lamina propria, but the architecture remains intact and intraepithelial eosinophils are not increased.

Terms such as EGIDs, eosinophilic gastritis, eosinophilic enteritis, and so forth should be reserved for biopsy specimens that show changes in addition to increased eosinophils, such as eosinophilic glandulitis/cryptitis, eosinophilic crypt abscesses, chronic architectural changes, and others (**Box 1**) (**Figs. 2–5**). Caution must be exercised when rendering these diagnoses as well, because normal biopsy tissue from children and adults may contain scattered small numbers of intraepithelial eosinophils.[7,9,14]

In general, markedly increased numbers of mucosal eosinophils are seen in biopsy specimens that also display other changes. Some specimens, however, exhibit indisputably increased numbers of eosinophils in the lamina propria with remarkably few, if any, other histologic alterations. In such cases, a diagnosis of marked mucosal eosinophilia versus eosinophilic gastritis, for example, might be used. Conversely, in general, mildly increased numbers of mucosal eosinophils are found in biopsy specimens that show few, if any, other remarkable changes. Eosinophil density, however, is not the only indicator of eosinophilic inflammation, and on occasion, although only mildly increased numbers of eosinophils are present, eosinophilic cryptitis/glandulitis or eosinophilic crypt or gland abscesses are found. The term *eosinophilic gastritis* or *eosinophilic enteritis*, therefore, is preferred as the diagnosis, even though the overall amount of eosinophilic inflammation is not remarkable. A relatively small amount of eosinophilic inflammation can be damaging because of the potent cytotoxins released by eosinophils.[1,2] Assessing eosinophil activation may not be as

---

Box 1
Histologic features of eosinophilic gastrointestinal disease

Mucosal eosinophilia

At all sites: increased numbers of eosinophils without any other pathology

Eosinophilic esophagitis

Increased numbers of intraepithelial eosinophils (peak count >15/HPF)

Degranulated eosinophils

Eosinophil microabscesses

Eosinophil surface layering

Marked basal layer hyperplasia

Elongated papillae

Lamina propria eosinophilia and fibrosis

Eosinophilic gastroenteritis/colitis

Increased number of mucosal eosinophils

Degranulated eosinophils

Intraepithelial eosinophils (surface and gland/crypt epithelium)

Eosinophil gland/crypt abscesses

Epithelial degenerative and regenerative changes

Foveolar/crypt hyperplasia

Villous atrophy in the small bowel

Minimal acute and chronic inflammation

Eosinophils in muscularis mucosa, submucosa, or both

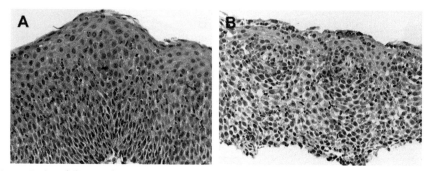

Fig. 2. Eosinophilic esophagitis. (*A*) Numerous intraepithelial eosinophils (peak count 123/HPF) and marked basal layer hyperplasia are seen. (*B*) Surface layering of eosinophils and spongiosis are present.

simple as finding extracellular granules, because trauma during tissue handling may cause eosinophil disruption.[7,16]

This approach should assist the pathologist in distinguishing for the clinician biopsy samples showing histopathology that may be at the upper range of normal from those showing more definitive and conclusive evidence of tissue damage associated with eosinophilic inflammation. It is hoped that this distinction will avoid overdiagnosis and underdiagnosis of EGIDs. The optimum communication occurs not in a pathology report but when pathologist and clinician review biopsy specimens together and jointly form a clinicopathologic diagnosis.

DIFFERENTIAL DIAGNOSIS

Diseases associated with GIT eosinophilic inflammation include infection, food allergies, medication reaction, connective tissue disease and vasculitis, inflammatory fibroid polyps, hypereosinophilic syndrome, inflammatory bowel disease, organ transplantation, allergic granulomatosis, chronic granulomatous disease, neoplasms such as Langerhans cell histiocytosis, lymphoma, and others.[4,5,17] When a specific cause for the eosinophilic inflammation cannot be identified, the disease is considered primary EGIDs. Examination of mucosal biopsy specimens may reveal infectious

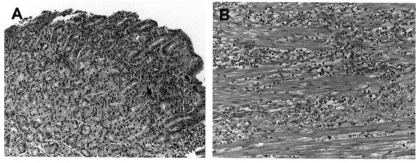

Fig. 3. Eosinophilic gastritis. (*A*) Extremely large numbers of eosinophils are seen mostly near the surface, with gland infiltration and destruction by eosinophils (eosinophilic glandulitis) (*arrow*). (*B*) Marked eosinophilic inflammation in the muscularis propria.

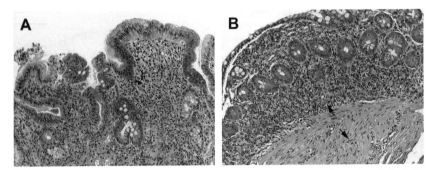

Fig. 4. Eosinophilic enteritis. (*A*) Duodenal bulb shows predominantly eosinophilic inflammation with marked architectural changes and reactive epithelial changes. This patient also had eosinophilic esophagitis. (*B*) Ileum intensely inflamed with eosinophils shows villous atrophy, crypt destruction (*upper arrow*), and numerous eosinophils in the muscularis mucosa (*lower arrow*).

organisms or vasculitis when the submuocsa is included, but in most cases, the histopathology is nonspecific.

EOSINOPHILIC ESOPHAGITIS

The pathology of EE is the best characterized of the EGIDs, probably because there is universal agreement that, in contrast to other sites in the GIT in which mucosal eosinophils are normally present, eosinophils are absent from or rarely found in normal esophageal epithelium (see **Fig. 2**). A recent consensus statement based on review of the EE literature[18] recommended that at least 15 intraepithelial eosinophils per HPF are required to diagnose EE, and a higher peak number is appropriate for research. In most cases of EE, in addition to numerous intraepithelial eosinophils, esophageal epithelium is altered and the changes include basal layer hyperplasia, elongated papillae, eosinophil microabscesses, and eosinophil surface layering.[19] Characteristically, the epithelial inflammation in EE involves the proximal and distal esophagus. The major differential diagnosis for EE is GERD. The histologic changes in GERD are usually confined to the distal esophagus, and the eosinophilic

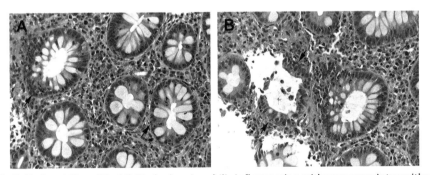

Fig. 5. Eosinophilic colitis. (*A*) Marked eosinophilic inflammation with numerous intraepithelial eosinophils creating eosinophilic cryptitis (*arrows*). (*B*) Eosinophilic cryptitis/crypt abscess (*arrows*). Pinworms were found in the biopsy samples in **Figs. 1** and **5** taken during colonoscopy.

inflammation, if present, is generally much less than in EE. Several studies, however, document that the histology of GERD may be indistinguishable from EE.[20,21] Primary EE is a clinicopathologic diagnosis that requires characteristic histology in addition to the proper clinical setting; histopathology or clinical data alone are not sufficient for diagnosis. Infection with parasites such as *Gnathostoma spinigerum*[22] and *Anisakis simplex*[23] has been implicated as a cause of EE.

EOSINOPHILIC GASTRITIS

A peak count of 8 eosinophils per HPF in antral gastric mucosa and 11/HPF in fundic gastric mucosa is normal in pediatric gastric biopsy specimens.[7] Increased numbers of eosinophils in the lamina propria; numerous eosinophils in the surface epithelium, gland epithelium, or both; in the lumen of glands, muscularis mucosa, and submucosa; and reactive and regenerative epithelial and gland architectural changes including gland distortion and dropout are all features of eosinophilic gastritis[5,24] (see **Fig. 3**). The pathologic changes may be patchy, and numerous biopsies may be necessary to identify the changes. In cases in which the mucosa is not inflamed, the diagnosis must be made by transmural biopsies or resections. Numerous eosinophils may be found in the muscularis propria or subserosa in those cases. Strictures and gastric outlet obstruction may occur with muscularis propria inflammation. Infection with the parasite *Eustoma rotundatum*[25] or with cytomegalovirus[12,26] has been associated with eosinophilic gastritis/EG. Few reports associate infection with *Helicobacter pylori* with gastric mucosal eosinophilia.[27]

EOSINOPHILIC ENTERITIS (EOSINOPHILIC DUODENITIS, EOSINOPHILIC JEJUNITIS, EOSINOPHILIC ILEITIS)

The peak number of eosinophils per HPF in normal pediatric mucosal biopsy specimens was reported as 26/HPF for duodenum and 28/HPF for ileum in one study[7] and 52/HPF for duodenum and 68/HPF for ileum in another study.[6] Changes characteristic of eosinophilic enteritis include (in addition to numerous eosinophils) crypt hyperplastic villous atrophy and epithelial cell necrosis (see **Fig. 4**). When submucosa is present, edema is commonly seen. Eosinophilic inflammation may be seen in muscularis mucosa, muscularis propria, and subserosa.[5,24]

EOSINOPHILIC COLITIS

Pathologists and clinicians must realize that although studies of normal biopsy tissue are scant, several studies of normal tissue from adults and children have documented that eosinophil density is greater in the right colon compared with the left colon[6,7,9] and that intraepithelial eosinophils may be more common in tissue from the right colon compared with the left colon in adults.[9] Therefore, biopsy samples from more than one site in the colon should be submitted separately and clearly marked according to site of origin. Increased numbers of mucosal eosinophils may be an early nonspecific finding of inflammatory bowel disease.[5] Eosinophilic colitis is characterized by increased numbers of eosinophils and other abnormalities, including crypt architectural changes, Paneth cell metaplasia in the distal colon, basal lymphoid aggregates and diffuse plasmacytosis, and eosinophils in the muscularis mucosa (see **Fig. 5**). Allergic proctocolitis is characterized by increased numbers of eosinophils in the lamina propria, surface and crypt epithelium, and muscularis mucosa, without significant architectural changes.[28] The lack of chronic changes may be a function of patient age because most affected patients are young.

SUMMARY

EGIDs have multiple possible etiologies. The histopathology in mucosal biopsy tissue is often characteristic but does not usually identify a specific etiology. More studies of normal biopsy tissue and tissue from patients who are known or suspected to have EGIDs, with clinicopathologic correlations, are required to more fully define the spectrum of histopathology in EGIDs.

REFERENCES

1. Rothenberg ME, Mishra A, Brandt EB, et al. Gastrointestinal eosinophils in health and disease. Adv Immunol 2001;78:291–328.
2. Zuo L, Rothenberg ME. Gastrointestinal eosinophilia. Immunol Allergy Clin North Am 2007;27:443–55.
3. Klein NC, Hargrove RL, Sleisenger MH, et al. Eosinophilic gastroenteritis. Medicine 1970;49:299–319.
4. Khan S, Orenstein SR. Eosinophilic gastroenteritis. Gastroenterol Clin North Am 2008;37:333–48.
5. Noffsinger A, Fenoglio-Preiser CM, Maru D, et al. Gastrintestinal diseases. An atlas of nontumor pathology. Washington, DC: American Registry of Pathology; 2007. Fascicle 5.
6. Lowichik A, Weinberg AG. A quantitative evaluation of mucosal eosinophils in the pediatric gastrointestinal tract. Mod Pathol 1996;9(2):110–4.
7. DeBrosse CW, Case JW, Putnam PE, et al. Quantity and distribution of eosinophils in the gastrointestinal tract of children. Pediatr Dev Pathol 2006;9(3):210–8.
8. Pacal RR, Gramlich TL, Parker KM, et al. Geographic variations in eosinophil concentration in normal colonic mucosa. Mod Pathol 1997;10(4):363–5.
9. Polydorides AD, Banner BF, Hannaway PJ, et al. Evaluation of site-specific and seasonal variation in colonic mucosal eosinophils. Hum Pathol 2008;39:832–6.
10. Lee CM, Changchien CS, Chen PC, et al. Eosinophilic gastroenteritis: 10 years experience. Am J Gastroenterol 1993;88:70–4.
11. Talley NJ, Shorter RG, Phillips SF, et al. Eosinophilic gastroenteritis: a clinicopathological study of patients with disease of the mucosa, muscle layer, and subserosal tissue. Gut 1990;31:54–8.
12. Whitington PF, Whitington GL. Eosinophilic gastroenteropathy in children. J Pediatr Gastroenterol Nutr 1988;7:379–85.
13. Chen M-J, Cheng-Hsin C, Shee-Chan L, et al. Eosinophilic gastroenteritis: clinical experience with 15 patients. World J Gastroenterol 2003;9(12):2813–6.
14. Winter HS, Antonioli DA, Fukagawa N, et al. Allergy-related proctocolitis in infants: diagnostic usefulness of rectal biopsy. Mod Pathol 1990;3:5–10.
15. Blanchard C, Wang N, Stringer KF, et al. Eotaxin-3 and a uniquely conserved gene-expression profile in eosinophilic esophagitis. J Clin Invest 2006;116: 536–47.
16. Kato M, Kephart GM, Talley NJ, et al. Eosinophil infiltration and degranulation in normal human tissue. Anat Rec 1998;252:418–25.
17. Talley NJ. Gut eosinophilia in food allergy and systemic and autoimmune diseases. Gastroenterol Clin North Am 2008;37:307–32.
18. Furuta GT, Liacouris CA, Collins MH, et al. Eosinophilic esophagitis in children and adults: a systematic review and consensus recommendations for diagnosis and treatment. Gastroenterology 2007;133:1342–63.
19. Walsh SV, Antonioli DA, Goldman H, et al. Allergic esophagitis in children. Am J Surg Pathol 1999;23:390–6.

20. Ngo P, Furuta GT, Antonioli DA, et al. Eosinophils in the esophagus—peptic or allergic eosinophilic esophagitis? Case series of three patients with esophageal eosinophilia. Am J Gastroenterol 2006;101:1666–70.
21. Rodrigo S, Abboud G, Oh D, et al. High intraepithelial eosinophil counts in esophageal squamous epithelium are not specific for esoinophilic esophagitis in adults. Am J Gastroenterol 2008;103:435–42.
22. Muller-Stover I, Richter J, Haussinger D. Infection with *Gnathostoma spinigerum* as a cause of eosinophilic oesophagitis. Deutsche Medizinishce Wochenschrift 2004;129:1973–5 [in German with English abstract].
23. Bircher AJ, Gysi B, Zenklusen HR, et al. Eosinophilic esophagitis associated with recurrent urticaria: is the worm *Anisakis simplex* involved? Schweizerische Medizinische Wochenschrift. Journal Suisse de Medecine 2000;130:1814–9 [in German with English abstract].
24. Fenoglio-Preiser CM, Noffsinger AE, Stemmermann GN, et al. Gastrointestinal pathology. An atlas and text. 3rd edition. Philadelphia: Lippincott Williams & Wilkins; 2008.
25. Johnstone JM, Morson BC. Eosinophilic gastroenteritis. Histopathology 1978;2: 335–48.
26. Takeyama J, Abukawa D, Miura K. Eosinophilic gastroenteritis with cytomegalovirus infection in an immunocompetent child. World J Gastroenterol 2007;14: 4653–4.
27. Papadopoulos AA, Tzathas C, Polymeros D, et al. Symptomatic eosinophilic gastritis cured with *Helicobacter pylori* eradication. Gut 2005;54:1822 [Letter].
28. Odze RD, Bines J, Leichtner AM, et al. Allergic proctocolitis in infants: a prospective clinicopathology biopsy study. Hum Pathol 1993;24:668–74.

Biomarkers for Nononcologic Gastrointestinal Diseases

Rohit Katial, MD[a,b,*]

KEYWORDS

- Gastrointestinal biomarkers • Eosinophilic esophagitis
- Mast cell markers • Eosinophil markers

Biomarkers are objectively measured indicators of normal and abnormal biologic processes and may vary with therapeutic interventions. The identification of such markers in blood or secretions to assess disease activity and response to therapy is of central importance in the search for noninvasive means to diagnose, track, and treat chronic inflammatory diseases. Although attractive, such an approach is fraught with issues of reproducibility, sensitivity, specificity, and variability. Additionally, the markers of interest must in some sense relate to clinical course, disease progression, therapeutic intervention, and disease severity. Unfortunately, little is currently known in this regard for most areas of inflammation. Biomarker research has progressed in the respiratory tract with the evaluation of both sputum and breath condensate for a variety of proteins, including cytokines, as well as for measurements of exhaled gases, such as nitric oxide in the setting of obstructive lung diseases. In other organs susceptible to inflammatory conditions, such as gastrointestinal diseases, the biomarker data center on detection of cancer. For nononcologic pathologic processes, little research has been done concerning biomarker data. This article reviews what is currently known about the use of biomarkers for gastrointestinal diseases, excluding tumor biology, and explores potential avenues that may prove interesting for further research. Since few data are available, the most plausible approach is first to review the basics of gastrointestinal immunity and the data surrounding mediators produced from cells involved in the gastrointestinal immune response.

[a] Department of Medicine, Division of Allergy and Immunology, National Jewish Health, 1400 Jackson Street, J329, Denver, CO 80206, USA
[b] Weinberg Clinical Research Unit, National Jewish Health, Denver, CO, USA
* Corresponding author. Department of Medicine, Division of Allergy and Immunology, National Jewish Health, 1400 Jackson Street, J329, Denver, CO 80206.
E-mail address: katialr@njc.org

Immunol Allergy Clin N Am 29 (2009) 119–127
doi:10.1016/j.iac.2008.09.012
0889-8561/08/$ – see front matter © 2009 Elsevier Inc. All rights reserved.

GASTROINTESTINAL MUCOSAL IMMUNITY

Complex multidirectional interactions take place in the gastrointestinal tract. These interactions involve, in a large part, interplay between innate immune responses, partly driven by the microbial flora, and the cells of the adaptive system, including dendritic cells, T lymphocytes, and B lymphocytes. A detailed discussion of the complexity of mucosal immunity is beyond the scope of this article, which focuses on the primary cells involved in the mucosal response, specifically the gut-associated lymphoid tissue.[1,2] The cells comprising the gut-associated lymphoid tissue include T and B lymphocytes, dendritic cells, and, in the lamina propria, eosinophils and mast cells. The latter are frequently increased in allergic diseases of the gastrointestinal tract. Additionally, there is recent evidence that dendritic cells play a key role in inducing in T cells a T regulatory phenotype resulting in increased production of transforming growth factor beta (TGF-β) and IL-10.[3] Exogenous antigens are sampled at the epithelial surface by specialized M cells that allow antigen entry into the gut and uptake by antigen presenting cells, leading to processing and presentation to T lymphocytes.[4] The lymphocytes traffic between Peyer patches and mesenteric lymph nodes and cycle back to the lamina propria.[5] Numerous cells are involved in this process and mature under the influence of cytokine and adhesion molecules (ie, CCL25, CXCL12, CCL28, interferon-gamma, IL-4, IL-10, and TGF-β), which leads to eventual expression of a variety of cell-surface markers, some of which may serve as biomarkers.[4]

MAST CELLS

Mast cells are important to a host of biologic processes, particularly the allergic response in the respiratory tract, but also the gastrointestinal allergic response to exogenous antigens, such as food proteins. Recently, researchers have found that the roles of mast cells extend beyond those associated with IgE-mediated reactions to include roles as modulators of both innate and adaptive immune responses, particularly in the mucosa.[6,7]

The mast cell is clearly central to IgE-mediated reactions, particular to food proteins. Briefly, antigen-specific IgE produced from B cells in the lamina propria coats the surface of mast cells. Secondary exposure to the sensitizing antigen results in cell degranulation with mediator release, to include leukotrienes, prostaglandins, histamine, proteases, heparin, tryptase, chymase, platelet-activating factor, monocyte chemotactic protein-1, -3, -4, and both T-helper 1 (Th1) and T-helper 2 (Th2) cytokines (tumor necrosis factor α, IL-1, IL-4, IL-6, IL-13, IL-18, IL-25).[8] In food-allergic patients, the presence of food allergen–specific IgE and a relevant history is frequently adequate to make the diagnosis. However, other gastrointestinal disease, where food proteins may contribute to underlying inflammation through other than an IgE-mediated mechanism, cannot easily be discerned based on the presence of allergen-specific IgE or patient history. In addition, the current diagnosis and monitoring of response to therapy in certain disorders, such as eosinophilic gastrointestinal diseases, hinge upon the demonstration of abnormal findings upon pathologic evaluation of gastrointestinal tissues obtained by biopsy or surgical resection. Therefore, the need for a less-invasive biomarker becomes essential. Mast cell mediators, an integral part of a complex system within the gastrointestinal tract, regulate expression of other receptors, which may contribute to gastrointestinal pathology. For example, tryptase can activate protease-activated receptor 2 on epithelial cells and this in turn can lead to release of proinflammatory mediators from nerve endings as well as increased intestinal water secretion via direct cellular mechanisms.[9] The protease-activated receptors contribute to gastrointestinal motility and dysmotility as seen in irritable bowel syndrome.[10] Additionally, these receptors play a role in regulating epithelial permeability by modulating tight junction proteins, thereby potentially increasing exposure of the submucosal immune system to food and bacterial products.[11,12] Protease-activated receptors have also been linked to prostaglandin products, some of which are released from mast cells.[13] Thus, measuring mediators that regulate protease-activated receptor expression and prostaglandin release may correlate with functional bowel disorders. Gecse and colleagues[14] studied diarrhea-predominant irritable bowel syndrome. Fecal enzymatic activity was assayed in healthy subjects and in patients with irritable bowel syndrome, ulcerative colitis, and acute infectious diarrhea. A threefold increase in fecal serine protease activity was seen in diarrhea-predominant irritable bowel syndrome patients compared with constipation-predominant irritable bowel or infectious diarrhea. These data suggest that colonic serine protease activity of diarrhea-predominant irritable bowel syndrome evokes a protease-activated receptor 2–mediated colonic epithelial barrier dysfunction and represents a new biomarker to distinguish diarrhea-predominant irritable bowel from infectious diarrhea and possibly inflammatory bowel disease (IBD) when combined with other stool inflammatory markers. Such data need further research to obtain clinical correlates.

Cell-surface markers on mast cells have also been studied in pathologic processes, such as systemic mastocytosis where affected patients develop gastrointestinal symptoms. Hahn and Hornick[15] quantitated and compared mast cells in mucosal biopsies from patients with mastocytosis involving the gastrointestinal tract, with mast cells in mucosal biopsies from a control group with diverse inflammatory gastrointestinal disorders. They sought to determine whether immunostaining for CD25 could be used to distinguish neoplastic from reactive mast cells in gastrointestinal biopsies. The investigators obtained 17 biopsies from 6 patients with mastocytosis, 17 from 5 patients with urticaria pigmentosa, and 157 biopsies from control cases including normal stomach, duodenum, terminal ileum, and colon, *Helicobacter pylori* gastritis, bile reflux gastropathy, peptic duodenitis, celiac disease, Crohn disease, ulcerative colitis, lymphocytic colitis, and collagenous colitis. Additionally, investigators obtained 20 biopsies from patients with irritable bowel syndrome, 8 from patients with parasitic infections, and 9 from those with eosinophilic gastroenteritis. Biopsies were stained for mast cell tryptase, c-kit (CD117), and CD25. Mast cells in all mastocytosis cases were positive for CD25, whereas gastrointestinal mucosal mast cells in all other control cases were negative for this marker. This study demonstrated that CD25 in gastrointestinal mucosal mast cells is specific for systemic mastocytosis with gastrointestinal involvement and can be used to confirm the diagnosis.

Mast cells may also produce such enzymes as matrix metalloproteinase (MMP) under inflammatory conditions. Di Girolamo studied tissue-based mast cells in the synovium of rheumatoid arthritis patients and demonstrated increased production and expression of MMP-9 in mast cells relative to healthy controls. Their observation suggests that MMP-9 is not stored in mast cells but is produced under conditions of inflammation.[16] MMPs are a family of metal-dependent enzymes responsible for the degradation and remodeling of the extracellular matrix and basement membrane that occurs during both normal physiologic activity and disease. It has been suggested that MMPs may also play a role in the pathogenesis of IBD by mediating mucosal breakdown in response to an enhanced inflammation. A newly published study demonstrates that elevated urinary MMP levels may be biomarkers of disease activity in patients with IBD. Ninety-five urine samples from 55 children and young adults with known or suspected IBD were collected. Urinary MMP levels were significantly elevated ($P < .0001$) in patients with IBD, as well as in each subgroup (Crohn disease or ulcerative colitis), relative to controls. Specifically, urinary MMP-2 and

MMP-9 levels were independent predictors of Crohn disease and ulcerative colitis ($P <$ .0001). These data are the first to demonstrate that urinary MMPs may represent novel noninvasive biomarkers for use in the evaluation of patients with IBD.[17] Kubben and colleagues[18] demonstrated elevated levels of MMP-9 in *H pylori*–infected gastric mucosa and showed a consistent decrease in tissue levels with *Helicobacter* eradication. Thus, MMP-9 is intriguing as a biomarker because it has been shown to correlate both in urine and tissue with pathologic disorders, although urine levels are more attractive because of the ease of collection.

Tryptase has been shown to enhance release of vascular endothelial growth factor (VEGF) in human osteoarthritis chondrocytes.[19] VEGF is a potent angiogenic, vascular permeability–enhancing, and calcium-dependent cytokine with overexpression in various inflammatory conditions, such as granulomatous inflammation, tissue repair, and ischemia. Griga and colleagues[20] evaluated serum levels of VEGF in IBD. Thirty-one patients with Crohn disease, 15 with ulcerative colitis, and 9 healthy volunteers were studied. The investigators observed significantly increased VEGF levels in patients with active Crohn disease and ulcerative colitis when compared with healthy controls. Because this is a serum marker, the ease of collection makes it an attractive marker for disease activity. However, larger numbers of patients need to be studied.

Eosinophilic esophagitis, as the name implies, is in part due to an abnormal accumulation of eosinophils. While the pathophysiology of eosinophilic esophagitis is quite complex and less clear than that of IgE-mediated food allergy, mast cell mediators, particularly the leukotriene byproducts of arachidonic acid metabolism, have been postulated as potential biomarkers. Gupta and colleagues[21] studied 12 children and 10 controls, measuring cysteinyl leukotrienes in esophageal specimens of subjects with eosinophilic esophagitis and found no difference. However, leukotriene levels were elevated in biopsies of tissue beyond the esophagus in affected subjects compared with those of controls. These data suggest the possibility that different chemotactic factors are operative in eosinophilic gastritis versus eosinophilic esophagitis and the leukotriene products may serve a role in defining differential involvement in the gastrointestinal tract for eosinophilic inflammation. The eosinophilic-based diseases are discussed in more detail below.

Although, mast cells are traditionally linked to IgE-mediated allergic disorders, they produce mediators that are involved with immune processes well beyond IgE. Mediators released from mast cells upon activation may directly contribute to disease pathogenesis or indirectly activate other enzymes that contribute to underlying inflammation, as shown in the reviewed data. As discussed above, some of these up-regulated proteins may ultimately serve as markers of disease activity and as a noninvasive tool to gauge response to therapy.

EOSINOPHILS

The distribution of eosinophils is not consistent throughout the gastrointestinal tract. However, under noninflammatory conditions the esophagus is the only privileged site without tissue-residing eosinophils. Accumulation of eosinophils within the lamina propria has been reported in IgE-mediated food allergy, gastroesophageal reflux disease, IBD, eosinophilic esophagitis, eosinophilic gastroenteritis, eosinophilic colitis, and the hypereosinophilic syndrome. Eosinophils are frequently detected based on both the presence of granular proteins (eosinophil peroxidase, major basic protein, eosinophil-derived neurotoxin, eosinophil cationic protein) and expression of cell-surface markers, such as CCR3 and IL-5 receptor.[22]

With eosinophilic esophagitis, as with the other four primary eosinophilic diseases, eosinophils intensively accumulate in tissue. Therefore, levels of peripheral blood eosinophils have been evaluated as a diagnostic and management tool. Unfortunately, the data vary widely with an incidence of increased peripheral blood eosinophil counts ranging between 10% and 100% depending upon the population being evaluated and the severity of the disease. One report by Gupta[23] evaluated pediatric patients with tissue-based eosinophilia and reported an incidence of 67% having increased peripheral eosinophil counts. Konikoff and colleagues[24] sought to identify biomarkers that correlated with disease activity and response to therapy in eosinophilic esophagitis patients. Forty-seven pediatric patients were evaluated by endoscopy for possible eosinophilic esophagitis. Blood samples were collected for peripheral blood eosinophil counts; eosinophil-derived neurotoxin; eotaxin-1, -2, and -3; and IL-5 levels. Stool samples were assayed for eosinophil-derived neurotoxin. Biomarker levels were correlated with esophageal eosinophil density, and differences in biomarker levels based on disease activity and treatment were determined. Blood eosinophils significantly correlated with esophageal eosinophil density and were increased in patients with active eosinophilic esophagitis versus controls. Noting the wide variability in peripheral eosinophil counts seen across studies in all eosinophilic esophagitis patients, it may be more plausible to study the counts in a less heterogenous group of patients by factoring in age, disease activity, and medications. Such a strategy may demonstrate improved sensitivity, improved specificity, and less variability for diagnosis and monitoring therapeutic response with peripheral eosinophil levels.

A multitude of cytokines, some produced by T cells, others by eosinophils themselves, have an impact on eosinophil survival, trafficking, or both. Two of the major ones are IL-5 and the eotaxins. IL-5, an eosinophilopoietin, prevents eosinophil apoptosis and results in cellular mobilization from bone marrow stores. Three eotaxins exist: 1, 2, and 3. Eotaxin-1 is the most potent chemoattractant for eosinophils. As mentioned above, Konikoff and colleagues[24] not only studied peripheral eosinophil counts but also evaluated plasma levels of eotaxin-1, -2, and -3 and of IL-5. The investigators reported increased levels of eotaxin-3 compared with those of healthy controls. Interestingly, blood eotaxin-1 and -2, and IL-5 did not show an increase in eosinophilic esophagitis patients, an indication that eotaxin-3 could serve as a viable noninvasive marker. Additional tissue-based studies have evaluated IL-4, IL-5, IL-10, IL-13, and tumor necrosis factor α and have shown increases compared with healthy controls. However, the studies were small and need further validation in highly characterized populations.[25,26]

Eosinophil granular proteins released after eosinophil activation have also been studied as markers of disease in the gastrointestinal tract. Saitoh and colleagues[27] examined fecal levels of eosinophil granule–derived proteins in IBD, and examined the extracellular release of these proteins. Forty-two patients with ulcerative colitis, 37 with Crohn disease, and 29 control subjects had stool samples collected. Fecal eosinophil cationic protein and eosinophil protein X (probably same protein as eosinophil-derived neurotoxin) concentrations were significantly increased in both active forms of IBD compared with inactive disease. These investigators concluded that the measurement of eosinophil granule–derived proteins in feces is useful for evaluating disease activity and predicting relapse in patients with IBD. However, the study by Konikoff[24] did not find a correlation between stool samples of eosinophil-derived neurotoxin and eosinophilic esophagitis biopsy samples, but rather found a correlation between blood eosinophil-derived neurotoxin levels and tissue, thus further work is needed in the area to reconcile the reported findings. Collectively, these data imply that some combination of blood levels of eosinophils, eosinophil-derived neurotoxin, and eotaxin-3 may have value as noninvasive biomarkers for monitoring eosinophilic esophagitis.

One study, in addition to evaluating cell counts, cellularly produced enzymes, and cytokines, looked at eosinophil cell surface activation marker CD25 in eosinophilic esophagitis tissue samples. Straumann and colleagues[28] studied the expression of CD25 in 8 subjects with a confirmed diagnosis of eosinophilic esophagitis, and in 10 controls. CD25 expression and the TH2 cytokines, IL-4, IL-5, IL-10, and IL-13, in esophageal, intestinal, and blood eosinophils were measured. Fifty-four percent of eosinophils infiltrating the inflamed esophageal mucosa of patients with eosinophilic esophagitis showed strong evidence of CD25 expression compared with 29% of eosinophils from noninflamed duodenum. Additionally, tissue IL-4, IL-5, and IL-13 were increased in the affected cohort. The blood eosinophils also demonstrated increased expression of IL-13 and, to a lesser degree, IL-5. Measuring a combination of eosinophil markers in concert with clinical outcomes has not been fully studied but such clinical data could lead the way to the development of a panel of markers that together could correlate to disease activity with greater specificity.

Hypereosinophilic syndrome is a poorly understood entity but clinically defined by peripheral eosinophil counts of more than 1500 cells per milliliter for longer than 6 months with no other cause for the elevation. Blood eosinophils from hypereosinophilic syndrome patients demonstrate increased expression of IL-13. However and more interestingly, blood eosinophils from hypereosinophilic syndrome patients express CD25, unlike blood eosinophils from eosinophilic esophagitis.[28] In eosinophilic esophagitis, tissue eosinophils express CD25 but circulating cells do not. In hypereosinophilic syndrome, a combination of CD25 and IL-13 in circulating cells may be a fruitful combination to evaluate as potential markers with greater disease specificity.

The other two primary eosinophilic gastrointestinal diseases, eosinophilic gastroenteritis and eosinophilic colitis, are similar in that no single test makes the diagnosis but increased circulating eosinophil counts and fecally secreted eosinophil-derived products may suggest the diagnosis.[29] Increased levels of eosinophil-derived neurotoxin in serum and urine were reported in eosinophilic colitis by Inamura and colleagues.[30] Additionally, for eosinophilic gastroenteritis, there is a suggestion that mast cells contribute to the pathogenesis and biopsy data reveal increased tryptase-positive cells compared with controls. Thus, as more data become available, it is possible that mast cell mediators may also serve as potential biomarkers in these eosinophilic diseases.[31]

T REGULATORY CELLS

Because the mucosal immune system encounters exogenous antigens in the gastrointestinal tract, the local immune response must be tightly regulated to avoid abnormal responses against dietary proteins and commensal organisms. In situations where there is a break in immunologic tolerance, one sees inflammation induced by food antigens or, in the case of IBD, possibly by an aberrant response against enteric flora.[32–34]

Recent evidence suggests that among the key cells involved in maintaining immune homeostasis in the gastrointestinal tract are the T lymphocytes of the regulatory phenotype, known as T regs. These cells are CD4+CD25+ and produce both IL-10 and TGF-β, which have an impact on the effector function of the antigen presenting and on other immune cells. Of the two cytokines, TGF-β is probably of greater importance in regulating gastrointestinal inflammation.[3,35]

Such immunologic observations raise a question: Can levels of TGF-β serve as a biomarker in either the tissue or blood compartments? While this question has not been extensively explored, investigations so far suggest that the answer may be yes. Pérez-Machado and colleagues[36] studied the generation of TGF-β1–producing cells (Th3 cells) in duodenal biopsies in 20 control children with no pathologic diagnosis, 30 children with multiple food allergy, 9 with celiac disease, and 6 with inflammatory enteropathies. Immunohistochemistry and in situ hybridization were used to localize TGF-β1 protein and mRNA in matched biopsies. The investigators found no significant Th1/Th2 skewing amongst mucosal lymphocytes in allergic children compared with controls, although celiac and inflammatory enteropathy patients showed increased Th1 responses. By contrast, the allergic children showed reduction of TGF-β1+ lymphocytes in both epithelial and lamina propria compartments. Reduction of TGF-β1 expression was also seen in mononuclear cells and epithelium in food allergy by immunohistochemistry and in situ hybridization. Contrary to expectations, the dominant mucosal abnormality in food-allergic children was not Th2 deviation but impaired generation of Th3 cells. This suggests that TGF-β–producing cells may help stratify patients whose inflammation is in part driven by food antigens compared with those where it is not. Additionally, Aceves and colleagues[37] performed quantitative immunohistochemical analysis of esophageal biopsy specimens from children with and children without eosinophilic esophagitis to evaluate levels of expression of TGF-β1 and its signaling molecule, phosphorylated SMAD2/3 (phospho-SMAD2/3). They studied biopsy specimens from 7 patients with eosinophilic esophagitis (5 strictured, 2 without), 7 with gastroesophageal reflux disease, and 7 normal patients. Eosinophilic esophagitis subjects demonstrated increased expression of TGF-β1 and its signaling molecule phospho-SMAD2/3 compared with gastroesophageal reflux disease and normal control patients. Additionally, esophageal biopsies in eosinophilic esophagitis demonstrated an increased expression of the vascular cell adhesion molecule 1. This raises the possibility that a combination of TGF and vascular cell adhesion molecule expression may assist in stratifying patients on the basis of disease severity or prognosis. Although, these are tissue-based markers, they open the door for further investigation in other compartments, such as fecal, blood, or urine, as possible biomarkers for disease severity.

SUMMARY

Disease management for all disciplines of medicine is moving toward noninvasive means of diagnosis and the use of objective methods for assessing response to therapy. Additionally, as molecular and assaying technologies improve, a systems-based biologic approach is being used to personalize diagnosis and treatment based on biomarkers, polymorphisms, and gene expression. Studies attempting to find markers of disease activity that meet the definition of true biomarkers have begun to emerge in gastrointestinal disorders. An ideal biomarker should correlate with disease state and severity, reflect changes in therapy, be noninvasive, and have a high level of sensitivity and specificity. Although, the discipline has clearly not reached these goals, significant advances have been made in measurement of blood, urine, stool, nasal, and tissue-based proteins that correlate with a variety of allergic gastrointestinal diseases. It is hoped that a set of markers will eventually be found to enable the tailoring of therapy for what is currently considered a heterogeneous group of diseases whose pathophysiology is not well understood.

ACKNOWLEDGMENTS

I wish to sincerely thank Ms. Diedre Versluis for her many hours of assistance in manuscript preparation.

REFERENCES

1. Mowat AM. Anatomical basis of tolerance and immunity to intestinal antigens. Nat Rev Immunol 2003;3(4):331–41.
2. Dubois B, Goubier A, Joubert G, et al. Oral tolerance and regulation of mucosal immunity. Cell Mol Life Sci 2005;62(12):1322–32.
3. Chen W, Perruche S, Li J. CD4+CD25+ T regulatory cells and TGF-beta in mucosal immune system: the good and the bad. Curr Med Chem 2007;14(21):2245–9.
4. Wershil BK, Furuta GT. Gastrointestinal mucosal immunity. J Allergy Clin Immunol. 2008;121(Suppl 2):S380–3.
5. Rescigno M, Urbano M, Valzasina B, et al. Dendritic cells express tight junction proteins and penetrate gut epithelial monolayers to sample bacteria. Nat Immunol 2001;2(4):361–7.
6. Heib V, Becker M, Taube C, et al. Advances in the understanding of mast cell function. Br J Haematol 2008;142(5):683–94.
7. Vilagoftis H, Befus AD. Rapidly changing perspective about mast cells at mucosal surfaces. Immunol Rev 2005;206:190–203.
8. Farhadi A, Fields JZ, Keshavarzian A. Mucosal mast cells are pivotal elements in inflammatory bowel disease that connect the dots: stress, intestinal hyperpermeability and inflammation. World J Gastroenterol 2007;13(22):3027–30.
9. Mall M, Gonska T, Thomas J, et al. Activation of ion secretion via proteinase-activated receptor-2 in human colon. Am J Physiol Gastrointest Liver Physiol 2002;282(2):G200–10.
10. Gloro R, Ducrotte P, Reimund JM. Protease-activated receptors: potential therapeutic targets in irritable bowel syndrome? Expert Opin Ther Targets 2005;9(5):1079–95.
11. Cenac N, Chin AC, Garcia-Villar R, et al. PAR2 activation alters colonic paracellular permeability in mice via IFN-gamma-dependent and -independent pathways. J Physiol 2004;558(Pt 3):913–25 [Epub 2004 Jan 11].
12. Bueno L, Fioramonti J. Protease-activated receptor 2 and gut permeability: a review. Neurogastroenterol Motil 2008;20(6):580–7.
13. Sekiguchi F, Takaoka K, Kawabata A. Proteinase-activated receptors in the gastrointestinal system: a functional linkage to prostanoids. Inflammopharmacology 2007;15(6):246–51.
14. Gecse K, Róka R, Ferrier L, et al. Increased faecal serine protease activity in diarrhoeic IBS patients: a colonic lumenal factor impairing colonic permeability and sensitivity. Gut 2008;57(5):591–9 [Epub 2008 Jan 14].
15. Hahn HP, Hornick JL. Immunoreactivity for CD25 in gastrointestinal mucosal mast cells is specific for systemic mastocytosis. Am J Surg Pathol 2007;31(11):1669–76.
16. Di Girolamo N, Indoh I, Jackson N, et al. Human mast cell-derived gelatinase B (Matrix Metalloproteinase-9) is regulated by inflammatory cytokines: role in cell migration. J Immunol 2006;177(4):2638–50.
17. Manfredi MA, Zurakowski D, Rufo PA, et al. Increased incidence of urinary matrix matelloproteinases as predictors of disease in pediatric patients with inflammatory bowel disease. Inflamm Bowel Dis 2008;14(8):1091–6.
18. Kubben FJ, Sier CF, Schram MT. Eradication of *Helicobacter pylori* infection favourably affects altered gastric mucosal MMP-9 levels. Helicobacter 2007;12(5):498–504.
19. Masuko K, Murata M, Xiang Y, et al. Tryptase enhances release of vascular endothelial growth factor from human osteoarthritic chondrocytes. Clin Exp Rheumatol 2007;25(6):860–5.

20. Griga T, Tromm A, Spranger J, et al. Increased serum levels of vascular endothelial growth factor in patients with inflammatory bowel disease. Scand J Gastroenterol 1998;33(5):504–8.
21. Gupta SK, Peters-Golden M, Fitzgerald JF, et al. Cysteinyl leukotriene levels in esophageal mucosal biopsies of children with eosinophillic inflammation: Are they all the same? Am J Gastroenterol 2006;10(5):1125–8.
22. Conus S, Simon HU. General laboratory diagnostics of eosinophilic GI diseases. Best Pract Res Clin Gastroenterol 2008;22(3):441–53.
23. Gupta SK. Noninvasive markers of eosinophilic esophagitis. Gastrointest Endosc Clin N Am 2008;18(1):157–67, xi.
24. Konikoff MR, Blanchard C, Kirby C, et al. Potential of blood eosinophils, eosinophil-derived neurotoxin, and eotaxin-3 as biomarkers of eosinophilic esophagitis. Clin Gastroenterol Hepatol 2006;4(11):1328–36 [Epub 2006 Oct 23].
25. Straumann A, Bauer M, Fischer B, et al. Idiopathic eosinophilic esophagitis is associated with a T(H) 2-type allergic inflammatory response. J Allergy Clin Immunol 2001;108(6):954–61.
26. Gupta SK, Fitzgerald JF, Kondratyuk T, et al. Cytokine expression in normal and inflamed esophageal mucosa: a study into the pathogenesis of allergic eosinophillic esophagitis. J Pediatr Gastrenterol Nutr 2006;42(1):22–6.
27. Saitoh O, Kojima K, Sugi K, et al. Fecal eosinophil granule-derived proteins reflect disease activity in inflammatory bowel disease. Am J Gastroenterol 1999;94(12):3513–20.
28. Straumann A, Kristi J, Conus S, et al. Cytokine expression in healthy and inflamed mucosa: probing the role of eosinophils in the digestive tract. Inflamm Bowel Dis 2005;11(8):720–6.
29. Rothenberg ME. Eosinophilic gastrointestinal disorders (EGID). J Allergy Clin Immunol 2004;113(1):11–28.
30. Inamura H, Tomita M, Okano A, et al. Serial blood and urine levels of EDN and ECP in eosinophilic colitis. Allergy 2003;58(9):959–60.
31. Chehade M, Magid MS, Mofidi S, et al. Allergic eosinophilic gastroenteritis with protein-losing enteropathy: intestinal pathology, clinical course, and long-term follow-up. J Pediatr Gastroenterol Nutr 2006;42(5):516–21.
32. Ohkusa T, Sato N, Ogihara T, et al. Fusobacterium varium localized in the colonic mucosa of patients with ulcerative colitis stimulates species-specific antibody. J Gastroenterol Hepatol 2002;17(8):849–53.
33. Linskens RK, Mallant-Hent RC, Groothuismink ZM, et al. Evaluation of serological markers to differentiate between ulcerative colitis and Crohn's disease: pANCA, ASCA and agglutinating antibodies to anaerobic coccoid rods. Eur J Gastroenterol Hepatol 2002;14:1013–8.
34. Landers CJ, Cohavy O, Misra R, et al. Selected loss of tolerance evidenced by Crohn's disease-associated immune responses to auto- and microbial antigens. Gastroenterology 2002;123(3):689–99.
35. Monteleone G, Pallone F, MacDonald TT. Smad7 in TGF-beta–mediated negative regulation of gut inflammation. Trends Immunol 2004;25(10):513–7.
36. Perez-Machado MA, Ashwood P, Thomson MA, et al. Reduced transforming growth factor-beta1-producing T cells in the duodenal mucosa of children with food allergy. Eur J Immunol 2003;33(8):2307–15.
37. Aceves SS, Newbury RO, Dohil R, et al. Esophageal remodeling in pediatric eosinophilic esophagitis. J Allergy Clin Immunol 2007;119(1):206–12.

Functional Role of Eosinophils in Gastrointestinal Inflammation

Simon P. Hogan, PhD

KEYWORDS

- Eosinophil • Esophagitis • Eosinophilic gastroenteritis
- Inflammatory bowel disease

Eosinophil accumulation in the gastrointestinal (GI) tract is a common feature of numerous GI disorders including classic immunoglobulin (Ig)E-mediated food allergy,[6] eosinophilic gastroenteritis (EGE),[7] allergic colitis,[8] eosinophilic esophagitis (EE),[9,10] inflammatory bowel disease (IBD),[11] and gastroesophageal reflux disease.[12,13] The function of eosinophils in GI inflammation remains an enigma. Eosinophils can potentially initiate GI antigen-specific immune responses by acting as antigen-presenting cells (**Fig. 1**). Eosinophils express major histocompatibility complex class II molecules and relevant costimulatory molecules (CD40, CD28, CD86, B7.1, and B7.2) and secrete an array of cytokines (interleukin [IL]-2, IL-4, IL-12, and IL-10) capable of promoting lymphocyte proliferation, activation, and helper T cell type 1 or type 2 polarization. In addition, eosinophils can have proinflammatory effects including the up-regulation of GI adhesion systems and the modulation of leukocyte trafficking, tissue remodeling, and cellular activation states by releasing cytokines (IL-2, IL-4, IL-5, IL-10, IL-12, IL-13, IL-16, IL-18, and transforming growth factor [TGF]-β), chemokines (RANTES [regulated on activation normal T-cell expressed and secreted] and eotaxin), and lipid mediators (platelet activating factor and leukotriene C4) (see **Fig. 1**). Finally, eosinophils can serve as major effector cells, inducing tissue damage and dysfunction by releasing toxic granule proteins (major basic protein [MBP], eosinophilic cationic protein [ECP], eosinophil peroxidase [EPO], and eosinophil-derived neurotoxin [EDN]) and lipid mediators.[14] Consistent with multifunctional capabilities, there is accumulating evidence in various eosinophilic GI disorders (EGIDs) that eosinophils may have a dual function (ie, end-stage effector and immunoregulatory).[1,14–18]

This work was supported in part by the Crohn's and Colitis Foundation of America.
This review article was largely adapted from other references previously published.[1–5]
Division of Allergy and Immunology, Department of Pediatrics, Cincinnati Children's Hospital Medical Center, 3333 Burnet Avenue, Cincinnati, OH 45229-3039, USA
E-mail address: simon.hogan@cchmc.org

Immunol Allergy Clin N Am 29 (2009) 129–140
doi:10.1016/j.iac.2008.10.004   immunology.theclinics.com

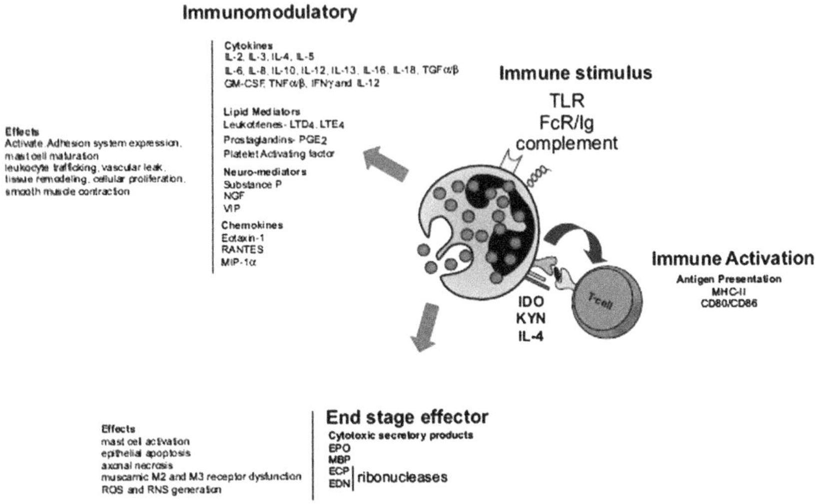

Fig.1. Eosinophil function in GI inflammation. Eosinophils are bilobed granulocytes with eosinophilic staining of secondary granules. The secondary granules contain four primary cationic proteins: eosinophil peroxidase (EPO), major basic protein (MBP), eosinophil cationic protein (ECP), and eosinophil-derived neurotoxin (EDN). All four proteins are cytotoxic molecules; in addition, ECP and EDN are ribonucleases. Eosinophils can be activated by immune stimulus by way of toll-like receptor (TLR), immunoglobulin, and complement. In addition to releasing their preformed cationic proteins, eosinophils can also release a variety of cytokines, chemokines, lipid mediators, and neuromodulators. Eosinophils activate T cells by serving as antigen-presenting cells. Eosinophils can also regulate T-cell polarization through synthesis of indoleamine 2,3-dioxygenase (IDO), an enzyme involved in oxidative metabolism of tryptophan, catalyzing the conversion of tryptophan to kynurenines (KYN), a regulator of T helper cell type 1 and 2 balance. Eosinophils generate an array of cytokines, chemokines, lipid mediators, and neuromodulators that regulate leukocyte trafficking, activation, and maturation; adhesion system expression; collagen synthesis; cellular proliferation; and mucus cell hypersecretion. Eosinophils can also act as an end-stage effector cell, secreting cationic proteins that can regulate mast cell function and generate reactive oxygen species (ROS), reactive nitrogen species (RNS), epithelial cell injury, and muscarnic receptor (M2 and M3) dysfunction. FcR, Fc receptor; GM-CSF, granulocyte-macrophage colony–stimulating factor; IFN, interferon; IL, interleukin; LT, leukotriene; MHC, major histocompatibility complex; MIP, macrophage inflammatory protein; PG, prostaglandin; RANTES, regulated on activation normal T-cell expressed and secreted; TGF, transforming growth factor; TNF, tumor necrosis factor; VIP, vasoactive intestinal peptide. (Adapted from Rothenberg ME, Hogan SP. The eosinophil. Annu Rev Immunol 2006;24:149; with permission.)

EOSINOPHIL-DERIVED CYTOKINES

Eosinophils can synthesize and secrete at least 35 important inflammatory and regulatory cytokines, chemokines, and growth factors. Those eosinophil-derived cytokines that have been quantified generally appear to be generated in relatively small amounts, suggesting an autocrine, paracrine, or juxtacrine role in regulating the function of the microenvironment. In some circumstances, however, eosinophils are the chief producers of cytokines such as TGF-β, which is linked with tissue remodeling in a variety of eosinophil-associated diseases such as asthma.[19] Eosinophils store their cytokines intracellularly as preformed mediators in crystalloid granules and small secretory vesicles.[20] This allows the immediate release of these mediators on eosinophil activation, instead of several hours or days required for other inflammatory cells. For example, the release of the chemokine RANTES was shown to occur within 60 to 120 minutes of eosinophil stimulation by interferon (IFN)-γ. This release of chemokines was related to rapid mobilization (within 10 minutes) of RANTES in small secretory vesicles that translocated this chemokine to the cell membrane before its release.[20–22]

Eosinophils contain a number of other granule-stored enzymes whose exact role in eosinophil function has not been defined.[23] They include acid phosphatase (large amounts of which have been isolated from eosinophils), collagenase, arylsulphatase B, histaminase, phospholipase D, catalase, nonspecific esterases, and vitamin B_{12}-binding protein. Eosinophils are also a source of matrix metalloproteinases (MMP), which have an important role in cell transmigration and inflammation,[24–28] although lesser amounts are produced from eosinophils than from monocytes, macrophages, and neutrophils. The intracellular location of matrix MMP-9 has been localized to perinuclear regions and not the crystalloid granules.[25]

EOSINOPHIL-DERIVED GRANULE CATIONIC PROTEINS

Eosinophils secrete an array of cytotoxic granule cationic proteins (MBP, ECP, EPO, and EDN) that are capable of inducing tissue damage and dysfunction.[17] Eosinophil granules contain a crystalloid core composed of MBP-1 (and MBP-2), and a matrix composed of ECP, EDN, and EPO.[17] MBP, EPO, and ECP are toxic to a variety of tissues, including heart, brain, and bronchial epithelium.[29–32] ECP and EDN are ribonucleases and have been shown to possess antiviral activity, and ECP causes voltage-insensitive, ion-selective toxic pores in the membranes of target cells, possibly facilitating the entry of other cytotoxic molecules.[33–36] ECP also has a number of additional noncytotoxic activities including suppression of T-cell proliferative responses and immunoglobulin synthesis by B cells, mast cell degranulation, and stimulation of airway mucus secretion and glycosaminoglycan production by human fibroblasts.[37] MBP has been shown to directly alter smooth muscle contraction responses by dysregulating vagal muscarinic M2 and M3 receptor function and to promote mast cell and basophil degranulation.[38–40] MBP has been recently implicated in regulating peripheral nerve plasticity.[41] EPO catalyzes the oxidation of pseudohalides (thyiocyanate), halides (chloride, bromide, and iodide), and nitric oxide (nitrite) to form highly reactive oxygen species (hypohalous acids), reactive nitrogen metabolites (nitric dioxide), and perioxynitrite-like oxidants, respectively. These molecules oxidize nucleophilic targets on proteins, promoting oxidative stress and subsequent cell death by apoptosis and necrosis.[42–44]

EOSINOPHIL DEGRANULATION

Eosinophils predominantly secrete their granule protein by regulated exocytosis and degranulation.[45] In a process of piecemeal degranulation, eosinophils selectively release components of their specific granules.[46] For example, activation of human eosinophils by IFN-γ promotes the mobilization of granule-derived RANTES to the cell periphery without inducing cationic protein release.[47,48] Regulated exocytosis occurs by the formation of a docking complex composed of soluble N-ethylmaleimide–sensitive factor attachment protein (SNAP) receptors located on the vesicle and the target membrane. It is postulated that receptor-coupled activation of eosinophils leads to rapid mobilization of cytoplasmic vesicles to the plasma membrane, leading to the formation of a SNAP receptor complex (VAMP-2/SNAP-23/syntaxin-4) and to subsequent mediator release.[45] The receptor-coupled activation of eosinophils may involve immunoglobulin, innate pattern recognition receptors (toll-like receptors [TLRs]), complement, or cytokine. Eosinophils express the Fc receptors (FcR) for IgA, IgD, IgG, and IgM.[49] CD32 (FcγRII) is constitutively expressed on resting human eosinophils,[50] and is up-regulated by IFN-γ.[51] Eosinophils do not constitutively express the FcγRI (CD 64) or the low-affinity FcγRIII (CD16); however, expression can be up-regulated by cytokines IFN-γ, complement (C5a), and platelet activating factor.[51] These receptors not only function as IgG receptors but also appear to have a role stimulating eosinophil survival, degranulation, and generation of leukotrienes.[52–55] Eosinophils express the IgA receptors (CD89).[56] Ex vivo studies have demonstrated that eosinophil degranulation can be induced by IgA-coated particles, suggesting that IgA receptor interaction induces eosinophil degranulation.[57] The expression or presence of the low-affinity IgE receptor (CD23) or the high-affinity IgE receptor on eosinophils remains controversial.[58] Eosinophils express complement receptors (CRs), including CR1 (CD35), CR3 (CD11b/CD18), C3a, CR4 (CD11c), C5a, CD103, and receptors for C1q.[49,59–61] CR1 is recognized by the complement fragments C3b, C4b, iC3b, and C1q. The expression of CR1 on eosinophils is regulated by certain stimuli including leukotriene B4, 15-hydroxyeicosatetraenoic acid, and 5- hydroperoxyeicosatetraenoic acid.[62] CR3 has also been shown to be expressed on eosinophils; CR3 interacts with a number of ligands, including iC3b and ICAM1, promoting eosinophil priming and degranulation.[63] Eosinophils have also been shown to express a number of TLRs, including TLR-1, TLR-2, TLR-4, TLR-5, TLR-6, TLR-7, TLR-8, TLR-9, and TLR-10.[64–66] The level of TLR expression on the eosinophils is low relative to other granulocytes such as neutrophils, except for relatively elevated levels of TLR-7/8.[64] Functional analysis using TLR-specific ligands revealed that TLR-7/8 ligands (R-848) induces eosinophil activation (superoxide production) and prolongs eosinophil survival. The expression of TLR-7/8 has been shown to be regulated by cytokines including IFN-γ.[64]

EOSINOPHILIC GASTROINTESTINAL DISORDERS

Eosinophil accumulation in the GI tract is a common feature of numerous GI disorders, including classic IgE-mediated food allergy,[6] EGE,[7] allergic colitis,[8] EE,[9,10] IBD,[11] and gastroesophageal reflux disease.[12,13]

Esophageal Disorders

A number of disorders are accompanied by eosinophil infiltration into the esophagus, including recurrent vomiting, parasitic and fungal infections, IBD, hypereosinophilic syndrome, esophageal leiomyomatosis, myeloproliferative disorders, carcinomatosis, periarteritis, allergic vasculitis, scleroderma, and drug injury.[67] Recently, there has been a significant amount of attention on the new and emerging eosinophil-associated esophageal disorder, EE. Patients who have primary EE commonly report symptoms that include vomiting, epigastric or chest pain, dysphagia, and respiratory obstructive problems.[68,69] In EE, eosinophil levels are generally 20 to 24 eosinophils per high-power field, reaching 200 eosinophils per high-power field in some cases, and are predominantly localized to the proximal and distal esophagus. In addition, esophageal tissues from patients who have EE demonstrate thickened mucosa with basal layer hyperplasia and papillary lengthening. EE has been associated with esophageal dysmotility. The etiology of the motor disturbances is unclear; however, recent esophageal ultrasound studies have revealed the presence of a dysfunctional muscularis mucosa in patients who have EE, providing a possible explanation for the impaired esophageal dysmotility.[70] Recently, investigators developed experimental models of

EE to begin to examine the contribution of eosinophils in EE. These studies have elegantly delineated an important contribution for the eosinophil-sensitive molecules IL-5 and IL-13 in the recruitment of eosinophils into the esophagus during experimental EE. Although the direct contribution of eosinophils to specific aspects of disease remains unclear, these investigators demonstrated an association between eosinophil numbers in the esophagus and epithelial cell hyperplasia, suggesting a pathophysiologic connection between eosinophils and the development of EE.

Small Bowel Disorders

EG and EGE present with a constellation of symptoms related to the degree and area of the GI tract affected; however, even patients who have isolated eosinophilic enteritis (eg, duodenitis) can have a range of GI symptoms. The mucosal form of EGE (the most common variant) is characterized by vomiting, abdominal pain (that can mimic acute appendicitis), diarrhea, blood loss in stools, iron-deficiency anemia, malabsorption, protein-losing enteropathy, and failure to thrive.[71] The muscularis form is characterized by infiltration of eosinophils predominantly in the muscularis layer, leading to thickening of the bowel wall, which may result in GI obstructive symptoms mimicking pyloric stenosis or other causes of gastric outlet obstruction. The serosal form occurs in a minority of patients who have EGE and is characterized by exudative ascites with higher peripheral eosinophil counts compared with the other forms.[72]

Histologic analysis of the small bowel from patients who have EGE reveals extracellular deposition of eosinophil granule constituents, and indeed, extracellular MBP and ECP are immunohistochemically detectable at elevated levels.[1] Further, Charcot-Leyden crystals, remnants of eosinophil degranulation, are commonly found on microscopic examination of stool samples. Electron microscopy studies have revealed ultrastructural changes in the secondary granules (indicative of eosinophil degranulation and mediator release) in duodenal samples from patients who have EGE. Patients who have EGE can have micronodules (with or without polyposis) noted on endoscopy, and these lesions often contain marked aggregates of lymphocytes and eosinophils.

In an effort to delineate the significance of eosinophil accumulation in eosinophil small bowel disorders, the author and colleagues[2] developed an experimental-model oral antigen–induced eosinophilic GI inflammation that mimics eosinophil-associated small bowel disease—in particular, EGE. Oral administration of the antigen ovalbumin to ovalbumin-sensitized mice induced a pronounced eosinophilic inflammation of the small intestine (duodenum, jejunum, and ileum). Oral antigen challenge induced a prominent cellular infiltrate comprising predominantly eosinophils. Increased eosinophil numbers were observed in various segments of the GI tract, including the esophagus, stomach, small intestine, and Peyer's patches. The oral antigen–challenged mice suffered from variable levels of reduced activity, increased respiratory rate, pilar erecti, and failure to thrive (cachexia). Postmortem GI examination of these mice revealed the presence of gastromegaly and evidence of gastric dysmotility.[73] Employing an in vivo gastric retention assay, the author and colleagues demonstrated impaired gastric emptying in oral allergen–challenged mice. In addition, morphometric analysis revealed a significant decrease in the villus/crypt ratio in the small intestine of oral allergen–challenged mice compared with control-challenged animals. Similarly, patients who have a variety of inflammatory GI disorders also present histologically with reduction in the intestinal villus/crypt ratio.[15] Employing eotaxin-1 (CCL11) deficient mice, the author and colleagues[2] demonstrated that intestinal eosinophilic inflammation induced by oral antigen challenge is dependent on CCL11. Furthermore, they showed that the cachexia and gastric dysmotility is dependent on CCL11 and eosinophils, suggesting that eosinophils contribute to marked GI pathology including villus/crypt shortening, gastric dysmotility, gastromegaly, and failure to thrive. Electron microscopy analysis revealed that eosinophils in the jejunum of oral antigen–challenged mice are in close proximity to damaged enteric nerves.[2] The enteric nerves contain swollen enlarged axonal chambers, with variable loss of internal organelles, including the dense core granules of Schwann cells. Of interest, these features, indicative of axonal necrosis, have been observed in patients with EGID.[74] Notably, studies examining full-thickness intestinal biopsies from pediatric patients who have persistent obstructive symptoms have revealed eosinophil infiltration into the myenteric plexus.[75]

Colonic Disorders

Eosinophils accumulate in the colon of patients who have a variety of disorders including eosinophilic colitis, infections (including pinworms and dog hookworms), drug reactions, vasculitis (eg, Churg-Strauss syndrome), and IBD.[3] IBD, Crohn's disease, and ulcerative colitis (UC) are chronic, relapsing, remitting GI diseases and, in specific subtypes, are characterized by an eosinophilic inflammation of the intestine.[76] Elevated levels of eosinophils have been observed in colonic biopsy samples from patients who have UC, and increased numbers of this cell and of eosinophil-derived granular proteins (MBP, ECP, EPO, and EDN) have been shown to correlate with morphologic changes to the GI tract, to disease severity, and to GI dysfunction.[77,78] Immunohistochemistry analysis of inflamed colonic mucosa of patients who have UC has revealed evidence of eosinophil activation and degranulation.[77] Eosinophils usually represent only a small percentage of the infiltrating leukocytes,[11] but their level has been proposed to be a negative prognostic indicator.[79]

Forbes and colleagues[80] previously employed a model of dextran sulfate sodium (DSS)-induced colitis to begin to examine the contribution of eosinophils in colonic epithelial injury. The model of DSS-induced colitis is a colonic epithelial injury model that is associated with a pronounced colonic eosinophilic inflammation. Electron microscopy studies revealed that the infiltrating eosinophils in the colon of DSS-treated mice appear to undergo cytolytic eosinophilic degranulation as evidenced by the presence of free eosinophilic granules in the extracellular spaces adjacent to these eosinophils.[80] Consistent with this observation, Forbes and colleagues[80] demonstrated elevated levels of colonic luminal EPO activity. Employing EPO-deficient mice and EPO antagonists, Forbes and colleagues[80] showed that some of the pathologic features of DSS-induced colitis were significantly attenuated in the absence of EPO activity, indicating a role for eosinophils and EPO in the pathogenesis of DSS-induced colonic injury.

EPO catalyzes the oxidation of halides and pseudohalides (chloride, bromide, and thyiocyanate) with the products of respiratory burst (molecular oxygen and hydrogen peroxide [H_2O_2]) to generate cytotoxic oxidants (3-bromotyrosine, 3-chlorotyrosine, and hypothyiocynite). These cytotoxic oxidants induce tissue damage and cell death.[81] EPO has also been shown to preferentially catalyze the oxidation of nitrite (NO_2^-), generating the highly toxic reactive nitrogen species (RNS) 3-nitrotyrosine and peroxynitrate.[43,44] Eosinophils and EPO have been shown to play an important role in RNS-mediated oxidative stress–induced tissue injury in asthma.[82,83] Clinical investigations have demonstrated elevated inducible nitric oxide synthase activity; nitric oxide, NO_2^-, and peroxynitrite ($ONOO^-$) production; and protein nitration (3-nitrotyrosine positive staining) in patients who have asthma compared with nonasthmatics.[44,83,84] Immunohistochemical analysis of bronchial tissue revealed eosinophils colocalized with 3-nitrotyrosine positive staining suggesting that eosinophil-derived EPO directly contributes to the generation of $ONOO^-$ and NO_2^- and, thus, protein nitration in asthma.[44] Notably, at physiologic levels of NO_2^- and in the presence of H_2O_2, eosinophils have been shown to promote protein nitration.[44] UC has also been shown to be associated with increased inducible nitric oxide synthase activity and nitric oxide and RNS production.[84] Furthermore, recent clinical studies have demonstrated an imbalance in secondary mucosal antioxidant pathways and in the production of reactive oxygen metabolites including H_2O_2, hypochlorous acid, and RNS in IBD.[85] It is possible that the release of EPO in the lumen during experimental UC leads to the generation of RNS and reactive oxygen metabolites and the subsequent development of the pathophysiologic features of the disease.

Clinical investigations have demonstrated increased levels of a number of other eosinophil granular proteins, including MBP, ECP, and EDN, in biopsy samples from patients who have colonic injury, strengthening a causal link to this granulocyte.[77,78] Furuta and colleagues,[86] employing the oxazalone model of experimental colitis, demonstrated a role for MBP in disease pathogenesis. Moreover, MBP-deficient mice were less susceptible to oxazolone-induced colitis compared with wild-type mice. In vitro analysis demonstrated that MBP promoted increased intestinal epithelial cell permeability. Notably, the increase in intestinal epithelial cell permeability was associated with the down-regulation of tight junction protein occludin-1 on colonic epithelial cells.[86] Clinical and experimental analysis has provided evidence of a casual link between increased intestinal permeability and susceptibility to IBD.[87] Further experimental analysis is required to fully delineate the contribution of eosinophil granule proteins in the pathogenesis of IBD.

Previous clinical investigations have also demonstrated collagen deposition in the intestinal biopsy samples from patients who have IBD.[88] The collagen deposition is thought to be primarily associated with cellular inflammation and TGF-β and insulin-like growth factor-I expression.[88] Furthermore, eosinophils have been linked to fibroblast activation and fibrosis and stricture formation in Crohn's disease.[89,90] There is evidence to suggest that eosinophils may be involved in remodeling and tissue repair through fibroblast stimulation by release of ECP and TGF-β.[91] Notably, clinical studies have previously demonstrated that the level of eosinophil activation is elevated in the quiescent phase of UC compared with the active phase.[92] Experimental DSS-induced colitis is characterized by extensive deposition of collagen in the colonic submucosa.[80] Notably, eosinophils are interspersed throughout the fibrotic layer, suggesting that eosinophils may contribute to collagen deposition. The mechanism causing collagen deposition is currently unknown; however, it is tempting to speculate that eosinophil-derived TGF-β contributes, at least in part, to colonic remodeling in IBD. Recent investigations have demonstrated that eosinophils produce TGF-β during chronic inflammation.[93,94] Further analysis is required to define the contribution of eosinophils to colonic remodeling.

SUMMARY

EGIDs are becoming more prevalent in the Western world. EGIDs are associated with a variety of nonspecific common GI symptoms and laboratory findings, making their diagnosis completely dependent on microscopic examination of GI biopsy samples, generally obtained during endoscopic evaluation. A variety of clinical and experimental models have revealed that eosinophils promote potent proinflammatory effects mediated by their ability to release their cytotoxic secondary granule constituents and a variety of lipid mediators and cytokines. Although much progress has been made, there is still a paucity of knowledge concerning the individual role of eosinophil-derived granule proteins and inflammatory mediators in EGIDs. It is hoped that further clinical and experimental investigation will unravel the individual role of eosinophil-derived mediators in the pathogenesis of EGIDs.

ACKNOWLEDGMENTS

The author would like to thank the numerous colleagues who contributed to the body of information presented in this review, including Drs. Elizabeth Forbes, Luqman Seidu, Marc Rothenberg, and Paul Foster. The author is also grateful to Lisa Roberts and Courtney Wilkens for their assistance with the manuscript preparation.

REFERENCES

1. Rothenberg ME, Mishra A, Brandt EB, et al. Gastrointestinal eosinophils in health and disease. Adv Immunol 2001;78:291–328.
2. Hogan SP, Rothenberg ME, Forbes E, et al. Chemokines in eosinophil-associated gastrointestinal disorders. Curr Allergy Asthma Rep 2004;4(1):74–82.
3. Rothenberg ME. Eosinophilic gastrointestinal disorders (EGID). J Allergy Clin Immunol 2004;113(1):11–28.
4. Hogan SP, Foster PS, Rothenberg ME. Experimental analysis of eosinophil-associated gastrointestinal diseases. Curr Opin Allergy Clin Immunol 2002;2:239–48.
5. Rothenberg ME, Mishra A, Brandt EB, et al. Gastrointestinal eosinophils. Immunol Rev 2001;179:139–55.
6. Moon A, Kleinman RE. Allergic gastroenteropathy in children. Ann Allergy Asthma Immunol 1995;74(1):5–12.
7. Keshavarzian A, Saverymuttu SH, Tai PC, et al. Activated eosinophils in familial eosinophilic gastroenteritis. Gastroenterology 1985;88(4):1041–9.
8. Sherman MP, Cox KL. Neonatal eosinophilic colitis. J Pediatr 1982;100(4):587–9.
9. Furuta GT. Eosinophils in the esophagus: acid is not the only cause. J Pediatr Gastroenterol Nutr 1998;26(4):468–71.
10. Fox VL, Nurko S, Furuta GT. Eosinophilic esophagitis. Gastrointest Endosc 2002;56:260–70.
11. Walsh RE, Gaginella TS. The eosinophil in inflammatory bowel disease. Scand J Gastroenterol 1991;26:1217–24.
12. Winter HS, Madara JL, Stafford RJ, et al. Intraepithelial eosinophils: a new diagnostic criterion for reflux esophagitis. Gastroenterology 1982;83(4):818–23.
13. Brown LF, Goldman H, Antonioli DA. Intraepithelial eosinophils in endoscopic biopsies of adults with reflux esophagitis. Am J Surg Pathol 1984;8(12):899–905.
14. Rothenberg ME. Eosinophilia. N Engl J Med 1998;338(22):1592–600.
15. Sampson HA. Food allergy. Part 1: immunopathogenesis and clinical disorders. J Allergy Clin Immunol 1999;103(5 Pt 1):717–28.
16. Furuta GT, Ackerman SJ, Wershil BK. The role of the eosinophil in gastrointestinal diseases. Curr Opin Gastroenterol 1995;11:541–7.
17. Gleich GJ, Adolphson CR. The eosinophilic leukocyte: structure and function. Adv Immunol 1986;39(177):177–253.
18. Weller PF. The immunobiology of eosinophils. N Engl J Med 1991;324:1110–8.
19. Kay AB, Phipps S, Robinson DS. A role for eosinophils in airway remodelling in asthma. Trends Immunol 2004;25(9):477–82.
20. Lacy P, Moqbel R. Eosinophil cytokines. Chem Immunol 2000;76:134–55.
21. Lacy P, Moqbel R. Eokines: synthesis, storage and release from human eosinophils. Mem Inst Oswaldo Cruz 1997;92(Suppl):H125–33.

22. Moqbel R, Lacy P. Eosinophil cytokines. In: Busse WW, Holgate ST, editors, Inflammatory mechanisms in asthma, vol. 117. New York: Marcel Dekker, Inc.; 1998. p. 227–46.
23. Spry CJF. Eosinophils. A comprehensive review and guide to the scientific and medical literature. Oxford (UK): Oxford Medical Publications; 1988.
24. Gauthier MC, Racine C, Ferland C, et al. Expression of membrane type-4 matrix metalloproteinase (metalloproteinase-17) by human eosinophils. Int J Biochem Cell Biol 2003;35(12):1667–73.
25. Ohno I, Ohtani H, Nitta Y, et al. Eosinophils as a source of matrix metalloproteinase-9 in asthmatic airway inflammation. Am J Respir Cell Mol Biol 1997;16(3):212–9.
26. Okada S, Kita H, George TJ, et al. Migration of eosinophils through basement membrane components in vitro: role of matrix metalloproteinase-9. Am J Respir Cell Mol Biol 1997;17(4):519–28.
27. Schwingshackl A, Duszyk M, Brown N, et al. Human eosinophils release matrix metalloproteinase-9 on stimulation with TNF-β. J Allergy Clin Immunol 1999;104(5):983–9.
28. Wiehler S, Cuvelier SL, Chakrabarti S, et al. p38 MAP kinase regulates rapid matrix metalloproteinase-9 release from eosinophils. Biochem Biophys Res Commun 2004;315(2):463–70.
29. Tai P-C, hayes DJ, Clark JB, et al. Toxic effects of eosinophil secretion products on isolated rat heart cells in vitro. Biochem J 1982;204:75–80.
30. Venge P, Dahl R, Hallgren R, et al. Cationic proteins of human eosinophils and their role in the inflammatory reaction. In: Mahmoud AAF, Austin KF, editors. The eosinophil in health and disease. New York: Grune and Stratton; 1980. p. 1131–42.
31. Frigas E, Loegering DA, Gleich GJ. Cytotoxic effects of the guinea pig eosinophil major basic protein on tracheal epithelium. Lab Invest 1980;42(1):35–43.
32. Gleich GJ, Frigas E, Loegering DA, et al. The cytotoxic properties of the eosinophil major basic protein. J Immunol 1979;123:2925.
33. Young JD, Peterson CG, Venge P, et al. Mechanism of membrane damage mediated by human eosinophil cationic protein. Nature 1986;321(6070):613–6.
34. Slifman NR, Loegering DA, McKean DJ, et al. Ribonuclease activity associated with human eosinophil-derived neurotoxin and eosinophil cationic protein. J Immunol 1986;137(9):2913–7.
35. Gleich GJ, Loegering DA, Bell MP, et al. Biochemical and functional similarities between human eosinophil-derived neurotoxin and eosinophil cationic protein: homology with ribonuclease. Proc Natl Acad Sci USA 1986;83(10):3146–50.
36. Rosenberg HF, Domachowske JB. Eosinophils, eosinophil ribonucleases, and their role in host defense against respiratory virus pathogens. J Leukoc Biol 2001;70(5):691–8.
37. Venge P, Bystrom J, Carlson M, et al. Eosinophil cationic protein (ECP): molecular and biological properties and the use of ECP as a marker of eosinophil activation in disease. Clin Exp Allergy 1999;29:1172–86.
38. Zheutlin LM, Ackerman SJ, Gleich GJ, et al. Stimulation of basophil and rat mast cell histamine release by eosinophil granule-derived cationic proteins. J Immunol 1984;133(4):2180–5.
39. Piliponsky AM, Pickholtz D, Gleich GJ, et al. Human eosinophils induce histamine release from antigen-activated rat peritoneal mast cells: a possible role for mast cells in late-phase allergic reactions. J Allergy Clin Immunol 2001;107(6):993–1000.
40. Jacoby DB, Costello RM, Fryer AD. Eosinophil recruitment to the airway nerves. J Allergy Clin Immunol 2001;107(2):211–8.

41. Morgan RK, Costello RW, Durcan N, et al. Diverse effects of eosinophil cationic granule proteins on IMR-32 nerve cell signaling and survival. Am J Respir Cell Mol Biol 2005;28:28.
42. Agosti JM, Altman LC, Ayars GH, et al. The injurious effect of eosinophil peroxidase, hydrogen peroxide, and halides on pneumocytes in vitro. J Allergy Clin Immunol 1987;79(3):496–504.
43. Wu W, Chen Y, Hazen SL. Eosinophil peroxidase, nitrates, protein tyrosyl residues. Implications for oxidative damage by nitrating intermediates in eosinophilic inflammatory disorders. J Biol Chem 1999;274(36):25933–44.
44. MacPherson JC, Comhair SA, Erzurum SC, et al. Eosinophils are a major source of nitric oxide-derived oxidants in severe asthma: characterization of pathways available to eosinophils for generating reactive nitrogen species. J Immunol 2001;166:5763–72.
45. Logan MR, Odemuyiwa SO, Moqbel R. Understanding exocytosis in immune and inflammatory cells: the molecular basis of mediator secretion. J Allergy Clin Immunol 2003;111(5):923–32.
46. Dvorak AM, Furitsu T, Letourneau L, et al. Mature eosinophils stimulated to develop in human cord blood mononuclear cell cultures supplemented with recombinant human interleukin-5. Part I. Piecemeal degranulation of specific granules and distribution of Charcot-Leyden crystal protein. Am J Pathol 1991;138(1):69–82.
47. Lacy P, Mahmudi-Azer S, Bablitz B, et al. Rapid mobilization of intracellularly stored RANTES in response to interferon-γ in human eosinophils. Blood 1999;94:23–32.
48. Bandeira-Melo C, Gillard G, Ghiran I, et al. EliCell: a gel-phase dual antibody capture and detection assay to measure cytokine release from eosinophils. J Immunol Methods 2000;244(1–2):105–15.
49. Giembycz MA, Lindsay MA. Pharmacology of the eosinophil. Pharmacol Rev 1999;51(2):213–340.
50. Hartnell A, Moqbel R, Walsh GM, et al. Fc gamma and CD1 1/CD 1 8 receptor expression on normal density and low density human eosinophils. Immunology 1990;69(2):264–70.
51. Hartnell A, Kay AB, Wardlaw AJ. IFN-γ induces expression of Fc γ RIII (CD16) on human eosinophils. J Immunol 1992;148(5):1471–8.
52. Kim JT, Schimming AW, Kita H. Ligation of Fc gamma RII (CD32) pivotally regulates survival of human eosinophils. J Immunol 1999;162(7):4253–9.
53. Kita H, Abu-Ghazaleh RI, Gleich GJ, et al. Regulation of Ig-induced eosinophil degranulation by adenosine 3',5'-cyclic monophosphate. J Immunol 1991;146(8):2712–8.
54. Cromwell O, Moqbel R, Fitzharris P, et al. Leukotriene C4 generation from human eosinophils stimulated with IgG–Aspergillus fumigatus antigen immune complexes. 1988;82(4):535–43.
55. Cromwell O, Wardlaw AJ, Champion A, et al. IgG-dependent generation of platelet-activating factor by normal and low density human eosinophils. 1990;145(11):3862–8.
56. Monteiro RC, Hostoffer RW, Cooper MD, et al. Definition of immunoglobulin-A receptors on eosinophils and their enhanced expression in allergic individuals. J Clin Invest 1993;92:1681–5.
57. Abu Ghazaleh R, Fujisawa T, Mestecky J, et al. IgA-induced eosinophil degranulation. J Immunol 1989;142(7):2393–400.
58. Kita H, Gleich GJ. Eosinophils and IgE receptors: a continuing controversy. Blood 1997;89(10):3497–501.

59. Walsh GM, Hartnell A, Moqbel R, et al. Receptor expression and functional status of cultured human eosinophils derived from umbilical cord blood mononuclear cells. Blood 1990;76(1):105–11.

60. DiScipio RG, Daffern PJ, Jagels MA, et al. A comparison of C3a and C5a-mediated stable adhesion of rolling eosinophils in postcapillary venules and transendothelial migration in vitro and in vivo. J Immunol 1999;162(2):1127–36.

61. Daffern PJ, Pfiefer PH, Ember JA, et al. C3a is a chemotaxin for human eosinophils but not for neutrophils. I. C3a stimulation of neutrophils is secondary to eosinophil activation. J Exp Med 1995;181:2119–27.

62. Fischer E, Capron M, Prin L, et al. Human eosinophils express CR1 and CR3 complement receptors for cleavage fragments of C3. 1986;97(2):297–306.

63. Koenderman L, Kuijpers TW, Blom M, et al. Characteristics of CR3-mediated aggregation in human eosinophils: effect of priming by platelet-activating factor. J Allergy Clin Immunol 1991;87(5):947–54.

64. Nagase H, Okugawa S, Ota Y, et al. Expression and function of toll-like receptors in eosinophils: activation by toll-like receptor 7 ligand. J Immunol 2003;171(8):3977–82.

65. Plotz SG, Lentschat A, Behrendt H, et al. The interaction of human peripheral blood eosinophils with bacterial lipopolysaccharide is CD14 dependent. Blood 2001;97(1):235–41.

66. Sabroe I, Jones EC, Usher LR, et al. Toll-like receptor (TLR)2 and TLR4 in human peripheral blood granulocytes: a critical role for monocytes in leukocyte lipopolysaccharide responses. J Immunol 2002;168(9):4701–10.

67. Ahmad M, Soetikno RM, Ahmed A. The differential diagnosis of eosinophilic esophagitis. J Clin Gastroenterol 2000;30(3):242–4.

68. Orenstein SR, Shalaby TM, Di Lorenzo C, et al. The spectrum of pediatric eosinophilic esophagitis beyond infancy: a clinical series of 30 children. Am J Gastroenterol 2000;95:1422–30.

69. Walsh SV, Antonioli DA, Goldman H, et al. Allergic esophagitis in children: a clinicopathological entity. Am J Surg Pathol 1999;23(4):390–6.

70. Fox VL, Nurko S, Teitelbaum JE, et al. High-resolution EUS in children with eosinophilic "allergic" esophagitis. Gastrointest Endosc 2003;57(1):30–6.

71. Kelly KJ. Eosinophilic gastroenteritis. J Pediatr Gastroenterol Nutr 2000; 30(Suppl):S28–35.

72. Talley NJ, Shorter RG, Phillips SF, et al. Eosinophilic gastroenteritis: a clinicopathological study of patients with disease of the mucosa, muscle layer, and subserosal tissues. Gut 1990;31(1):54–8.

73. Hogan SP, Mishra A, Brandt EB, et al. A pathological function for eotaxin and eosinophils in eosinophilic gastrointestinal inflammation. Nat Immunol 2001; 2(4):353–60.

74. Dvorak AM, Onderdonk AB, McLeod RS, et al. Ultrastructural identification of exocytosis of granules from human gut eosinophils in vivo. Int Arch Allergy Immunol 1993;102(1):33–45.

75. Schappi MG, Smith VV, Milla PJ, et al. Eosinophilic myenteric ganglionitis is associated with functional intestinal obstruction. Gut 2003;52:752–5.

76. Hendrickson BA, Gokhale R, Cho JH. Clinical aspects and pathophysiology of inflammatory bowel disease. Clin Microbiol Rev 2002;15(1):79–94.

77. Carvalho AT, Elia CC, de Souza HS, et al. Immunohistochemical study of intestinal eosinophils in inflammatory bowel disease. J Clin Gastroenterol 2003;36(2):120–5.

78. Jeziorska M, Haboubi N, Schofield P, et al. Distribution and activation of eosinophils in inflammatory bowel disease using an improved immunohistochemical technique. J Pathol 2001;194(4):484–92.

79. Desreumaux P, Nutten S, Colombel JF. Activated eosinophils in inflammatory bowel disease: do they matter? Am J Gastroenterol 1999;94(12):3396–8.
80. Forbes E, Murase T, Yang M, et al. Immunopathogenesis of experimental ulcerative colitis is mediated by eosinophil peroxidase. J Immunol 2004;172: 5664–75.
81. Kruidenier L, Verspaget HW. Oxidative stress as a pathogenic factor in inflammatory bowel disease—radicals or ridiculous? Aliment Pharmacol Ther 2002;16: 1997–2015.
82. Saleh D, Ernst P, Lim S, et al. Increased formation of the potent oxidant peroxynitrite in the airways of asthmatic patients is associated with induction of nitric oxide synthase: effect of inhaled glucocorticoid. Faseb J 1998;12(11):929–37.
83. Massaro AF, Mehta S, Lilly CM, et al. Elevated nitric oxide concentrations in isolated lower airway gas of asthmatic subjects. Am J Respir Crit Care Med 1996;153:1510–4.
84. Kimura H, Hokari R, Miura S, et al. Increased expression of an inducible isoform of nitric oxide synthase and the formation of peroxynitrite in colonic mucosa of patients with active ulcerative colitis. Gut 1998;42(2):180–7.
85. Kruidenier L, Kuiper I, van Duijn W, et al. Imbalanced secondary mucosal antioxidant response in inflammatory bowel disease. J Pathol 2003;201:17–27.
86. Furuta GT, Nieuwenhuis EE, Karhausen J, et al. Eosinophils alter colonic epithelial barrier function: role for major basic protein. Am J Physiol Gastrointest Liver Physiol 2005;289(5):G890–7.
87. Laukoetter MG, Nava P, Nusrat A. Role of the intestinal barrier in inflammatory bowel disease. World J Gastroenterol 2008;14(3):401–7.
88. Lawrance IC. Inflammation location, but not type, determines the increase in TGF-B1 and IGF-1 expression and collagen deposition in IBD intestine. Inflamm Bowel Dis 2001;7:16–26.
89. Gelbmann CM, Mestermann S, Gross V, et al. Strictures in Crohn's disease are characterised by an accumulation of mast cells colocalised with laminin but not with fibronectin or vitronectin. Gut 1999;45(2):210–7.
90. Xu X, Rivkind A, Pikarsky A, et al. Mast cells and eosinophils have a potential profibrogenic role in Crohn disease. Scand J Gastroenterol 2004;39(5):440–7.
91. Levi-Schaffer F, Garbuzenko E, Rubin A, et al. Human eosinophils regulate human lung-and skin-derived fibroblast properties in vitro: a role for transforming growth factor β (TGF-β). 1999;96:9660–5.
92. Lampinen M, Ronnblom A, Amin K, et al. Eosinophil granulocytes are activated during the remission phase of ulcerative colitis. Gut 2005;54(12):1714–20.
93. Schmid-Grendelmeier P, Altznauer F, Fischer B, et al. Eosinophils express functional IL–13 in eosinophilic inflammatory diseases. J Immunol 2002;169: 1021–7.
94. Ohkawara Y, Tamura G, Iwasaki T, et al. Activation and transforming growth factor-β production in eosinophils by hyaluronan. Am J Respir Cell Mol Biol 2000;23:444–51.

Chemotactic Factors Associated with Eosinophilic Gastrointestinal Diseases

Carine Blanchard, PhD, Marc E. Rothenberg, MD, PhD*

KEYWORDS

- Eosinophil • Gastrointestinal • Chemokine
- Cytokine • Pathogenesis

Eosinophils are residents of the gastrointestinal (GI) tract. A high eosinophil accumulation in the GI tract without a known cause (eg, infection, inflammatory bowel disease) is observed in eosinophilic GI diseases (EGID). Known chemokines and chemotactic factors associated with this eosinophilic infiltration are presented in this article.

CHEMOKINES INVOLVED IN THE HEALTHY GASTROINTESTINAL TRACT
Eosinophils in the Healthy Gastrointestinal Tract

Under normal conditions, most tissues have low levels of eosinophils. Some organs are rich in eosinophils, however, such as the GI tract, spleen, lymph nodes, thymus, mammary glands, and uterus. Interestingly, although present in these multiple tissues, only GI eosinophils are associated with a marked degranulation.[1] At baseline, in healthy patients or normal mice, eosinophils are present in the lamina propria throughout the GI tract from the stomach to the colon.[1,2] Eosinophils are not found, however, in Peyer's patches or intraepithelial locations.[3-6] Because eosinophils can infiltrate these sites in EGID, the knowledge of the distribution of eosinophils and the chemokines responsible for their presence in the GI tract at baseline is essential to identify

This work was supported by in part by the American Heart Association 0625296B (CB); the Thrasher Research Fund NR-0014 (CB); the PHS Grant P30 DK0789392 (CB); the NIH AI079874-01 (CB), AI070235, AI45898, and DK076893 (MER); the Food Allergy and Anaphylaxis Network (MER); Campaign Urging Research for Eosinophil Disorders; the Buckeye Foundation (MER); and the Food Allergy Project (MER).
Division of Allergy and Immunology, Department of Pediatrics, Cincinnati Children's Hospital Medical Center, 3333 Burnet Avenue, MLC 7028, Cincinnati, OH 45229–3039, USA
* Corresponding author.
E-mail address: rothenberg@cchmc.org (M.E. Rothenberg).

a possible cause of EGID.[1-3] DeBrosse and colleagues[2] have shown an increasing level of eosinophils from the esophagus to the colon with barely any eosinophils detected in the esophagus. In the lamina propria, a maximum of 8 eosinophils per high power field (HPF) were noted in the antrum, 11 in the fundus, up to 26 in the duodenum. Finally, up to 50 eosinophils per HPF were seen in the colon with a high variability inside the different colon segments and between individuals.[2]

Chemokine Receptor Expression

The intestinal tract expresses numerous chemokines at baseline (eg, eotaxin-1 and -2, RANTES). In addition to the expression of chemokines in the GI tract, eosinophils expressed numerous chemokine receptors (ie, CCR3, CCR1 constitutively, and CXCR2, CXCR3, CXCR6 when activated with interleukin [IL]-5). Blood eosinophils are under a continual chemotactic gradient originating from the GI tract. The fine balance between the chemokine released, the density of receptor, and the adhesion molecules expression determine the entry of eosinophils in the gut tissue. Eosinophils highly express CCR3; the role for CCR3 and CCR3 ligands in GI eosinophilia has been studied in animal model using gene-deficient mice (**Fig. 1**A).

Chemokine Expression and Involvement in the Gastrointestinal Eosinophils at Baseline

Murine models have convincingly demonstrated that eosinophilic infiltration is not dependent on the colonic flora or the endotoxin load of the gut as assessed by the high eosinophil level observed in prenatal mice.[7] Germ-free mice have normal levels of GI eosinophils. Eotaxin-1 and -2 are constitutively expressed in a variety of tissues, but are expressed at high levels in the GI tract.[7-10] Interestingly, eotaxin-3 mRNA is not detected at baseline in the GI tract using Northern blot.[11] The use of animals deficient in the eotaxin genes has enlightened the field regarding the baseline chemotactic signals responsible for baseline eosinophilia in the gut. For example, it has been shown that the intestine of eotaxin-1–deficient mice is almost completely devoid of eosinophils suggesting that the baseline intestinal eosinophilia is the consequence of the constitutive expression of this chemokine.[7,12] Similar results were observed in CCR3-deficient mice (deficient for the receptor of eotaxin-1), which have a decreased eosinophil level in the jejunum at baseline (1.3 versus 9 eosinophils per HPF). The residual presence of eosinophils in the GI tract of the CCR3-deficient mice (1.3 per HPF) and eotaxin-1–deficient mice (0.3 per villus) suggests a modest involvement of other chemotactic factors for eosinophils in the jejunum.[12-14]

CHEMOTACTIC FACTORS IN EOSINOPHILIC GASTROINTESTINAL DISEASES

In EGID, the eosinophils number is elevated in one or more segment of the esophago-gastrointestinal tract.

Known Stimulus in Eosinophilic Gastrointestinal Diseases Responsible for the Induction of Chemotactic Signal

Th2 disease
EGID inflammation is believed to be driven by CD4+ Th2 cells.[15,16] These cells are the key component in the production of IL-4, -13, -5, and -10, and the control of allergic inflammation responses. IL-4 and -13 are responsible for Th2 cell production and IgE by B cells and IL-5 controls eosinophil production, activation, and survival. Interestingly, resident eosinophils have different cytokine expression patterns under inflammatory or noninflammatory conditions,[15] and esophageal eosinophils from

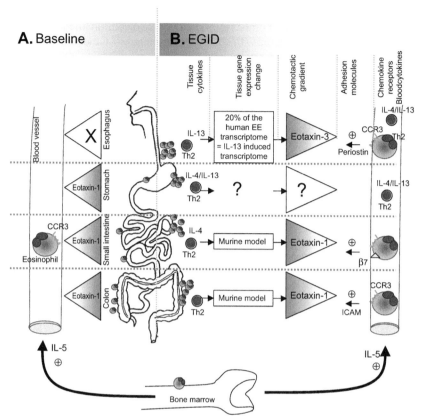

Fig. 1. Chemotactic factors involved in eosinophil infiltration in the GI tract. (*A*) Hematopoietic cells are present at baseline in all segments of the GI tract. The distribution of eosinophils differs from one segment to another. Basal IL-5 level allows maturation and survival of eosinophils. In the esophagus, no eosinophils are seen; however, the eosinophil levels in the tissue increase from the stomach to the colon. Eotaxin-1 expression in the GI tract and CCR3 expression on the eosinophils are involved in the baseline eosinophilia. (*B*) Eosinophil infiltration in EGID has been associated with Th2 diseases and increased Th2 cytokine production (IL-4, IL-13), and has been shown in eosinophilic esophagitis, eosinophilic gastroenteritis, and eosinophilic gastritis patients. CCR3 expressed on eosinophils have been shown critical for intestinal and esophageal eosinophilic diseases. The eotaxins 1 and 3 are responsible in part for EGID in the intestines and the esophagus, respectively. Others molecules, such the adhesion molecules B7 integrin and intercellular adhesion molecule, have been shown to be involved in eosinophilic gastroenteritis and EC models but no data document their role eosinophilic esophagitis and eosinophilic gastritis.

eosinophilic esophagitis (EE) patients express relatively high levels of Th2 cytokines.[15,16] Th2 cytokines have been shown to regulate the expression of a large variety of chemokines in vitro.

Chemotactic factors in eosinophilic esophagitis
Murine models have demonstrated that IL-5 maintains the systemic eosinophil levels needed for esophageal eosinophilia accumulation.[7,17] Eosinophil accumulation has been shown to be CCL11–eotaxin-1 and CCR3 dependent using the respective KO

mice.[18,19] Remarkably, eosinophils are still infiltrating the esophagus of CD2-IL-5tg–CCL11KO mice, suggesting that other factors may be involved.[7] In human EE, eotaxin-3 expression strongly correlates with eosinophils numbers.[19] Other factors, such as chemokines, extracellular matrix component (periostin), or adhesion molecules, may facilitate the entry of eosinophils in esophageal tissue.[19–21] Lymphocytes, mast cells, and dendritic cells are also increased in EE and microarray analysis has revealed the presence of multiple other chemokines overexpressed in EE patients, such as CXCL1, IL-8, and CXCL6,[19] although eotaxin-3 is the most strongly up-regulated gene of the EE transcriptome. Additionally, IL-13 has recently been shown to induce 20% of the EE transcriptome, and more particularly to induce eotaxin-3 expression in primary esophageal epithelial cells.[16]

Chemotactic factors in eosinophilic gastritis and gastroenteritis

The paucity of studies on the molecular pathogenesis of eosinophilic gastritis and eosinophilic gastroenteritis is striking. In clinical studies, increased secretion of IL-4 and IL-5 by peripheral blood T cells has been reported in patients with eosinophilic gastroenteritis.[22] Similarly, in the duodenum, lamina propria mononuclear cells are more primed to secrete Th2 cytokines in EGID compared with control patients when stimulated with milk proteins.[23] The allergic component of eosinophilic gastroenteritis and eosinophilic gastritis is also emphasized by the increased atopy rate in EGID[24] and by the increased presence of tissue mast cells in human and murine models of allergic diarrhea, suggesting a critical role for mast cells in the development of EGID symptoms.[25] In mice, the overexpression of eotaxin-1 by epithelial cells is sufficient to induce intestinal eosinophilia in eotaxin-deficient mice, suggesting a possible role for eotaxin-1 in small bowel eosinophilia.[17]

Interestingly, RANTES expression strongly correlates with eosinophilia levels in food allergy model in mice (OVA)[26] and, like eotaxin-1, RANTES mRNA is highly expressed in the jejunum of mice.[26] RANTES is also expressed at baseline in the human GI tract and may contribute to hematopoietic cell recruitment at baseline and in EGID.[23] It is also increased in the colon of atopic dermatitis patients[27] and in a rat colitis model.[28] No studies on RANTES-deficient mice have determined the ultimate role of this cytokine in eosinophil recruitment at baseline and in EGID.

Chemotactic factors in eosinophilic colitis

Eosinophilic colitis is divided into allergic and nonallergic colitis, but is usually not an IgE-associated disease. Although the exact causes of the disease are still unknown, T-cell function has been suggested in human studies.[23] T cell has also been shown to transfer the disease in a murine model of ovalbumin-induced colonic inflammation. The development of the intestinal inflammation model was strongly associated with the transcription factor STAT6, involved in the signaling of IL-13 and -4.[29] These cytokines (IL-13 and -4) have been implicated in this model and may drive Th2-induced chemokine expression (eg, eotaxins). Using an experimental GI allergy model, an essential role for eotaxin-1 in regulating eosinophil-associated GI pathology has been demonstrated.[30]

Additionally, a critical role for eotaxin-1 in the development of eosinophilia in dextran sodium sulfate-induced colitis suggests a possible role for this cytokine in eosinophilic-associated colonic diseases.[31]

Murine Models of Eosinophilic Gastrointestinal Diseases: Knowledge Gained and Limitation

It is compelling to note the paucity of murine models that characterize or reproduce the human EGIDs. EGID is a relatively common disease and very few formal models exist. As a consequence, molecular mechanisms involved in human EGID are still not well understood.

In addition, the imperfect overlap between the murine and human chemokines and chemokine receptor genetic map may reveal some discrepancies between murine models and human diseases. Eotaxin-3, not expressed in mice,[32] and highly involved in human EE, is one example of such a limitation.

Cellular Localization of the Chemokines Involved in Eosinophils Chemoattraction in Eosinophilic Gastrointestinal Diseases

Because of the various structures present in the GI tract, the cell types involved in the production of these chemokines are quite different. From the top to the bottom, the esophageal epithelial cell has been shown to overexpress eotaxin-3. In the stomach, no study has formally defined the chemokine or the source of chemokines responsible for the eosinophilic accumulation. In the small intestine, eotaxin-1 is expressed by inflammatory cells (mononuclear cell at the neck of the crypt in mice). Finally, in the human colon, eotaxin-1 is expressed by inflammatory cells[33] and epithelial cells. RANTES mRNA was found expressed by intraepithelial lymphocytes and subepithelial lamina propria.[34]

Paradox of Eotaxin-1, -2, and -3

Still, a conundrum exists: eotaxin-1, -2, and -3 can be regulated by the same Th2 stimuli in vitro and all interact with the same receptor CCR3. Studies suggest that a tissue and cell specificity of the expression of these chemokines, in addition to a different kinetic expression and affinity for CCR3, influences the course of asthma pathogenesis. The individual role of these chemokines in the different GI segments requires further study. The global paucity of information regarding the involvement of these chemokines in murine models and in human EGID studies indicates that the baseline eotaxin-1 highly expressed in the GI tract might promote most of the tissue-dwelling eosinophils. In lower eosinophilic GI disease, eotaxin-1 might be the main chemotactic signal, whereas eotaxin-3 is the key player in upper EGID (esophagus) (see **Fig. 1**B).

Other Molecules (Adhesion Molecules, Integrins) Involved in Cell Recruitment in Eosinophilic Gastrointestinal Diseases

Although chemokine and chemokine receptors are essential for the recruitment of eosinophils, a critical role in eosinophil GI infiltration has been attributed to integrins. Colonic eosinophils express the integrins alphaL, alphaM, and β_2, counterreceptors for the intercellular adhesion molecule-1. Using intercellular adhesion molecule-1–deficient mice and anti–intercellular adhesion molecule-1 neutralizing antibodies, Forbes and colleagues[35] showed that hapten-induced colonic eosinophilic inflammation is critically dependent on intercellular adhesion molecule-1, suggesting that β_2 integrin and intercellular adhesion molecule-1 are key components to eosinophil recruitment into the colon during GI inflammation associated with colonic injury.

The intestinal eosinophilia induced by the eotaxin-1 intestine transgene has been shown to be dependent on the β_7 integrin.[36] β_7 integrin has been shown to be important for eosinophil recruitment to the intestinal tract under inflammatory conditions in an intestinal allergy model where β_7 gene-deficient mice displayed impaired eosinophilia compared with wild-type mice without affecting blood eosinophilia.[37]

Similarly, scattered studies have suggested that leukotriene receptor antagonists are able to improve EGID clinical symptoms,[38] although their effect on the eosinophil level is controversial.[38–42]

Finally, in EE it has recently been shown that the extracellular matrix protein periostin, an IL-13–induced gene that is highly overexpressed in EE patients compared with control biopsy samples, correlates with eosinophil numbers in the biopsies. Interestingly, in experimental EE, periostin-deficient mice have decreased eosinophil recruitment to the esophagus. A direct role of periostin on eosinophil adhesion was shown. This study suggests that periostin may facilitate eosinophil infiltration in the esophagus of EE patients.[21]

SUMMARY

Although studies indicate that Th2 cytokines, (IL-5, -13, -4), and chemokines (eotaxins) are involved in pathogenesis, allergen elimination and corticosteroids are still the gold standard therapy for EGID. Anti–IL-5 therapy has been used in EE and hypereosinophilic syndrome–associated EGID.[43–46] It is envisioned that molecular diagnostics, similar to the approach currently being taken to classify cancer,[19] where therapeutic approaches and outcomes can be predicted, will be applied to EGID and become useful for diagnosis and prediction of therapeutic responsiveness and prognosis. It is important to note that the mechanisms by which any therapeutic intervention improves EGID pathologic symptoms have not been established, highlighting the value of translational research aiming to develop optimal EGID therapy. It is anticipated that mechanism-based therapeutic intervention (eg, antieotaxin, CCR3 antagonists, anti–IL-5, and anti–IL-13) will prove to be successful therapies for EGID.

REFERENCES

1. Kato M, Kephart GM, Talley NJ, et al. Eosinophil infiltration and degranulation in normal human tissue. Anat Rec 1998;252:418–25.
2. DeBrosse CW, Case JW, Putnam PE, et al. Quantity and distribution of eosinophils in the gastrointestinal tract of children. Pediatr Dev Pathol 2006;9:210–8.
3. Mishra A, Hogan SP, Brandt EB, et al. Peyer's patch eosinophils: identification, characterization, and regulation by mucosal allergen exposure, interleukin-5, and eotaxin. Blood 2000;96:1538–44.
4. Rothenberg ME. Eosinophilic gastrointestinal disorders (EGID). J Allergy Clin Immunol 2004;113:11–28.
5. Rothenberg ME, Mishra A, Brandt EB, et al. Gastrointestinal eosinophils. Immunol Rev 2001;179:139–55.
6. Rothenberg ME, Mishra A, Brandt EB, et al. Gastrointestinal eosinophils in health and disease. Adv Immunol 2001;78:291–328.
7. Mishra A, Hogan SP, Lee JJ, et al. Fundamental signals that regulate eosinophil homing to the gastrointestinal tract. J Clin Invest 1999;103:1719–27.
8. Rothenberg ME, Luster AD, Lilly CM, et al. Constitutive and allergen-induced expression of eotaxin mRNA in the guinea pig lung. J Exp Med 1995;181:1211–6.
9. Garcia-Zepeda EA, Combadiere C, Rothenberg ME, et al. Human monocyte chemoattractant protein (MCP)-4 is a novel CC chemokine with activities on monocytes, eosinophils, and basophils induced in allergic and nonallergic inflammation that signals through the CC chemokine receptors (CCR)-2 and -3. J Immunol 1996;157:5613–26.
10. Zimmermann N, Hogan SP, Mishra A, et al. Murine eotaxin-2: a constitutive eosinophil chemokine induced by allergen challenge and IL-4 overexpression. J Immunol 2000;165:5839–46.

11. Kitaura M, Suzuki N, Imai T, et al. Molecular cloning of a novel human CC chemo-kine (eotaxin-3) that is a functional ligand of CC chemokine receptor 3. J Biolumin Chemilumin 1999;274:27975–80.

12. Matthews AN, Friend DS, Zimmermann N, et al. Eotaxin is required for the base-line level of tissue eosinophils. Proc Natl Acad Sci U S A 1998;95:6273–8.

13. Gurish MF, Humbles A, Tao H, et al. CCR3 is required for tissue eosinophilia and lar-val cytotoxicity after infection with *Trichinella spiralis*. J Immunol 2002;168:5730–6.

14. Humbles AA, Lu B, Friend DS, et al. The murine CCR3 receptor regulates both the role of eosinophils and mast cells in allergen-induced airway inflammation and hyperresponsiveness. Proc Natl Acad Sci U S A 2002;99:1479–84.

15. Straumann A, Kristl J, Conus S, et al. Cytokine expression in healthy and inflamed mucosa: probing the role of eosinophils in the digestive tract. Inflamm Bowel Dis 2005;11:720–6.

16. Blanchard C, Mingler MK, Vicario M, et al. IL-13 involvement in eosinophilic esophagitis: transcriptome analysis and reversibility with glucocorticoids. J Allergy Clin Immunol 2007;120:1292–300.

17. Mishra A, Hogan SP, Brandt EB, et al. IL-5 promotes eosinophil trafficking to the esophagus. J Immunol 2002;168:2464–9.

18. Mishra A, Rothenberg ME. Intratracheal IL-13 induces eosinophilic esophagitis by an IL-5, eotaxin-1, and STAT6-dependent mechanism. Gastroenterology 2003;125:1419–27.

19. Blanchard C, Wang N, Stringer KF, et al. Eotaxin-3 and a uniquely conserved gene-expression profile in eosinophilic esophagitis. J Clin Invest 2006;116: 536–47.

20. Blanchard C, Wang N, Rothenberg ME. Eosinophilic esophagitis: pathogenesis, genetics, and therapy. J Allergy Clin Immunol 2006;118:1054–9.

21. Blanchard C, Mingler MK, MacBride M, et al. Periostin facilitates eosinophil tissue in-filtration in allergic lung and esophageal responses. Mucosal Immunology 2008;1: 289–96.

22. Jaffe JS, James SP, Mullins GE, et al. Evidence for an abnormal profile of interleukin-4 (IL-4), IL-5, and gamma-interferon (gamma-IFN) in peripheral blood T cells from patients with allergic eosinophilic gastroenteritis. J Clin Immunol 1994;14:299–309.

23. Beyer K, Castro R, Birnbaum A, et al. Human milk-specific mucosal lymphocytes of the gastrointestinal tract display a TH2 cytokine profile. J Allergy Clin Immunol 2002;109:707–13.

24. Katz AJ, Twarog FJ, Zeiger RS, et al. Milk-sensitive and eosinophilic gastroenter-opathy: similar clinical features with contrasting mechanisms and clinical course. J Allergy Clin Immunol 1984;74:72–8.

25. Brandt EB, Strait RT, Hershko D, et al. Mast cells are required for experimental oral allergen-induced diarrhea. J Clin Invest 2003;112:1666–77.

26. Lee JB, Matsumoto T, Shin YO, et al. The role of RANTES in a murine model of food allergy. Immunol Invest 2004;33:27–38.

27. Yamada H, Izutani R, Chihara J, et al. RANTES mRNA expression in skin and colon of patients with atopic dermatitis. Int Arch Allergy Immunol 1996;111(Suppl 1): 19–21.

28. Ajuebor MN, Hogaboam CM, Kunkel SL, et al. The chemokine RANTES is a cru-cial mediator of the progression from acute to chronic colitis in the rat. J Immunol 2001;166:552–8.

29. Kweon MN, Yamamoto M, Kajiki M, et al. Systemically derived large intestinal CD4(+) Th2 cells play a central role in STAT6-mediated allergic diarrhea. J Clin Invest 2000;106:199–206.

30. Hogan SP, Mishra A, Brandt EB, et al. A critical role for eotaxin in experimental oral antigen-induced eosinophilic gastrointestinal allergy. Proc Natl Acad Sci USA 2000;97:6681–6.
31. Forbes E, Murase T, Yang M, et al. Immunopathogenesis of experimental ulcerative colitis is mediated by eosinophil peroxidase. J Immunol 2004;172:5664–75.
32. Pope SM, Fulkerson PC, Blanchard C, et al. Identification of a cooperative mechanism involving interleukin-13 and eotaxin-2 in experimental allergic lung inflammation. J Biol Chem 2005;280:13952–61.
33. Wagsater D, Lofgren S, Hugander A, et al. Analysis of single nucleotide polymorphism in the promoter and protein expression of the chemokine eotaxin-1 in colorectal cancer patients. World J Surg Oncol 2007;5:84.
34. Mazzucchelli L, Hauser C, Zgraggen K, et al. Differential in situ expression of the genes encoding the chemokines MCP-1 and RANTES in human inflammatory bowel disease. J Pathol 1996;178:201–6.
35. Forbes E, Hulett M, Ahrens R, et al. ICAM-1-dependent pathways regulate colonic eosinophilic inflammation. J Leukoc Biol 2006;80:330–41.
36. Mishra A, Hogan SP, Brandt EB, et al. Enterocyte expression of the eotaxin and interleukin-5 transgenes induces compartmentalized dysregulation of eosinophil trafficking. J Biol Chem 2002;277:4406–12.
37. Brandt EB, Zimmermann N, Muntel EE, et al. The alpha4bbeta7-integrin is dynamically expressed on murine eosinophils and involved in eosinophil trafficking to the intestine. Clin Exp Allergy 2006;36:543–53.
38. Quack I, Sellin L, Buchner NJ, et al. Eosinophilic gastroenteritis in a young girl: long term remission under Montelukast. BMC Gastroenterol 2005;5:24.
39. Attwood SE, Lewis CJ, Bronder CS, et al. Eosinophilic oesophagitis: a novel treatment using Montelukast. Gut 2003;52:181–5.
40. Daikh BE, Ryan CK, Schwartz RH. Montelukast reduces peripheral blood eosinophilia but not tissue eosinophilia or symptoms in a patient with eosinophilic gastroenteritis and esophageal stricture. Ann Allergy Asthma Immunol 2003;90:23–7.
41. Gupta SK, Peters-Golden M, Fitzgerald JF, et al. Cysteinyl leukotriene levels in esophageal mucosal biopsies of children with eosinophilic inflammation: are they all the same? Am J Gastroenterol 2006;101:1125–8.
42. Urek MC, Kujundzic M, Banic M, et al. Leukotriene receptor antagonists as potential steroid sparing agents in a patient with serosal eosinophilic gastroenteritis. Gut 2006;55:1363–4.
43. Garrett JK, Jameson SC, Thomson B, et al. Anti-interleukin-5 (mepolizumab) therapy for hypereosinophilic syndromes. J Allergy Clin Immunol 2004;113:115–9.
44. Sutton SA, Assa'ad AH, Rothenberg ME. Anti-IL-5 and hypereosinophilic syndromes. Clin Immunol 2005;115:51–60.
45. Stein ML, Collins MH, Villanueva JM, et al. Anti-IL-5 (mepolizumab) therapy for eosinophilic esophagitis. J Allergy Clin Immunol 2006;118:1312–9.
46. Simon D, Braathen LR, Simon HU. [Anti-interlekuin-5 therapy for eosinophilic diseases.]. Hautarzt 2007;58:122, 124–7 [in German].

The Role of Lymphocytes in Eosinophilic Gastrointestinal Disorders

Mirna Chehade, MD[a,b,]*, Hugh A. Sampson, MD[b]

KEYWORDS

- Eosinophilic esophagitis • Eosinophilic gastroenteritis
- Lymphocyte • helper T cell • Food allergy

Eosinophilic gastrointestinal disorders (EGIDs) encompass a variety of disorders named after the organ of involvement with inflammation and eosinophilia and its resultant symptoms. EGIDs include specific entities such as eosinophilic esophagitis (EoE), eosinophilic gastroenteritis (EG), and eosinophilic colitis.[1] Although the pathogenesis of EGIDs is still poorly understood, dietary food antigens have been shown to cause EGIDs through several short-term clinical studies. Various clinical trials of food elimination resulted in various degrees of clinical response and histologic improvement. These trials included amino acid–based formula therapy[2–4] and elimination of suspected allergens based on testing[5] or elimination of six major allergens.[6] Reintroduction of the foods resulted in reoccurrence of symptoms,[2] proving a causative relationship of EGIDs to food antigens. This relationship of EGIDs with food allergy points to a potential breach of oral tolerance in EGIDs and to a potentially important role played by lymphocytes in responding to the oral food antigens. In this article, the concept of oral tolerance is discussed briefly, focusing on the role of regulatory T lymphocytes in the process. Discussion then centers on the available evidence for the role that lymphocytes play in the induction and pathogenesis of EGIDs, focusing specifically on T lymphocytes carrying the type 2 helper T-cell phenotype (T_H2), which is important in mediating allergic phenomena. The authors also summarize available evidence for a potential breach in oral tolerance in EGIDs. Among the EGIDs, EoE

[a] Pediatric Gastroenterology and Nutrition, Box 1198, Mount Sinai School of Medicine, One Gustave L. Levy Place, New York, NY 10029, USA
[b] Pediatric Allergy and Immunology, Box 1198, Mount Sinai School of Medicine, One Gustave L. Levy Place, New York, NY 10029, USA
* Corresponding author. Pediatrics, Box 1198, Mount Sinai School of Medicine, One Gustave L. Levy Place, New York, NY
E-mail address: mirna.chehade@mssm.edu (M. Chehade).

Immunol Allergy Clin N Am 29 (2009) 149–158
doi:10.1016/j.iac.2008.10.006   immunology.theclinics.com
0889-8561/08/$ – see front matter © 2009 Elsevier Inc. All rights reserved.

and EG are particularly discussed because they have been the most extensively studied and the most challenging subsets of EGIDs to clinicians and researchers alike.

ORAL TOLERANCE

The gastrointestinal tract is the largest immunologic organ in the body. Despite the large extent of dietary antigenic exposure, only a small percentage of individuals develop food allergy, which is due to the development of oral tolerance to dietary proteins. Oral tolerance refers to a state of active inhibition of immune responses to an antigen by means of prior exposure to that antigen through the oral route.[7]

Normally, dietary proteins that escape gastrointestinal luminal digestion and processing come in contact with the intestinal epithelium and the underlying mucosal immune system in various ways. Dietary antigens can be sampled by intestinal dendritic cells that extend processes into the lumen.[8] Particulate antigens can be taken up by microfold cells overlying Peyer's patches and delivered to dendritic cells in the subepithelial dome region and then to underlying B-cell follicles of the Peyer's patches.[9,10] Immunoglobulin (Ig)A switching occurs in these cells, mediated by transforming growth factor (TGF)-β–secreting T cells, hence contributing to oral tolerance.[11] Soluble dietary antigens may cross the intestinal epithelium through transcellular or paracellular routes to encounter T lymphocytes or macrophages in the lamina propria.[12,13] In addition to dendritic cell–presenting antigens, intestinal epithelial cells are thought to act as nonprofessional antigen-presenting cells given that they constitutively express major histocompatibility complex class II molecules on their basolateral membranes[14,15] and present antigen to primed T cells.

After the dietary antigen is in contact with immune cells, oral tolerance can be induced by two mechanisms, depending on the quantity of antigen (**Fig. 1**). High-dose oral tolerance is mediated by lymphocyte anergy,[16] which occurs through T-cell receptor ligation in the absence of costimulatory signals[17] or by lymphocyte deletion, which occurs by means of Fas-mediated apoptosis (see **Fig. 1B**).[18] Low-dose tolerance is mediated by regulatory T cells. In addition to CD8[+] T cells[19,20] and natural killer T cells,[21] various types of regulatory CD4[+] T cells play a role in low-dose tolerance.[22–24] These cells include T_H3 cells, which mediate suppression through secreted TGF-β,[25,26] T regulatory cells 1 that mediate suppression through secreted interleukin (IL)-10,[27] and CD4[+]CD25[+] cells that mediate suppression possibly through surface-bound TGF-β (see **Fig. 1C**).[28,29] A breach in any of these mechanisms has been demonstrated to result in loss of oral tolerance to an antigen in animal models and is hypothesized to lead to food allergies in humans.[30]

EOSINOPHILIC ESOPHAGITIS
Lymphocytes are Increased in Number in Eosinophilic Esophagitis

Rare intraepithelial lymphocytes are normally found in the esophagus of healthy individuals.[31–33] These cells were historically referred to as squiggle cells by histopathologists because of their irregular nuclear contours resulting from their intermingling with esophageal epithelial cells, as seen by microscopic examination of hematoxylin and eosin–stained sections of the esophageal mucosa.[33] Squiggle cells were found to be T lymphocytes.[32,33] In the esophageal epithelial layer, suppressor T cells (CD8[+]) are more frequent than helper T cells (CD4[+]);[31,34] whereas in the esophageal lamina propria, lymphocytes are comprised mainly of helper T cells.[34]

The number of esophageal intraepithelial T lymphocytes is increased in patients who have EoE compared with healthy control subjects, as demonstrated by immunohistochemical staining for CD3[+] cells.[31,35,36] Both CD4 and CD8 subsets of the T lymphocytes were found to be increased in EoE, with maintenance of CD8

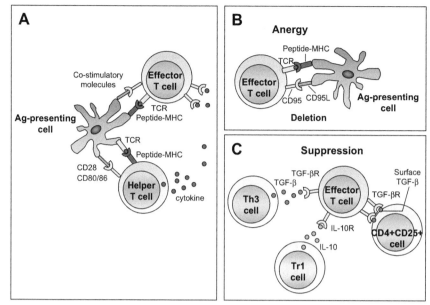

Fig. 1. Mechanisms of oral tolerance. (*A*) Generation of an immune response. (*B*) High-dose tolerance. (*C*) Low-dose tolerance. Ag, antigen; MHC, major histocompatibility complex; TCR, T-cell receptor; Tr1, T regulatory cells 1. (*Modified from* Chehade M, Mayer L. Oral tolerance and its relation to food hypersensitivities. J Allergy Clin Immunol 2005;115(1):3–12; with permission.)

predominating over CD4 cells.[31,35] The number of lymphocytes and their characterization into subsets in the esophageal subepithelial lamina propria of patients who have EoE have not been examined.

As for B lymphocytes, although absent from the esophageal epithelium in healthy individuals,[31] some were shown to be present in the subepithelial lamina propria along with helper T cells.[34] In EoE, B lymphocytes were found to infiltrate the esophageal epithelium, as demonstrated by immunohistochemical staining for the B-cell marker CD20, albeit in very small numbers.[31]

The Role of Lymphocytes in Induction and Pathogenesis of Eosinophilic Esophagitis

To examine whether lymphocytes play a role in the induction of EoE, Mishra and colleagues[37] used a murine model of EoE created by intranasal instillation of *Aspergillus fumigatus* antigen, which resulted in pulmonary and esophageal eosinophilia. Lymphocytes were found to be increased in the esophagus of *Aspergillus*-treated mice compared with saline-treated mice.[38] Specifically, a twofold increase in B cells and a fourfold to fivefold increase in CD4$^+$ and CD8$^+$ T lymphocytes were found. B and T lymphocytes were detected in the mucosal and submucosal regions of the esophagus. When *RAG-1* gene–deficient mice lacking B and T cells were intranasally challenged with *Aspergillus* antigen, no esophageal infiltration was found, indicating an important role for lymphocytes in EoE induction. Using B cell–deficient mice (IgH6) and T cell–deficient mice (Foxn1), the investigators were able to demonstrate that T cells, rather than B cells, were important in the induction of esophageal eosinophilia. Within T cells, CD4$^+$ rather than CD8$^+$ cells were shown to be important: CD4-deficient mice were moderately protected from the induction of EoE, whereas CD8α-deficient mice developed unaltered EoE.

In humans, the role of lymphocytes in the induction of EoE is less clear. B lymphocyte function in EoE has not been examined. Although slightly increased in number in the esophagus of EoE patients, it is not known whether these B cells bear IgE and hence contribute to the pool of IgE-positive cells (most of which are thought to be mast cells) found in the esophagus of patients who have EoE. B lymphocytes are known to be capable of holding antigens to their surface for recognition by specific T lymphocytes along with major histocompatibility complex class II molecules.[39] The potential role of B cells in antigen presentation in EoE remains to be tested.

The role of T lymphocytes, especially CD4 cells in the induction of EoE in humans, has not been directly investigated. Various descriptive studies, however, point to T_H2 adaptive immunity in EoE. The role of T_H2 cytokines in the induction of EoE was demonstrated by Mishra and colleagues[40] in a murine model of EoE. Intratracheal delivery of the T_H2 cytokine IL-13 to mice induces dose-dependent esophageal eosinophilia by an IL-5 and STAT6–dependent mechanism. These results strongly implicate T_H2-associated immune responses in the pathogenesis of EoE, indicating that the T_H2 phenotype in EoE is potentially crucial in its pathogenesis in humans.

In humans, aside from the many clinical short-term therapeutic studies linking the induction of EoE to food allergens[2,3,5] and therefore pointing to a T_H2 type of immune response, various investigators have examined the predominant cytokines in the peripheral blood and the esophagus of patients who have EoE and found them to be consistent with a T_H2 phenotype.

In the peripheral circulation, Bullock and colleagues[41] examined cytokine expression by peripheral blood mononuclear cells (PBMCs) and found that children who had active EoE had an increased percentage of $CD4^+$ T cells expressing IL-5 compared with nonatopic control subjects. This percentage was lower in EoE patients in remission than in patients who had active disease. Straumann and colleagues[36] stimulated PBMCs of EoE patients with phytohemagglutinin, a nonspecific stimulant, and measured resultant cytokine secretion by the PBMCs. Increased release of the T_H2 cytokine IL-13 was found in 40% of the patients studied. Yamazaki and colleagues[42] conducted similar experiments using stimulation with specific allergens. PBMCs from 15 adult patients who had EoE were incubated in vitro with food allergen extracts and aeroallergen extracts. Food extracts consisted of milk, egg, soy, wheat, and peanut. Compared with healthy control subjects, PBMCs from EoE patients secreted significantly more of the T_H2 cytokine IL-5, IL-13, or both in response to various allergens, even in the absence of clear-cut sensitization to the allergens when serum levels of allergen-specific IgE were measured. Whether the T_H2 response is secondary to the concomitant atopic features of the patients remains unknown, because 73% of the EoE patients in the study had concurrent allergic disease, a finding common to patients who have EoE.[43,44] A study comparing EoE patients with non-EoE allergic control subjects is needed to confirm these findings.

In the esophagus, increased levels of the T_H2 cytokine IL-5 in biopsy samples of patients who had EoE were found, whether assayed at the messenger RNA (mRNA) level by real-time polymerase chain reaction (RT-PCR) or at the protein level using immunohistochemical staining of esophageal sections.[36,45] Using microarray analysis, mRNA for IL-4 and IL-13, two other T_H2 cytokines, were not detected or up-regulated in the esophagus of patients who had EoE.[46] Using RT-PCR, a more sensitive technique, esophageal IL-13 was found to be increased in patients who had EoE compared with control subjects.[47] IL-13, in turn, likely plays an important role in EoE pathogenesis: when stimulated with IL-13 in vitro, esophageal epithelial cells produce high levels of eotaxin-3,[47] a highly induced chemokine in EoE that is shown to regulate eosinophil responses in vitro[48] and to correlate with the severity of esophageal eosinophilia in EoE.[46]

Identification of the specific inflammatory cells producing the T_H2 cytokines just described, however, has not been done. As a result, we do not know the exact extent of the lymphocytes' contribution to the production of these T_H2 cytokines, especially given that other immune cells can also secrete these cytokines. For example, when esophageal eosinophils of patients who had EoE were examined for T_H2 cytokine expression using immunohistochemical staining, 60% of these cells were found to express IL-4 and IL-13.[49] Further studies addressing the specific contribution of esophageal lymphocytes to the production of T_H2 cytokines, especially in response to specific dietary allergens, need to be performed.

No studies addressing regulatory T cells and their corresponding cytokines such as TGF-β in EoE have been published. The coexistence of EoE in patients who have other diseases such as celiac disease[50,51] and Crohn's disease (Mirna Chehade, MD, Hugh A. Sampson, MD, unpublished data, 2008), both characterized by a predominant T_H1 rather than a T_H2 phenotype, points to the potential importance of abnormal regulatory cell function leading to the development of these diseases in the same patient and warrants further study.

EOSINOPHILIC GASTROENTERITIS

Lymphocytes are Increased in Number in Eosinophilic Gastroenteritis

Jaffe and colleagues[52] counted the number of lymphocytes in gastric biopsy samples of patients who had EG characterized by moderate to severe gastric eosinophilia. A twofold to threefold increase in the number of T cells was found in gastric biopsy samples of patients who had EG compared with normal gastric tissue in control subjects using immunohistochemical staining. No further differentiation into CD4+ and CD8+ cells was performed. B cells were found only in the rare benign lymphoid aggregates and were absent in the epithelium and lamina propria of EG patients and control subjects. As with EoE, these findings also indicate a more prominent role for T lymphocytes and adaptive immunity than for humoral immunity in EG.

The Role of Lymphocytes in Induction and Pathogenesis of Eosinophilic Gastroenteritis

Using a murine model of EG, Hogan and colleagues[53] demonstrated that gastrointestinal eosinophil accumulation was antigen induced and associated with a T_H2 phenotype. Oral challenge of allergen-sensitized mice with enteric-coated beads containing the allergen resulted in marked serum allergen–specific IgE, increased splenic T lymphocyte secretion of the T_H2 cytokines IL-4 and IL-5 following in vitro allergen restimulation, and increased eosinophil accumulation in the blood and small intestine compared with placebo-challenged mice. Therefore, the accumulation of gastrointestinal eosinophils may be antigen induced and associated with a T_H2 phenotype.

In patients who have EG, mRNA levels for IL-5 are slightly increased in gastric mucosal biopsy samples compared with those of control subjects when assayed by RT-PCR. In contrast, mRNA for the T_H1 cytokine interferon (IFN)-γ was undetectable in the stomach of EG patients but demonstrable in that of normal control subjects.[52] These results point to a T_H2 phenotype in EG in humans, as demonstrated for EoE. Similar to EoE, the cellular sources of the cytokines studied were not specifically determined, resulting in a lack of a direct evidence for the degree of tissue T lymphocyte contribution to this phenotype.

In the peripheral circulation, the role of T cells was more directly investigated in patients who had EG. T-cell synthesis of IL-5 was increased in patients who had EG compared with control subjects, especially the CD4 subset.[52] When stimulated nonspecifically with the mitogen phytohemagglutinin, production of the T_H2 cytokines IL-4 and IL-5 was found to be markedly elevated in EG patients compared with control subjects.[52] Mitogen-stimulated synthesis of the T_H1 cytokine IFN-γ by CD4 cells was normal. These results again point to a T_H2 phenotype and suggest a role for T lymphocytes in the pathogenesis of EG.

Beyer and colleagues[54] examined cytokine secretion by tissue lymphocytes in response to specific allergens in patients who had EG. In this study, duodenal biopsy specimens from patients who had EG and milk-induced symptoms and from control individuals were minced and cultured in vitro with nonspecific mitogens (phytohemagglutinin, phorbol myristate acetate, and irradiated PBMCs) or with milk proteins (α-casein, β-casein, α-lactalbumin, and β-lactoglobulin). Polyclonal expansion of mucosal T cells using mitogens resulted in predominantly T_H1 cells from the duodenum of EG patients and control subjects. After stimulation with milk proteins, milk-specific mucosal T-cell lines could be established from most patients who had EG but from none of the control subjects. In contrast to nonspecific polyclonal expansion, milk-specific expansion showed a clear T_H2 cytokine profile, with T lymphocytes releasing predominantly IL-5 and IL-13 following in vitro restimulation with milk proteins. These results show that intestinal allergen-specific T lymphocytes release T_H2 cytokines following allergen stimulation, potentially playing an important role in the pathogenesis of EG.

In both studies,[52,54] the T_H1 proinflammatory cytokine IFN-γ was also found to be excessively produced by peripheral blood and intestinal T lymphocytes of patients who had EG following in vitro stimulation, although to a much lesser extent than the T_H2 cytokines.

Equally important in Beyer and colleagues'[54] study was the lack of production of the regulatory cytokines TGF-β and IL-10 by duodenal milk-specific T lymphocytes of patients who had milk-allergic EG when stimulated in vitro with milk proteins.[54] These findings point to a lack of a tolerogenic response by lymphocytes in response to food allergens in patients who have EG and warrant further investigation for future therapeutic dietary interventions.

SUMMARY

EGIDs appear to be antigen-driven diseases, with an increase in the number of T lymphocytes detectable in the tissue involved with inflammation and eosinophilia. Ex vivo examination reveals a T_H2-predominant phenotype of involved tissues using biopsy samples or following antigenic stimulation of peripheral or tissue lymphocytes. The exact role of these lymphocytes in the induction and pathogenesis of EGIDs in patients is still not confirmed, however. Although T lymphocytes were shown in murine models to have an essential role in induction of EoE, little is known about their exact role in human EGIDs. More studies are needed to determine sites of antigen absorption, inductive sites for T lymphocytes, and homing molecules for these T lymphocytes back to the diseased tissues. These studies will help tailor development of targeted therapies for EGIDs. In addition, the contribution of T lymphocytes in the pathogenesis and severity of EGIDs still needs to be fully investigated. The T_H2 cytokine IL-13 was shown to be important in disease pathogenesis in human EoE; however, the extent of T-lymphocyte contribution to the production of this cytokine and other T_H2 cytokines still needs to be elucidated. Furthermore, the effect of elevated T_H2 cytokines on tissue eosinophilia needs to be studied. Results from these studies may help determine whether concomitant therapies are needed in some patients, especially when using therapies specifically targeting eosinophils. Finally, mechanisms leading to a breach of oral tolerance in patients who have EGIDs are still preliminary. So far, we know only that tissue antigen–specific T cells from patients who have EG do not produce T regulatory cytokines on in vitro restimulation. Because the sensitization potential for dietary antigens cannot be identified using standard diagnostic techniques (eg, prick skin tests or serum food allergen–specific IgE levels), the potential for achieving tolerance to these foods cannot be predicted in patients who have EGIDs. Therefore, studies dissecting mechanisms of oral tolerance and subsequent ways to monitor for the development of tolerance in patients who have EGIDs are crucial, because they may help dictate timing of dietary antigen re-introduction in patients on restricted diets and thus improve the quality of life of patients suffering from these diseases.

REFERENCES

1. Rothenberg ME. Eosinophilic gastrointestinal disorders (EGID). J Allergy Clin Immunol 2004;113(1):11–28.
2. Kelly KJ, Lazenby AJ, Rowe PC, et al. Eosinophilic esophagitis attributed to gastroesophageal reflux: improvement with an amino acid-based formula. Gastroenterology 1995;109(5):1503–12.
3. Markowitz JE, Spergel JM, Ruchelli E, et al. Elemental diet is an effective treatment for eosinophilic esophagitis in children and adolescents. Am J Gastroenterol 2003;98(4):777–82.
4. Chehade M, Magid MS, Mofidi S, et al. Allergic eosinophilic gastroenteritis with protein-losing enteropathy: intestinal pathology, clinical course, and long-term follow-up. J Pediatr Gastroenterol Nutr 2006;42(5):516–21.
5. Spergel JM, Beausoleil JL, Mascarenhas M, et al. The use of skin prick tests and patch tests to identify causative foods in eosinophilic esophagitis. J Allergy Clin Immunol 2002;109(2):363–8.
6. Kagalwalla AF, Sentongo TA, Ritz S, et al. Effect of six-food elimination diet on clinical and histologic outcomes in eosinophilic esophagitis. Clin Gastroenterol Hepatol 2006;4(9):1097–102.
7. Chase M. Inhibition of experimental drug allergy by prior feeding of the sensitizing agent. Proc Soc Exp Biol 1946;61:257–9.
8. Rescigno M, Urbano M, Valzasina B, et al. Dendritic cells express tight junction proteins and penetrate gut epithelial monolayers to sample bacteria. Nat Immunol 2001;2(4):361–7.
9. Sicinski P, Rowinski J, Warchol JB, et al. Poliovirus type 1 enters the human host through intestinal M cells. Gastroenterology 1990;98(1):56–8.
10. Shreedhar VK, Kelsall BL, Neutra MR. Cholera toxin induces migration of dendritic cells from the subepithelial dome region to T- and B-cell areas of Peyer's patches. Infect Immun 2003;71(1):504–9.
11. Kraehenbuhl JP, Neutra MR. Transepithelial transport and mucosal defense II: secretion of IgA. Trends Cell Biol 1992;2(6):170–4.
12. Walker WA, Isselbacher KJ. Uptake and transport of macromolecules by the intestine. Possible role in clinical disorders. Gastroenterology 1974;67(3):531–50.
13. Warshaw AL, Walker WA, Isselbacher KJ. Protein uptake by the intestine: evidence for absorption of intact macromolecules. Gastroenterology 1974;66(5):987–92.
14. Mason DW, Dallman M, Barclay AN. Graft-versus-host disease induces expression of Ia antigen in rat epidermal cells and gut epithelium. Nature 1981;293(5828):150–1.

15. Scott H, Solheim BG, Brandtzaeg P, et al. HLA-DR-like antigens in the epithelium of the human small intestine. Scand J Immunol 1980;12(1):77–82.
16. Whitacre CC, Gienapp IE, Orosz CG, et al. Oral tolerance in experimental autoimmune encephalomyelitis III. Evidence for clonal anergy. J Immunol 1991;147(7): 2155–63.
17. Appleman LJ, Boussiotis VA. T cell anergy and costimulation. Immunol Rev 2003; 192:161–80.
18. Chen Y, Inobe J, Marks R, et al. Peripheral deletion of antigen-reactive T cells in oral tolerance. Nature 1995;376(6536):177–80.
19. Mayer L, Shlien R. Evidence for function of Ia molecules on gut epithelial cells in man. J Exp Med 1987;166(5):1471–83.
20. Bland PW, Warren LG. Antigen presentation by epithelial cells of the rat small intestine. II. Selective induction of suppressor T cells. Immunology 1986;58(1): 9–14.
21. Trop S, Samsonov D, Gotsman I, et al. Liver-associated lymphocytes expressing NK1.1 are essential for oral immune tolerance induction in a murine model. Hepatology 1999;29(3):746–55.
22. Chen Y, Inobe J, Weiner HL. Induction of oral tolerance to myelin basic protein in CD8-depleted mice: both CD4+ and CD8+ cells mediate active suppression. J Immunol 1995;155(2):910–6.
23. Barone KS, Jain SL, Michael JG. Effect of in vivo depletion of CD4+ and CD8+ cells on the induction and maintenance of oral tolerance. Cell Immunol 1995; 163(1):19–29.
24. Garside P, Steel M, Liew FY, et al. CD4+ but not CD8+ T cells are required for the induction of oral tolerance. Int Immunol 1995;7(3):501–4.
25. Chen Y, Kuchroo VK, Inobe J, et al. Regulatory T cell clones induced by oral tolerance: suppression of autoimmune encephalomyelitis. Science 1994;265(5176):1237–40.
26. Meade R, Askenase PW, Geba GP, et al. Transforming growth factor-beta 1 inhibits murine immediate and delayed type hypersensitivity. J Immunol 1992; 149(2):521–8.
27. Groux H, O'Garra A, Bigler M, et al. A CD4+ T-cell subset inhibits antigen-specific T-cell responses and prevents colitis. Nature 1997;389(6652):737–42.
28. Zhang X, Izikson L, Liu L, et al. Activation of CD25(+)CD4(+) regulatory T cells by oral antigen administration. J Immunol 2001;167(8):4245–53.
29. Nakamura K, Kitani A, Strober W. Cell contact-dependent immunosuppression by CD4(+)CD25(+) regulatory T cells is mediated by cell surface-bound transforming growth factor beta. J Exp Med 2001;194(5):629–44.
30. Chehade M, Mayer L. Oral tolerance and its relation to food hypersensitivities. J Allergy Clin Immunol 2005;115(1):3–12.
31. Lucendo AJ, Navarro M, Comas C, et al. Immunophenotypic characterization and quantification of the epithelial inflammatory infiltrate in eosinophilic esophagitis through stereology: an analysis of the cellular mechanisms of the disease and the immunologic capacity of the esophagus. Am J Surg Pathol 2007;31(4): 598–606.
32. Mangano MM, Antonioli DA, Schnitt SJ, et al. Nature and significance of cells with irregular nuclear contours in esophageal mucosal biopsies. Mod Pathol 1992; 5(2):191–6.
33. Cucchiara S, D'Armiento F, Alfieri E, et al. Intraepithelial cells with irregular nuclear contours as a marker of esophagitis in children with gastroesophageal reflux disease. Dig Dis Sci 1995;40(11):2305–11.

34. Geboes K, De Wolf-Peeters C, Rutgeerts P, et al. Lymphocytes and Langerhans cells in the human oesophageal epithelium. Virchows Arch A Pathol Anat Histopathol 1983;401(1):45–55.
35. Teitelbaum JE, Fox VL, Twarog FJ, et al. Eosinophilic esophagitis in children: immunopathological analysis and response to fluticasone propionate. Gastroenterology 2002;122(5):1216–25.
36. Straumann A, Bauer M, Fischer B, et al. Idiopathic eosinophilic esophagitis is associated with a T(H)2-type allergic inflammatory response. J Allergy Clin Immunol 2001;108(6):954–61.
37. Mishra A, Hogan SP, Brandt EB, et al. An etiological role for aeroallergens and eosinophils in experimental esophagitis. J Clin Invest 2001;107(1):83–90.
38. Mishra A, Schlotman J, Wang M, et al. Critical role for adaptive T cell immunity in experimental eosinophilic esophagitis in mice. J Leukoc Biol 2007;81(4):916–24.
39. Pierce SK, Morris JF, Grusby MJ, et al. Antigen-presenting function of B lymphocytes. Immunol Rev 1988;106:149–80.
40. Mishra A, Rothenberg ME. Intratracheal IL-13 induces eosinophilic esophagitis by an IL-5, eotaxin-1, and STAT6-dependent mechanism. Gastroenterology 2003;125(5):1419–27.
41. Bullock JZ, Villanueva JM, Blanchard C, et al. Interplay of adaptive Th2 immunity with eotaxin-3/c-C chemokine receptor 3 in eosinophilic esophagitis. J Pediatr Gastroenterol Nutr 2007;45(1):22–31.
42. Yamazaki K, Murray JA, Arora AS, et al. Allergen-specific in vitro cytokine production in adult patients with eosinophilic esophagitis. Dig Dis Sci 2006;51(11):1934–41.
43. Simon D, Marti H, Heer P, et al. Eosinophilic esophagitis is frequently associated with IgE-mediated allergic airway diseases. J Allergy Clin Immunol 2005;115(5):1090–2.
44. Liacouras CA, Spergel JM, Ruchelli E, et al. Eosinophilic esophagitis: a 10-year experience in 381 children. Clin Gastroenterol Hepatol 2005;3(12):1198–206.
45. Gupta SK, Fitzgerald JF, Kondratyuk T, et al. Cytokine expression in normal and inflamed esophageal mucosa: a study into the pathogenesis of allergic eosinophilic esophagitis. J Pediatr Gastroenterol Nutr 2006;42(1):22–6.
46. Blanchard C, Wang N, Stringer KF, et al. Eotaxin-3 and a uniquely conserved gene-expression profile in eosinophilic esophagitis. J Clin Invest 2006;116(2):536–47.
47. Blanchard C, Mingler MK, Vicario M, et al. IL-13 involvement in eosinophilic esophagitis: transcriptome analysis and reversibility with glucocorticoids. J Allergy Clin Immunol 2007;120(6):1292–300.
48. Kitaura M, Suzuki N, Imai T, et al. Molecular cloning of a novel human CC chemokine (Eotaxin-3) that is a functional ligand of CC chemokine receptor 3. J Biol Chem 1999;274(39):27975–80.
49. Straumann A, Kristl J, Conus S, et al. Cytokine expression in healthy and inflamed mucosa: probing the role of eosinophils in the digestive tract. Inflamm Bowel Dis 2005;11(8):720–6.
50. Verzegnassi F, Bua J, De Angelis P, et al. Eosinophilic oesophagitis and coeliac disease: is it just a casual association? Gut 2007;56(7):1029–30.
51. Quaglietta L, Coccorullo P, Miele E, et al. Eosinophilic oesophagitis and coeliac disease: is there an association? Aliment Pharmacol Ther 2007;26(3):487–93.
52. Jaffe JS, James SP, Mullins GE, et al. Evidence for an abnormal profile of interleukin-4 (IL-4), IL-5, and gamma-interferon (gamma-IFN) in peripheral blood T cells from patients with allergic eosinophilic gastroenteritis. J Clin Immunol 1994;14(5):299–309.

53. Hogan SP, Mishra A, Brandt EB, et al. A critical role for eotaxin in experimental oral antigen-induced eosinophilic gastrointestinal allergy. Proc Natl Acad Sci U S A 2000;97(12):6681–6.
54. Beyer K, Castro R, Birnbaum A, et al. Human milk-specific mucosal lymphocytes of the gastrointestinal tract display a TH2 cytokine profile. J Allergy Clin Immunol 2002;109(4):707–13.

The Role of the High-Affinity IgE Receptor, FcεRI, in Eosinophilic Gastrointestinal Diseases

Eleonora Dehlink, MD, PhD[a,b], Edda Fiebiger, PhD[a,*]

KEYWORDS

- Fc-reception • Food allergy • Th2 mucosa
- Gastrointestinal inflammation

Primary eosinophilic gastrointestinal disorders (EGIDs) are a heterogeneous group of diseases that include eosinophilic esophagitis (EoE), eosinophilic gastritis, eosinophilic gastroenteritis, eosinophilic enteritis, and eosinophilic colitis. The unifying hallmark and diagnostic marker of EGIDs is an eosinophil-rich inflammatory infiltrate of the gastrointestinal mucosa, in the absence of known causes for eosinophilia. The etiology of EGIDs is not yet fully understood. The pathogenesis, however, seems to involve a complex interplay of genetic predisposition, exposure to food and environmental allergens, and IgE-mediated activation of the immune system.[1–4] Accumulating evidence relates EGIDs to the group of immune disorders, such as IgE-mediated allergy, mediated by T helper type 2 cells. This article describes a possible role of IgE-mediated immune-activation via the high-affinity receptor for IgE, FcεRI, in the pathogenesis of primary EGIDs.

This work was supported in part by the Children's Digestive Health and Nutrition Foundation Young Investigator Award of the North American Society for Pediatric Gastroenterology, Hepatology & Nutrition and the Gerber Foundation (to Dr. Fiebiger) and the Austrian Program for Advanced Research and Technology of the Austrian Academy of Sciences (Dr. Dehlink).

[a] Division of Gastroenterology and Nutrition, Children's Hospital Boston, Harvard Medical School, 300 Longwood Avenue, Enders 724, Boston, MA 02115, USA
[b] Department of Pediatrics and Adolescent Medicine, Medical University of Vienna, Waehringer Guertel 18-20, 1090 Vienna, Austria
* Corresponding author.
E-mail address: edda.fiebiger@childrens.harvard.edu (E. Fiebiger).

Immunol Allergy Clin N Am 29 (2009) 159–170
doi:10.1016/j.iac.2008.09.004
0889-8561/08/$ – see front matter © 2009 Elsevier Inc. All rights reserved.

immunology.theclinics.com

EOSINOPHILIC GASTROINTESTINAL DISORDERS AS IgE-MEDIATED ALLERGIC DISEASES?—PROS AND CONS

Several lines of evidence support the concept of EGIDs as some form of allergic disorder. A majority of patients with EGIDs have concomitant IgE-mediated allergies to food and aeroallergens, making a possible causal relation between EGIDs, especially EoE, and IgE-mediated allergies a pertinent subject of discussion. EoE has been increasingly confused with erosive esophagitis in the adult gastrointestinal (GI) world. A growing body of data shows a strong association with allergic sensitizations and atopic illnesses. Positive skin-prick tests to common environmental and food allergens are seen in up to 79% of children with EoE.[5] In a recent case series of 23 adults with EoE, 82% had serum IgE specific for one or more food allergens, and 78% had allergic diseases, mainly allergic rhinitis.[6] Atopic disorders in general seem to be more prevalent in patients with EoE compared with the total population. In an Australian cohort of 45 children with EoE, 55.56% also had atopic eczema, 66.67% had asthma, and 93.33% had allergic rhinitis.[7] A study in adults previously diagnosed with EoE revealed that 68% had a present or past history of allergic illnesses, rhinitis being the most common, and 77% had sensitizations to aeroallergens.[8] Food allergens in particular have been shown to be causally linked with EoE. For most patients, elimination of foods based on allergy testing or an elemental diet abolished symptoms and reversed histologic pathologies.[9–11] The sensitization spectrum to food allergens in children with EoE is comparable to that for the general pediatric population, with milk, egg, soy, peanut, and wheat being most common.[5,12] As is typical in a "classic" allergy, the sensitization pattern in adult EoE patients seems to shift toward dietary allergens cross-reactive with aeroallergens, such as carrot, tomato, and wheat.[6,8] While classic IgE-mediated anaphylaxis is generally rare in EGIDs patients, a single study reported a history of anaphylaxis in 24% of children with EoE, a rate 100 times that of the general population.[7]

Further evidence of a close pathophysiological link between "classic" IgE-mediated allergic disorders and EGIDs is the finding that allergic inflammation of the respiratory system during allergen season is accompanied by eosinophil infiltration of the gastrointestinal mucosa. Eosinophilic inflammation of the esophageal mucosa[13] and duodenal mucosa[14] has been found in patients with respiratory tract allergy during the pollen season. Some EoE patients even experience a seasonal variation in symptoms and esophageal inflammation, depending on the environmental allergen burden.[15] In children newly diagnosed with EoE, the intensity of esophageal eosinophilia was higher in the summer than during the winter months, further emphasizing a role of seasonal environmental allergens in the pathogenesis of EoE.[16]

Most strikingly, EGIDs patients have been shown to benefit from IgE-targeted therapy. In nine adult patients with eosinophilic gastroenteritis and a history of atopy, treatment with anti-IgE antibodies (omalizumab) significantly decreased symptom scores, serum IgE levels, and allergen skin test wheal and erythema responses. Absolute blood eosinophil counts as well as tissue eosinophila in the duodenum and the gastric antrum also declined.[17]

While evidence in support of pathogenetic implications of IgE-mediated allergies for EoE is accumulating, limited data are available for primary eosinophilic gastritis, enteritis, and gastroenteritis. Some investigators report atopy and increased serum IgE levels to food proteins in a majority of their EoE patients and resolution of symptoms upon elimination of the causal allergen or elemental diet.[4] In eosinophilic colitis, IgE does not seem to play a role, and radioallergosorbent and skin-prick tests are characteristically negative.[4,18]

IgE-mediated mechanisms play a role in up to 79% of EoE patients and a considerable subgroup of patients with other EGIDs, but such mechanisms are likely only one component in the complex pathophysiology of EGIDs.[4,12] In contrast, a substantial group of patients with EGIDs are not atopic.[4,12] They show no measurable allergen-specific serum IgE, have negative skin-prick tests, and no symptoms temporally related to allergen exposure. Still, many patients without elevated specific serum IgE respond to elimination of certain foods or an elemental diet. In these patients, T cell–mediated mechanisms, consistent with the delayed-type food hypersensitivity, have been suggested by several studies. Peripheral blood T cells from patients with allergic eosinophilic gastroenteritis have been described to be of the T helper type 2 (Th-2) phenotype.[19] Beyer and colleagues[20] reported a Th-2 skew in milk-specific T cell lines from the duodenal lamina propria of children with and without milk-specific IgE who had been diagnosed with eosinophilic gastroenteritis. Blood lymphocytes of positively challenged children with milk- and soy-protein induced enterocolitis proliferated upon in vitro stimulation with soy, cow's milk, and egg white.[21] In a murine model, induction of experimental EoE was accompanied by an increase in B- and T-lymphocyte subpopulations in the esophagus, and mice lacking adaptive immunity or deficient in T cells were protected from disease.[22] In the absence of measureable serum IgE, a proposal has emerged that a local population of IgE-producing B cells or cell-bound IgE in resident mucosal immune cells may play a role. However, such a population has not yet been identified in EGID patients.

In summary, clinical and experimental data suggest that IgE sensitizations and atopic illnesses are highly associated with EGIDs, but whether they are causally linked or just concomitant disorders is not clear yet. Nevertheless, because the majority of patients feature IgE sensitizations and allergy to food and environmental allergens, local IgE-mediated mechanisms are highly likely to play a role. Available data suggest that EGIDs are positioned between purely IgE-mediated, immediate-type allergies and cellular-mediated delayed-type Th-2 responses. Based on these pieces of evidence, we hypothesize that the high-affinity IgE receptor, FcεRI, plays a role in the pathogenesis of EGIDs.

THE HIGH-AFFINITY RECEPTOR FOR IgE, FcεRI

FcεRI is one of the key molecules in the pathophysiology of allergic reactions.[23–25] As a multimeric cell surface receptor, FcεRI shares with other immune recognition receptors the overall structure of a ligand-binding immunoglobulin domain–containing protein (α-chain) associated with signaling subunits that regulate cellular activation (β- and γ-chains) (**Fig. 1**).[24,26,27] FcεRI binds its ligand, the Fc part of IgE, monovalently via its α-chain. IgE binding per se does not lead to activation of immune cells. The extremely stable IgE-receptor complex on the surface of peripheral blood and tissue cells should rather be pictured as a loaded gun waiting for contact with IgE-specific antigens, which trigger the allergic cascade.

Activation of the immune system via FcεRI is dependent on multivalent crosslinking of FcεRIα-bound specific IgE. FcεRIα, however, only contains the IgE-binding site. Signaling events are initiated via immunoreceptor tyrosine-based activation motifs of the signaling subunits, the β- and γ-chains. A rather uncommon feature of FcεRI is that this receptor complex is expressed in different isoforms in a manner dependent on cell type and species. FcεRI can be expressed either as a tetrameric or a trimeric isoform. Tetrameric FcεRI, composed of the ligand-binding α-chain, one β-chain, and a pair of disulphide-linked γ-subunits ($FcεRI\alpha\beta\gamma_2$), is found on the surface of immune-effector cells, such as basophils and mast cells in rodents and humans (see **Fig. 1**). In

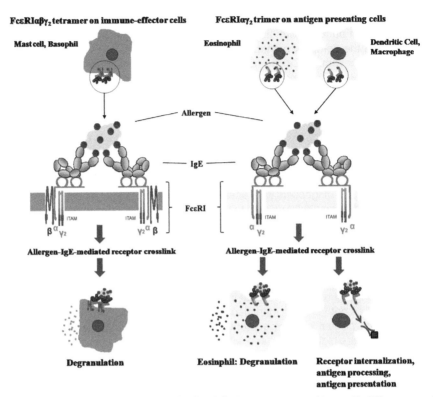

Fig.1. IgE-FcεRI–mediated activation of cells of the immune system. Human FcεRI is expressed on mast cells and basophils in its tetrameric isoform (FcεRIαβγ$_2$) (*left panel*). Eosinophils, dendritic cells, and macrophages express the trimeric isoform of the receptor (FcεRIαγ$_2$) (*right panel*). Allergens activate immune cells by crosslinking FcεRI complexes loaded with specific IgE. The IgE-binding α-chain associates with the signaling subunits, β and γ. Each immunoreceptor tyrosine-based activation motif (ITAM) of the signaling subunits uses phosphotyrosin-based activation to induce degranulation of mast cells, basophils, and eosinophils. Dendritic cells and macrophages internalize allergen-IgE complexes after FcεRI crosslinking and shuttle them toward antigen presentation to elicit T helper cell responses.

the absence of β-transcripts, humans express a trimeric version of FcεRI on many cells of the innate and adaptive immune systems, including eosinophils and antigen-presenting cells (APCs).

The best-described regulator of FcεRI surface expression levels is the receptor's natural ligand, IgE. Binding of monomeric IgE to FcεRIα stabilizes the receptor at the cell surface as an IgE-FcεRI complex. This stabilization enhances surface expression of the receptor on immune-effector cells, as well as on APCs. The mechanism of this stabilization is not completely understood. Receptor surface stability seems to depend solely on the length of the stalk region of the FcεRIα chain.[28] In vivo, the cell surface density of FcεRI is thus tightly correlated with serum IgE levels. Allergic individuals show enhanced surface expression of the receptor on peripheral blood basophils, monocytes, and dendritic cells. Along the same line, treatment with anti-IgE monoclonal antibodies, such as omalizumab, not only decreases serum IgE but also FcεRI-surface expression on peripheral blood cells.[29,30] Lower levels of surface FcεRI consecutively render immune cells less sensitive to allergen stimuli, as shown by a significant increase in the allergen dose required for in vitro basophil activation following omalizumab therapy of eosinophilic gastroenteritis patients.[17]

With regards to EGIDs, it is important to stress that FcεRI expression on eosinophils also correlates with serum IgE concentrations.[31] Furthermore, gene-expression profile analysis in EoE shows elevated levels of FcεRI.[32] This review argues for a role of FcεRI-mediated immune activation in the gastrointestinal mucosa of EGID patients. Beyond the defined role of tetrameric FcεRI on mast cells and basophils in type I allergic reactions, we hypothesize that expression of trimeric FcεRI on human eosinophils and APCs is critically involved in the pathology of EGIDs.

IgE AND IgE-BINDING STRUCTURES IN THE GASTROINTESTINAL MUCOSA

The gastrointestinal immune system must balance its ability to respond to pathogens while remaining unresponsive to food and environmental antigens and the commensal microbiota.[33] Distortion of this delicate immune equilibrium in the gastrointestinal tract can result in a break of oral tolerance and precipitate inappropriate immune reactions,[34] including immediate hypersensitivity and EGIDs. The lines of defense against pathogens in the gastrointestinal tract include immunoglobulins, such as IgE. IgE antibodies are secreted into the gastrointestinal mucous by B cells of the lamina propria to immediately sense invading pathogens. In parallel with the falling numbers of parasite infections in industrialized countries, the specificity of the IgE repertoire has shifted from pathogens toward innocuous environmental antigens over the past century. This shift is reflected in the rising numbers of patients suffering from IgE-mediated allergies to airborne and food allergens.[35-37]

Once an individual is sensitized to an allergen, allergen-specific IgE can be found in the serum, and is also secreted into various body fluids lining mucous membranes. Nasal fluid from children with respiratory allergies,[14] bronchoalveolar lavage from asthmatics[38] and stool of food-allergic patients[39] contain allergen-specific IgE. Whether or not the saliva or stool of patients suffering from EGIDs also contains IgE remains to be analyzed.

IgE signals the presence of specific ligands at the mucosal surface to the mucosal immune system via IgE receptors. In addition to FcεRI, the high-affinity IgE receptor, humans express two other surface receptors for IgE in the gastrointestinal tract: the low-affinity IgE receptor, FcεRII or CD23, and galectin-3. Intestinal epithelial cells constitutively express the low-affinity IgE receptor CD23.[40,41] So far, no data exist on the expression of FcεRI or galectin-3 on intestinal epithelial cells. FcεRI is, however, expressed on many immune-effector cells and APCs abundant in the mucosa throughout the gastrointestinal tract (see below). Here, we will focus on IgE-mediated FcεRI activation, which we believe to be critical in the pathology of EGIDs. Note that a detailed, comparative analysis of the nature and expression levels of IgE-binding structures in the gastrointestinal tract of healthy subjects and patients suffering from EGIDs is lacking so far. Detailed information on IgE-receptor expression in the gastrointestinal tracts of healthy subjects and diseased subjects will shed new light on mechanisms of IgE-mediated immune activation in EGIDs.

IgE TRANSPORT IN THE GASTROINTESTINAL TRACT

The common consensus is that CD23 acts as a transport receptor for IgE sampling in the gastrointestinal mucosa.[42,43] IgE-mediated activation of the gastrointestinal immune system via CD23 has been studied in detail because intestinal epithelial cells constitutively express this receptor in mice as well as in humans.[23,40] Intestinal epithelial cells use CD23 to mediate transepithelial crossing of intact IgE-allergen complexes.[44,45] Once these complexes bridge the barrier, they activate subepithelial mast cells and initiate immediate allergic responses in the gastrointestinal mucosa.[39] Besides transcytosis of IgE-antigen complexes, engagement of CD23 induces the release of IL-8 and CCL20 from intestinal epithelial cells.[46] These chemokines are capable of recruiting effector cells of late-phase allergic reactions and APCs. Strikingly, IL-8 is also one of the most important eosinophil chemoattractant cytokines.[47] The role of CD23 thus seems to extend to that of a pure transcytosis receptor at the gastrointestinal mucosal surface. CD23-triggered release of chemoattractants upon allergen exposure could contribute to the formation of the eosinophil-rich infiltrates characteristic of EGIDs.

While the role of CD23 in the gastrointestinal mucosa has been established, no reports on FcεRI expression on epithelial cells exist. It is therefore rather unlikely that FcεRI is a transcytosis receptor in intestinal epithelial cells. However, humans abundantly express FcεRI in the mucosa throughout the gastrointestinal tract on APCs, such as Langerhans cells and dendritic cells.[48,49] In the oral mucosa, Langerhans cells constitutively express FcεRI in atopic and nonatopic patients.[50] Langerhans cells are also found in the esophageal epithelium.[51] Humans constitutively express FcεRI in dendritic cells of the esophagus, the stomach, and the small intestine (Dehlink and colleagues, unpublished observation). Dendritic cells are not simply resident cells in the lamina propria of the gastrointestinal tract. They are able to open tight junctions of the epithelial cell barrier and send out projections into the intestinal lumen to monitor the antigenic environment of the gastrointestinal tract and sample noninvasive luminal bacteria.[52,53] It is tempting to speculate that FcεRI on these dendritic cell protrusions functions as a transport receptor for IgE or IgE-antigen complexes into the lamina propria of the gastrointestinal tract in healthy or diseased subjects. This hypothesis remains to be investigated.

Transepithelial shuttling of IgE and IgE-antigen complexes is yet only one possible task of FcεRI on immune cells in the gastrointestinal mucosa. The extremely stable monovalent, high-affinity interaction of IgE with FcεRIα allows us to speculate about another trafficking mechanism. FcεRIα on blood cells could serve as a sponge for IgE anywhere in the organism and drag IgE from the periphery into mucosal tissues. This mechanism could be particularly important in EGIDs where lesions are typically described by high cell counts of eosinophils. These eosinophils could use surface FcεRI[54,55] to enrich tissue IgE in the lamina propria of the gastrointestinal tract. Higher levels of tissue IgE would consequently lower the threshold for immune activation by specific allergens. In other allergic diseases, such as atopic dermatitis, high levels of IgE-occupied APCs have been described in eczematous skin.[56] An answer is urgently needed for the question of whether the same holds true for EGIDs.

ACTIVATION OF TETRAMERIC FcεRIαβγ$_2$ IN THE GASTROINTESTINAL MUCOSA—CONSEQUENCES FOR EOSINOPHILIC GASTROINTESTINAL DISORDERS

Tetrameric FcεRIαβγ$_2$ is a marker for mast cells and basophils (see **Fig. 1**), which are classic effector cells of immediate type (type I) allergic reactions. The binding of multivalent allergen to adjacent IgE-loaded FcεRI complexes on the cell surface leads to aggregation of neighboring receptors. Cross-linking of FcεRI initiates cell activation via immunoreceptor tyrosine-based activation motifs, which are present in one copy in the β- chain as well as in each of the γ-chains in FcεRIαβγ$_2$.[48,57,58] In mast cells and basophils, this activation occurs within minutes after antigen contact and results in degranulation of preformed cytoplasmatic granules. Inflammatory mediators, such as histamine and serine proteases, are secreted into the extracellular space. This results in the typical clinical manifestation of the early phase of allergic reactions, and causes the characteristic signs and symptoms of immediate-type hypersensitivity reactions, as in allergic rhinitis, asthma, IgE-mediated food allergies, or anaphylaxis.

FcεRI-dependent activation of mast cells also induces the synthesis of proinflammatory cytokines, chemokines, and lipid mediators. These mediators are involved in the late-phase allergic response, which is seen several hours after the initial allergen contact. Late-phase reactions are characterized by the recruitment of inflammatory cells, such as neutrophils, eosinophils, APCs, lymphocytes, and macrophages, to the site of allergen encounter.[59–61]

Tissue specimens of EoE patients, besides having elevated eosinophil levels, display characteristics of inflammatory lesions of type I allergy. Increased numbers of IgE-bearing cells and activated mucosal mast cells are found[62] and the mucosa is heavily infiltrated by lymphocytes and APCs.[63] Although "classic" immediate hypersensitivity reactions and anaphylaxis to food or airborne allergens are rarely seen in EGID patients, the finding of increased activated mast cell counts in EoE lesions[62] strengthens our hypothesis that FcεRI-mediated immune activation plays a role in the pathology of EGIDs. However, the immunologic mechanisms underlying EGIDs seem to be more subtle and multifarious.

ACTIVATION OF TRIMERIC FcεRIαγ_2 IN THE GASTROINTESTINAL MUCOSA—CONSEQUENCES FOR EOSINOPHILIC GASTROINTESTINAL DISORDERS

Humans constitutively express the trimeric isoform, FcεRIαγ_2, on professional APCs in the GI tract, like dendritic cells and Langerhans cells. These professional APCs have the unique ability to elicit primary immune responses toward foreign antigens. Such an event is required for the adaptive immune response that characterizes delayed type Th-2–mediated immune responses considered central in the pathogenesis of EGIDs. This type of immune activation requires that an exogenous antigen enter the cell where it is processed rapidly to generate antigenic peptides. These peptides are then presented on major histocompatibility complex class II molecules at the APC surface for recognition by T cells of the adaptive immune system. The expression of FcεRIαγ_2 on APCs in the human gastrointestinal tract and possible consequences for IgE-mediated immune activation as observed in EGIDs are discussed below.

Dendritic cells in the gastrointestinal tract monitor the gastrointestinal lumen. As mentioned earlier, dendritic cells of the intestinal mucosa reach through the epithelial cell layer with periscopelike protrusions for direct access to the antigenic environment of the intestinal lumen.[52,53] Phagocytosis and macropinocytosis are key features of dendritic cells that ensure efficient antigen uptake. In addition to fluid phase antigen uptake, resting dendritic cells can use surface receptors, like FcεRIαγ_2, for uptake of antigen. Receptor-mediated antigen uptake is a mechanism that allows the elicitation of efficient immune responses toward minor amounts of antigen.[64,65] Surrogate ligands that enter the dendritic cell through receptor-mediated uptake are presented to T cells 100- to 1000- fold more efficiently when compared with soluble antigen.[48,65] This mechanism could explain the strong immune responses observed once sensitization to antigens and the production of antigen-specific IgE has occurred in a patient.

In their immature state, dendritic cells reside at sites of antigen exposure, such as the mucosal surfaces or the skin. These dendritic cells have a high capacity to endocytose and process exogenous antigens. Upon exposure to innate stimuli (eg, Toll-like receptor ligands), dendritic cells undergo a process of functional maturation that includes the termination of antigen uptake, the migration from the periphery to secondary lymphoid organs, the up-regulation of surface major histocompatibility complex and costimulatory molecules, and the secretion of cytokines, such as IL-12. Mature dendritic cells are able to productively present previously captured antigenic material to naïve T cells. Cognate contact with CD4$^+$ T cells in lymphoid organs leads to CD40 ligand (CD40L)–dependent activation of dendritic cells. The stimulation of regulatory T cells is also dependent on dendritic cells.[64,65] Detailed insight into IgE-mediated antigen presentation events in the gastrointestinal tract and consequences for the gastrointestinal T-cell repertoire is thus critical to our understanding of how the gastrointestinal system balances immune responses.

Trimeric FcεRI on primary human peripheral blood dendritic cells can, in principle, function as an antigen uptake receptor for major histocompatibility complex class II–mediated antigen presentation.[66] Thus, it is fair to assume that FcεRI may function the same way when expressed on dendritic cells located in the intestinal mucosa. FcεRI expression on mucosal dendritic cells and loading with IgE might result in "allergic sensitization" of patients with EGIDs. The inflammatory conditions in EGID patients might also allow non–professional APCs, such as macrophages and monocytes, to present allergen in a major histocompatibility complex class II–dependent fashion after FcεRI-mediated antigen uptake. Under inflammatory conditions, eosinophils can express major histocompatibility complex class II molecules and turn into non–professional APCs.[67,68] It is thus tempting to speculate that antigen presentation by eosinophils contributes to the Th-2 phenotype of EGIDs. In EGIDs, APCs could engage the gastrointestinal immune system via IgE-FcεRI–dependent antigen presentation and that way initiate and sustain the self-perpetuating cycle that leads to chronic immune activation and aggravation of the disease.

IgE-INDEPENDENT ACTIVATION OF FcεRI IN THE GASTROINTESTINAL MUCOSA—IMPLICATIONS FOR EOSINOPHILIC GASTROINTESTINAL DISORDERS

Thus far, we described solely IgE-mediated FcεRI-activation events and their potential role in EGIDs. FcεRI-mediated immune activation can also occur in an IgE-independent manner. We therefore next want to discuss mechanisms of IgE-independent FcεRI activation with regards to EGIDs. Such mechanisms might be particularly relevant for the pathology of EGIDs in patients lacking elevated serum IgE levels or symptoms attributable to specific allergens. Two IgE-independent mechanisms of FcεRI-mediated immune activation have been described: (1) receptor crosslinking via galectin-3 and (2) receptor crosslinking via anti-FcεRIα IgG autoantibodies.

Galectin-3, formerly known as epsilon binding protein (εBP), is a β-galactose–containing oligosaccharide that binds to IgE, FcεRI, or both.[23,69] Galectin-3 is commonly known as a marker for tumor progression,[70] but has also been shown to activate mast cells and basophils in the absence as well as in the presence of IgE.[69,71] Whether galectin-3 is able to activate trimeric FcεRI as expressed by human APCs remains to be determined. In view of reports on elevated mast cell numbers in EGID patients,[62] this oligosaccharide is an interesting candidate for modulating mast cell responses in the absence of IgE in EGID patients.

IgG autoantibodies with specificity for the alpha subunit of FcεRI (FcεRIα) are described to activate FcεRI-expressing cells by crosslinking the receptor via their Fab portion. In 30% of patients with chronic idiopathic urticaria, such antibodies are responsible for pseudoallergic reactions in absence of defined allergens.[72–75] Recently, these autoantibodies were also described in patients with asthma.[76] It is possible that anti-FcεRIα autoantibodies play a role in EGIDs as well. In conclusion, this pathway of FcεRI activation allows for the novel speculation that autoimmune events may play a role in EGIDs in the absence of specific IgE sensitizations.

SUMMARY

We have discussed the possible contribution of the high-affinity IgE receptor, FcεRI, in the pathology of EGIDs. The hypothesis that FcεRI is indeed a critical structure in triggering eosinophilic inflammation in EGIDs is supported several ways. Numerous case reports and clinical studies have pointed out the strong association between EGIDs and atopic diseases. Gene expression profiling of EoE patients showed up-regulation of FcεRI. The inflammatory infiltrate in EGIDs is characterized by eosinophils, mast cells, and dendritic cells. Those cells abundantly express FcεRI. Most strikingly, anti-IgE therapy in patients with eosinophilic gastroenteritis improves symptoms and down-regulates FcεRI expression. It is therefore highly likely that FcεRI is critically involved in the pathology of EGIDs. However, there is still much ground to cover and primary data to collect. A better understanding of the role of FcεRI in IgE-mediated as well as IgE-independent immune activation will, we hope, point toward new therapeutic directions to combat EGIDs.

REFERENCES

1. Furuta GT. Emerging questions regarding eosinophil's role in the esophago-gastrointestinal tract. Curr Opin Gastroenterol 2006;22:658–63.
2. Hogan SP. Recent advances in eosinophil biology. Int Arch Allergy Immunol 2007; 143(Suppl 1):3–14.
3. Hogan SP, Rothenberg ME. Eosinophil function in eosinophil-associated gastrointestinal disorders. Curr Allergy Asthma Rep 2006;6:65–71.
4. Rothenberg ME. Eosinophilic gastrointestinal disorders (EGID). J Allergy Clin Immunol 2004;113:11–28.
5. Assa'ad AH, Putnam PE, Collins MH, et al. Pediatric patients with eosinophilic esophagitis: an 8-year follow-up. J Allergy Clin Immunol 2007;119:731–8.
6. Roy-Ghanta S, Larosa DF, Katzka DA. Atopic characteristics of adult patients with eosinophilic esophagitis. Clin Gastroenterol Hepatol 2008;6:531–5.
7. Sugnanam KK, Collins JT, Smith PK, et al. Dichotomy of food and inhalant allergen sensitization in eosinophilic esophagitis. Allergy 2007;62:1257–60.
8. Simon D, Marti H, Heer P, et al. Eosinophilic esophagitis is frequently associated with IgE-mediated allergic airway diseases. J Allergy Clin Immunol 2005;115:1090–2.
9. Markowitz JE, Spergel JM, Ruchelli E, et al. Elemental diet is an effective treatment for eosinophilic esophagitis in children and adolescents. Am J Gastroenterol 2003;98:777–82.
10. Spergel JM. Eosinophilic esophagitis in adults and children: evidence for a food allergy component in many patients. Curr Opin Allergy Clin Immunol 2007;7:274–8.
11. Spergel JM, Shuker M. Nutritional management of eosinophilic esophagitis. Gastrointest Endosc Clin N Am 2008;18:179–94.
12. Assa'ad A. Eosinophilic esophagitis: association with allergic disorders. Gastrointest Endosc Clin N Am 2008;18:119–32.
13. Onbasi K, Sin AZ, Doganavsargil B, et al. Eosinophil infiltration of the oesophageal mucosa in patients with pollen allergy during the season. Clin Exp Allergy 2005;35: 1423–31.
14. Magnusson J, Lin XP, Dahlman-Hoglund A, et al. Seasonal intestinal inflammation in patients with birch pollen allergy. J Allergy Clin Immunol 2003;112:45–50.
15. Fogg MI, Ruchelli E, Spergel JM. Pollen and eosinophilic esophagitis. J Allergy Clin Immunol 2003;112:796–7.
16. Wang FY, Gupta SK, Fitzgerald JF. Is there a seasonal variation in the incidence or intensity of allergic eosinophilic esophagitis in newly diagnosed children? J Clin Gastroenterol 2007;41:451–3.

17. Foroughi S, Foster B, Kim N, et al. Anti-IgE treatment of eosinophil-associated gastrointestinal disorders. J Allergy Clin Immunol 2007;120:594–601.

18. Sicherer SH. Clinical aspects of gastrointestinal food allergy in childhood. Pediatrics 2003;111:1609–16.

19. Jaffe JS, James SP, Mullins GE, et al. Evidence for an abnormal profile of interleukin-4 (IL-4), IL-5, and gamma-interferon (gamma-IFN) in peripheral blood T cells from patients with allergic eosinophilic gastroenteritis. J Clin Immunol 1994;14: 299–309.

20. Beyer K, Castro R, Birnbaum A, et al. Human milk-specific mucosal lymphocytes of the gastrointestinal tract display a TH2 cytokine profile. J Allergy Clin Immunol 2002;109:707–13.

21. Van Sickle GJ, Powell GK, McDonald PJ, et al. Milk- and soy protein-induced enterocolitis: evidence for lymphocyte sensitization to specific food proteins. Gastroenterology 1985;88:1915–21.

22. Mishra A, Schlotman J, Wang M, et al. Critical role for adaptive T cell immunity in experimental eosinophilic esophagitis in mice. J Leukoc Biol 2007;81:916–24.

23. Gould HJ, Sutton BJ. IgE in allergy and asthma today. Nat Rev Immunol 2008;8: 205–17.

24. Kraft S, Kinet JP. New developments in FcepsilonRI regulation, function and inhibition. Nat Rev Immunol 2007;7:365–78.

25. von Bubnoff D, Novak N, Kraft S, et al. The central role of FcepsilonRI in allergy. Clin Exp Dermatol 2003;28:184–7.

26. Call ME, Wucherpfennig KW. Common themes in the assembly and architecture of activating immune receptors. Nat Rev Immunol 2007;7:841–50.

27. Call ME, Wucherpfennig KW. The T cell receptor: critical role of the membrane environment in receptor assembly and function. Annu Rev Immunol 2005;23:101–25.

28. Kubota T, Mukai K, Minegishi Y, et al. Different stabilities of the structurally related receptors for IgE and IgG on the cell surface are determined by length of the stalk region in their alpha-chains. J Immunol 2006;176:7008–14.

29. Prussin C, Griffith DT, Boesel KM, et al. Omalizumab treatment downregulates dendritic cell FcepsilonRI expression. J Allergy Clin Immunol 2003;112:1147–54.

30. Saini SS, MacGlashan DW Jr, Sterbinsky SA, et al. Down-regulation of human basophil IgE and FC epsilon RI alpha surface densities and mediator release by anti-IgE-infusions is reversible in vitro and in vivo. J Immunol 1999;162:5624–30.

31. Sihra BS, Kon OM, Grant JA, et al. Expression of high-affinity IgE receptors (Fc epsilon RI) on peripheral blood basophils, monocytes, and eosinophils in atopic and nonatopic subjects: relationship to total serum IgE concentrations. J Allergy Clin Immunol 1997;99:699–706.

32. Blanchard C, Wang N, Stringer KF, et al. Eotaxin-3 and a uniquely conserved gene-expression profile in eosinophilic esophagitis. J Clin Invest 2006;116:536–47.

33. Macdonald TT, Monteleone G. Immunity, inflammation, and allergy in the gut. Science 2005;307:1920–5.

34. Chehade M, Mayer L. Oral tolerance and its relation to food hypersensitivities. J Allergy Clin Immunol 2005;115:3–12.

35. Partridge MR. Asthma: 1987–2007. What have we achieved and what are the persisting challenges? Prim Care Respir J 2007;16:145–8.

36. Shurin MR, Smolkin YS. Immune-mediated diseases: Where do we stand? Adv Exp Med Biol 2007;601:3–12.

37. Vanderheyden AD, Petras RE, DeYoung BR, et al. Emerging eosinophilic (allergic) esophagitis: increased incidence or increased recognition? Arch Pathol Lab Med 2007;131:777–9.

38. Wilson DR, Merrett TG, Varga EM, et al. Increases in allergen-specific IgE in BAL after segmental allergen challenge in atopic asthmatics. Am J Respir Crit Care Med 2002;165:22–6.
39. Li H, Nowak-Wegrzyn A, Charlop-Powers Z, et al. Transcytosis of IgE-antigen complexes by CD23a in human intestinal epithelial cells and its role in food allergy. Gastroenterology 2006;131:47–58.
40. Kaiserlian D, Lachaux A, Grosjean I, et al. CD23/FC epsilon RII is constitutively expressed on human intestinal epithelium, and upregulated in cow's milk protein intolerance. Adv Exp Med Biol 1995;371B:871–4.
41. Kaiserlian D, Lachaux A, Grosjean I, et al. Intestinal epithelial cells express the CD23/Fc epsilon RII molecule: enhanced expression in enteropathies. Immunology 1993;80:90–5.
42. Tu Y, Perdue MH. CD23-mediated transport of IgE/immune complexes across human intestinal epithelium: role of p38 MAPK. Am J Physiol Gastrointest Liver Physiol 2006;291:G532–8.
43. Tu Y, Salim S, Bourgeois J, et al. CD23-mediated IgE transport across human intestinal epithelium: inhibition by blocking sites of translation or binding. Gastroenterology 2005;129:928–40.
44. Bevilacqua C, Montagnac G, Benmerah A, et al. Food allergens are protected from degradation during CD23-mediated transepithelial transport. Int Arch Allergy Immunol 2004;135:108–16.
45. Yu LC, Yang PC, Berin MC, et al. Enhanced transepithelial antigen transport in intestine of allergic mice is mediated by IgE/CD23 and regulated by interleukin-4. Gastroenterology 2001;121:370–81.
46. Li H, Chehade M, Liu W, et al. Allergen-IgE complexes trigger CD23-dependent CCL20 release from human intestinal epithelial cells. Gastroenterology 2007;133:1905–15.
47. Lampinen M, Carlson M, Hakansson LD, et al. Cytokine-regulated accumulation of eosinophils in inflammatory disease. Allergy 2004;59:793–805.
48. Maurer D, Fiebiger E, Ebner C, et al. Peripheral blood dendritic cells express FceRI as a complex composed of FceRIa- and FceRIg-chains and can use this receptor for IgE-mediated allergen presentation. J Immunol 1996;157:607–13.
49. Wang B, Rieger A, Kilgus O, et al. Epidermal Langerhans cells from normal human skin bind monomeric IgE via Fc epsilon RI. J Exp Med 1992;175:1353–65.
50. Allam JP, Novak N, Fuchs C, et al. Characterization of dendritic cells from human oral mucosa: a new Langerhans' cell type with high constitutive FcepsilonRI expression. J Allergy Clin Immunol 2003;112:141–8.
51. Terris B, Potet F. Structure and role of Langerhans' cells in the human oesophageal epithelium. Digestion 1995;56(Suppl 1):9–14.
52. Niess JH, Brand S, Gu X, et al. CX3CR1-mediated dendritic cell access to the intestinal lumen and bacterial clearance. Science 2005;307:254–8.
53. Niess JH, Reinecker HC. Lamina propria dendritic cells in the physiology and pathology of the gastrointestinal tract. Curr Opin Gastroenterol 2005;21:687–91.
54. Gounni AS, Lamkhioued B, Ochiai K, et al. High-affinity IgE receptor on eosinophils is involved in defence against parasites. Nature 1994;367:183–6.
55. Kayaba H, Dombrowicz D, Woerly G, et al. Human eosinophils and human high affinity IgE receptor transgenic mouse eosinophils express low levels of high affinity IgE receptor, but release IL-10 upon receptor activation. J Immunol 2001; 167:995–1003.
56. Klubal R, Osterhoff B, Wang B, et al. The high-affinity receptor for IgE is the predominant IgE-binding structure in lesional skin of atopic dermatitis patients. J Invest Dermatol 1997;108:336–42.

57. Kinet JP. The high-affinity IgE receptor (Fc epsilon RI): from physiology to pathology. Annu Rev Immunol 1999;17:931–72.
58. Turner H, Kinet JP. Signalling through the high-affinity IgE receptor Fc epsilonRI. Nature 1999;402:B24–30.
59. Galli SJ, Kalesnikoff J, Grimbaldeston MA, et al. Mast cells as "tunable" effector and immunoregulatory cells: recent advances. Annu Rev Immunol 2005;23:749–86.
60. Kinet JP. The essential role of mast cells in orchestrating inflammation. Immunol Rev 2007;217:5–7.
61. Metz M, Maurer M. Mast cells—key effector cells in immune responses. Trends Immunol 2007;28:234–41.
62. Kirsch R, Bokhary R, Marcon MA, et al. Activated mucosal mast cells differentiate eosinophilic (allergic) esophagitis from gastroesophageal reflux disease. J Pediatr Gastroenterol Nutr 2007;44:20–6.
63. Teitelbaum JE, Fox VL, Twarog FJ, et al. Eosinophilic esophagitis in children: immunopathological analysis and response to fluticasone propionate. Gastroenterology 2002;122:1216–25.
64. Mellman I. Antigen processing and presentation by dendritic cells: cell biological mechanisms. Adv Exp Med Biol 2005;560:63–7.
65. Trombetta ES, Mellman I. Cell biology of antigen processing in vitro and in vivo. Annu Rev Immunol 2005;23:975–1028.
66. Maurer D, Ebner C, Reininger B, et al. The high affinity IgE receptor (FceRI) mediates IgE-dependent allergen presentation. J Immunol 1995;154:6285–90.
67. Shi HZ. Eosinophils function as antigen-presenting cells. J Leukoc Biol 2004;76:520–7.
68. Shi HZ, Humbles A, Gerard C, et al. Lymph node trafficking and antigen presentation by endobronchial eosinophils. J Clin Invest 2000;105:945–53.
69. Liu FT, Hsu DK. The role of galectin-3 in promotion of the inflammatory response. Drug News Perspect 2007;20:455–60.
70. Liu FT, Rabinovich GA. Galectins as modulators of tumour progression. Nat Rev Cancer 2005;5:29–41.
71. Liu FT. Regulatory roles of galectins in the immune response. Int Arch Allergy Immunol 2005;136:385–400.
72. Fiebiger E, Hammerschmid F, Stingl G, et al. Anti-FcepsilonRIalpha autoantibodies in autoimmune-mediated disorders. Identification of a structure-function relationship. J Clin Invest 1998;101:243–51.
73. Fiebiger E, Maurer D, Holub H, et al. Serum IgG autoantibodies directed against the alpha chain of Fc epsilon RI: a selective marker and pathogenetic factor for a distinct subset of chronic urticaria patients? J Clin Invest 1995;96:2606–12.
74. Grattan CE. Autoimmune urticaria. Immunol Allergy Clin North Am 2004;24:163–81.
75. Hide M, Francis DM, Grattan CE, et al. Autoantibodies against the high-affinity IgE receptor as a cause of histamine release in chronic urticaria. N Engl J Med 1993;328:1599–604.
76. Sun RS, Chen XH, Liu RQ, et al. Autoantibodies to the high-affinity IgE receptor in patients with asthma. Asian Pac J Allergy Immunol 2008;26:19–22.

Epithelial Function in Eosinophilic Gastrointestinal Diseases

Sophie Fillon, PhD[a,c], Zachary D. Robinson, MS[a,c], Sean P. Colgan, PhD[b,c], Glenn T. Furuta, MD[a,c,*]

KEYWORDS

- Eosinophils • Epithelium • Gastrointestinal
- Inflammation • Pathogenesis

Under normal conditions, eosinophils are absent in the esophagus but exist in varying numbers along the rest of the gastrointestinal tract, particularly in the lamina propria.[1,2] For unknown reasons, eosinophils over the last decade have been increasingly associated with a wide variety of intestinal symptoms. Because of this, their histologic brilliance has created more than just a glancing comment limited to the bedside or the bottom of a pathology report. The enigmatic role of eosinophils in the pathophysiology of gastrointestinal diseases is becoming not only interesting but also increasingly relevant. In particular, because of the close anatomical proximity of eosinophils and epithelial cells and since many of the symptoms associated with eosinophilic gastrointestinal diseases can be attributed to epithelial dysfunction, an increasing number of studies seek to better define this eosinophil/epithelial cell relationship.

EOSINOPHILIC GASTROINTESTINAL DISEASES AND THE ROLE OF THE EPITHELIUM

EGIDs are a heterogeneous group of diseases characterized by gastrointestinal symptoms and large numbers of eosinophils in the intestinal tract. EGIDs include eosinophilic esophagitis (EoE), eosinophilic gastroenteritis, and eosinophilic colitis. For the

Research for this article was supported by a gift from the Campaign for Urgent Research on Eosinophilic Diseases.

[a] Section of Pediatric Gastroenterology, Hepatology and Nutrition, University of Colorado Denver School of Medicine, 13123 East 16th Avenue, B290, Aurora, CO 80045, USA
[b] Mucosal Inflammation Program, Division of Gastroenterology, University of Colorado Denver School of Medicine, 13123 East 16th Avenue, B290, Aurora, CO 80045, USA
[c] Division of Gastroenterology, University of Colorado Denver, School of Medicine, 12700 East 19th Avenue, B146, Aurora, CO 80045
* Corresponding author.
E-mail address: Furuta.glenn@tchden.org (G. T. Furuta).

Immunol Allergy Clin N Am 29 (2009) 171–178
doi:10.1016/j.iac.2008.09.003   immunology.theclinics.com

diagnosis of EGIDs to be confirmed, other causes of gastrointestinal eosinophilia must be ruled out. (See the articles by Putnam; Franciosi and Liacouras; and Fleischer and Atkins elsewhere in this issue for related discussion.) Original descriptions of EGIDs separated patients into subtypes according to the anatomic location of their eosinophilia (ie, mucosal, muscular, and serosal disease). Mucosal biopsies are normally taken from the most superficial gastrointestinal surface. Thus, researchers have little data to help understand the precise relationships eosinophils share with other resident cells in this complex immunologic microenvironment. However, studies of the gastrointestinal tract and other organs are now beginning to paint a picture of how eosinophils and epithelial cells interact to produce symptoms consistent with EGIDs. For instance, eosinophil products have been associated with barrier dysfunction, a problem that is increasingly associated with the pathogenesis of a wide variety of inflammatory bowel diseases. Eosinophil relationships with other resident cells, including fibroblasts, mast cells, lymphocytes, and nerves, are not discussed here, but have been reviewed recently.[3–5]

EOSINOPHIL MIGRATION TO MUCOSAL SURFACES DIFFERS AMONG ORGANS

The movement of eosinophils to mucosal surfaces, in particular toward the epithelium, is complex and appears to be organ specific. (See the article by Blanchard and Rothenberg on this topic elsewhere in this issue.) The exact mechanisms driving eosinophils and epithelial cells together are likely unique to different organs. For instance, while the lung relies on IL-5 to drive eosinophils into its mucosa, skin eosinophilia appears to be under the control of the chemokine receptor CCR3. In murine studies of esophageal inflammation, IL-5 is critical to chemotaxis, whereas gastric eosinophilia is eotaxin-1 dependent. Finally, baseline intestinal eosinophilia appears to be eotaxin dependent since eotaxin-deficient mice have fewer intestinal eosinophils than control mice do. Studies with intercellular adhesion molecule 1 (ICAM-1)–deficient mice and ICAM-neutralizing antibodies in a dextran sulfate sodium colitis model demonstrated the β2-integrin/ICAM-1 dependency of colonic eosinophilic inflammation.[6] Thus, studies regarding the relationship of eosinophils and epithelium need to be viewed with respect to the organ-specific homing signals. Data suggest that a diversity of regulatory mechanisms for the different gastrointestinal microenvironments may ultimately influence future therapeutic interventions.

INFLUENCE OF EOSINOPHILS ON EPITHELIAL FUNCTION
Eosinophils Possess the Ability to Synthesize and Release Potent Biological Mediators

Eosinophils contain a number of preformed granule proteins, including major basic protein (MBP), eosinophilic cationic protein, eosinophilic peroxidase, and eosinophil-derived neurotoxin, which can be released into the tissue microenvironment. While disease-specific patterns of tissue eosinophil degranulation have not yet been identified, a growing body of literature demonstrates evidence of degranulation within murine models of gastrointestinal inflammation and human diseases.

In addition, eosinophils synthesize and release numerous cytokines (IL-2, IL-4, IL-5, IL-10, IL-12, IL-13, IL-16, IL-18, transforming growth factor [TGF] α and β) chemokines (RANTES [regulated on activation, normal T expressed and secreted] and eotaxins), and lipid mediators (platelet activating factor and leukotriene C4).[7] Previous work demonstrated that these cytokines are capable of inducing a number of different immune responses in inflammatory diseases, such as asthma, atopic dermatitis, rhinitis, and inflammatory bowel diseases.[3] IL-5 is particularly critical to eosinophil growth, chemotaxis, and activation. IL-13 functions as an eosinophil chemoattractant to perpetuate eosinophilic inflammation.[8] Eosinophils are also a source of profibrotic cytokines and fibrogenic mediators implicated in airway remodeling, such as IL-11, IL-17, IL-17E (IL-25), TGF-α, TGF-β1, and matrix metalloproteinase 9 (MMP-9). IL-11, a member of the IL-6 family of cytokines, has fibrogenic potential. Its expression within the airways has been localized mainly to epithelial cells and MBP-positive eosinophils.

Chronic skin lesions in atopic dermatitis are also associated predominantly with TGF-β1 and IL-11 expression produced mainly by eosinophils. This observation further supports the concept that these cells might be involved in the development of structural remodeling in the injured skin of patients with atopic dermatitis.[9]

Eosinophilic Mediators Impact Epithelial Cells

While direct evidence of the eosinophil's impact on the epithelium is difficult to ascertain in vivo and in human studies, a number of in vitro studies have shown that eosinophils can significantly influence epithelial structure and function. The degree of inflammation may be critical in how eosinophils influence the epithelium. For instance, our previous work demonstrated that at concentrations of three eosinophils per epithelial cell, eosinophils diminished epithelial barrier function. This loss of barrier was found to be linked to the highly charged granule protein, MBP. Application of MBP to the basolateral surface led to diminished barrier and MBP-null mice are relatively protected from barrier dysfunction when compared with wild-type mice.[10] In contrast, recent work suggests that at very low eosinophil/epithelial ratios (eg, 0.01), eosinophils may in fact benefit epithelial barrier function.[11] These contrasting results may partially explain the pathologic role of large numbers of eosinophils observed during disease states and the physiologic role of low numbers that could address the innate functions of eosinophils in a healthy state.

Eosinophils may also exhibit autocrine functions during inflammation. Eosinophil-derived cytokines appear to be generated in small amounts, suggesting an autocrine, paracrine, or juxtacrine role in regulating the function of the surrounding microenvironment.[3] Eotaxins (-1, -2, and -3) are very potent eosinophil chemoattractants. Their secretion by eosinophils indicates their ability to initiate and perpetuate an inflammatory response.[12]

Increased mucosal eosinophil and granule protein deposition has been described in a number of gastrointestinal diseases also associated with altered epithelial barrier dysfunction, including food allergic enteropathy and inflammatory bowel diseases. Eosinophil-derived granule proteins are detected in lavage fluid and in the mucosa of patients with inflammatory bowel diseases and EGIDs. As stated previously, eosinophil-derived MBP has been shown in a coculture model to alter colonic epithelial barrier function.[10]

Eosinophils produce significant levels of TGF-β linked to a variety of eosinophil-associated diseases, including asthma.[13] Human studies have demonstrated that anti–IL-5 reduces levels of airway eosinophils expressing TGF-β, as well as levels of airway remodeling assessed by bronchial biopsies. Moreover, murine models of airway remodeling have provided important insight into potential mechanisms by which TGF-β activation of the Smad-2/3 signaling pathway may contribute to airway remodeling.[14] Some patients with EoE and dense eosinophilia in their esophagus demonstrate evidence of remodeling and fibrosis with isolated strictures, long-segment narrowing, and esophageal fragility.[15,16]

Eosinophil-derived granule proteins have also been associated with damage to the airway epithelium, and hypersecretion of mucus.[17] For instance, in many asthmatic patients, eosinophils are the main inflammatory cells present adjacent to the airway epithelium. Bronchoalveolar lavage fluid from asthmatics contains elevated numbers of eosinophils and concentrations of MBP. Increased MBP levels in bronchoalveolar lavage fluid positively correlates with bronchial hyperreactivity in asthmatic patients.[17] Bronchoalveolar lavage was performed on 17 subjects with mild atopic asthma (9 symptomatic, 8 asymptomatic) and on 14 nonasthmatic control subjects (6 hay fever, 8 nonatopic). A significant increase in the eosinophil count and the concentration of MBP in bronchoalveolar lavage fluid in the symptomatic asthmatics was observed. Moreover, there was a significant correlation between the amounts of MBP recovered and the percentage of eosinophils in the bronchoalveolar lavage. These changes were more marked when asthmatics with airway hyperreactivity were compared with subjects with normoreactive airways. Furthermore, there was a significant increase in the percentage of epithelial cells in the hyperreactive asthmatics. This study supports the hypothesis that bronchial hyperresponsiveness is secondary to epithelial cell damage mediated at least in part through eosinophil-derived granule products.[18]

Moreover, other eosinophil products are known to stimulate epithelial proliferation. Choe and colleagues[19] showed that, when stretch forces were applied to the airway epithelium, coculture with eosinophils up-regulated epithelial cell airway remodeling genes. In this system, in which human bronchial epithelial cells were layered on a collagen gel embedded with human lung fibroblasts, activated eosinophils and stretch forces increased epithelial thickness, production of mucus, cilia growth, and evidence of tight junctions. This experiment suggests that mechanical strain affects airway wall remodeling synergistically with eosinophilic inflammation.

Another recent study addressed the impact of eosinophils on primary cultures of human bronchial epithelial cells. Pegorier and colleagues[20] demonstrated that when primary cultured human bronchial epithelia cells as well as normal human bronchial epithelial cells were exposed to subcytotoxic concentrations of MBP and eosinophilic peroxidase, there was up-regulation of endothelin-1, TGF-α, TGF-β1, platelet-derived growth factor β, epidermal growth factor receptor, MMP-9, fibronectin, and tenascin genes. In addition, ex vivo modeling of human airway demonstrated that the addition of activated eosinophils to a matrix of fibroblasts and bronchial epithelial cells led to a significant increase in epithelial thickness. Moreover, eosinophil-derived IL-1α and TGF-β expression participated in this response, thus promoting a role for eosinophils in disruption of extracellular matrices leading to tissue remodeling and fibrosis.[21] In summary, a growing body of work demonstrates that eosinophil products influence the synthesis of bioactive molecules by epithelial cells that alter the extracellular matrix composition.

Tissue eosinophilia and eosinophilic granule proteins are found in biopsies of atopic dermatitis lesions.[22] Moreover, studies in an atopic dermatitis mouse model have shown that tissue eosinophilia correlates with skin hypertrophy and increased thickness of the epidermal and dermal layers, suggesting the involvement of a repair process as a result of exposure to the cytotoxic effects of MBP and eosinophilic cationic protein.[23] Eosinophils are an important source of MMP-9, known to have an important role in cell migration and inflammation.[24–26] The MMP-9 have relevance to chronic structural airway changes in asthma. They can be generated by structural and inflammatory cells and have the ability to degrade proteoglycans and enhance airway fibrosis and smooth muscle proliferation through their ability to release and activate latent, matrix-bound growth factors.[27]

Translational and in vitro studies suggest that eosinophils may play a role in the generation of mucus. For instance, rhinopulmonary epithelia associated with mucosal eosinophils have goblet cell hyperplasia and metaplasia, indicative of accelerated mucus production.[28] In support of this association, exposure of human airway epithelial cells to supernatants derived from activated eosinophils leads to increased mucin production. Eosinophil-derived TGF-α and the activation of epidermal growth factor receptor participate in this response.[29] Finally, in murine ovalbumin-induced airway eosinophilic inflammation, use of CCR3 monoclonal antibody reduces both eosinophil recruitment to the lung and mucus production.[30,31]

Recent clinical observations have led to the speculation that eosinophils may lead to epithelial dysfunction in EoE.[32,33] In support of this hypothesis, Mishra and colleagues[34] showed that, in an aeroallergen model of EoE, there is a significant IL-5–dependent accumulation of collagen in the lamina propria and epithelial mucosa. IL-5–deficient mice show reduced basal layer thickness and diminished lamina propria collagen deposition as compared with wild-type mice. An increased level of IL-5 was detected in the esophagus of EoE patients and in the corresponding animal model. The investigators also observed increased expression of IL-5, TGF-β1 and mucin 5AC in biopsies from EoE patients and in experimental EoE. The Δdbl-GATA mice are mice unable to produce eosinophils, which are deficient of eosinophils, showed a significant reduction of esophageal remodeling compared with wild-type mice after allergen challenge. In summary, these data provide evidence that eosinophils and IL-5 participate in esophageal remodeling.

EPITHELIA'S IMPACT ON EOSINOPHILS
Epithelial Function

The epithelium is a cellular interface between the external environment and the inside of the body. This interface is limited to a single cell layer except in the esophagus, which has a stratified squamous epithelium. While this monolayer of cells is also protected by a variety of unique organ-specific innate molecules, such as mucous, trefoil factors, defensins, and antibodies, its protective role is not limited to its barrier function alone. In addition, the epithelium serves as a potent reservoir of cytokines and lipid mediators and is functionally active in chloride secretion, which, in a healthy state, cleanses the epithelial surface. When these functions are disrupted or dysregulated, disease develops. For instance, the loss of barrier in the gut leads to bleeding, protein loss, and exposure of the immunologically primed lamina propria to potentially noxious luminal contents. When proinflammatory cytokines, such as TNF-α, are produced in excess, the mucosa is infiltrated with polymorphonuclear cells, resulting in crypt abscess formation. Finally, excess chloride secretion leads to diarrhea with resultant dehydration.

Epithelial Impact on Eosinophils

As mentioned previously, and in the article elsewhere in this issue by Blanchard and Rothenberg, the intestinal epithelia is capable of releasing a number of chemokines, such as eotaxins-1, -2, and -3, that direct eosinophils to specific parts of the gastrointestinal tract. In addition, epithelia promote eosinophil survival by releasing epithelial-derived granulocyte macrophage colony stimulating factor, which delays apoptosis. Neurotrophin levels are known to be increased in bronchoalveolar lavage fluid during allergic asthma. Hahn and colleagues[35] investigated the role of neurotrophins as inflammatory mediators in eosinophil-epithelial cell interactions during the allergic immune response. The investigators demonstrated the neurotrophin expression by immunohistochemistry and ELISA in the lung of a mouse model of chronic experimental asthma. For this study, investigators also performed coculture experiments with airway epithelial cells and bronchoalveolar lavage fluid eosinophils. Hahn and colleagues observed that neurotrophin levels increased during chronic allergic airway inflammation, and that airway epithelial cells were the major source of members of the neurotrophin family, such as nerve growth factor and brain-derived neurotrophic factor within the inflamed lung. Epithelial neurotrophin production was up-regulated by IL-1β, TNF-α, and T helper 2 cytokines. Lung eosinophils expressed the brain-derived neurotrophic factor and nerve growth factor receptors, and coculture with airway epithelial cells resulted in increased epithelial neurotrophin production and prolonged eosinophil survival. In summary, the study shows that, during allergic inflammation, airway epithelial cells express increased amounts of nerve growth factor and brain-derived neurotrophic factor, which promote the survival of tissue eosinophils. Controlling epithelial neurotrophin production might be an important therapeutic target to prevent allergic airway eosinophilia. This study suggests the presence of an autocrine pathway through which epithelial cells contribute to eosinophil accumulation on the mucosal surface of the asthmatic lung.

Experiments in animal models have shown that intratracheal administration of the cytokine IL-13 induces dose-dependent eosinophil recruitment in the mouse esophagus but not in the stomach. Intratracheal IL-13 induced esophageal epithelial hyperplasia. However, this recruitment is absent in IL-5–deficient mice and the ability of IL-13 to induce EoE was abolished in STAT6-deficient mice (mice deficient in signal transducers and activators of transcription proteins 6). Furthermore, IL-13–induced EoE was significantly diminished in eotaxin-1–deficient mice. As such, IL-13 delivery to the lung in the mouse induces EoE by an eotaxin-1, IL-5, and STAT6-dependent mechanism. These data further establish a close connection between respiratory and esophageal inflammation.[36]

SUMMARY

As EGIDs present an increasing health care burden to clinicians, our understanding of contribution of eosinophils to the pathogenesis of these diseases is still in its infancy. The intimate anatomic proximity of eosinophils and epithelial cells permits the speculation that eosinophil-epithelial cross talk, as studied in other diseases (eg, asthma and atopic dermatitis), contributes to EGID pathogenesis. Future studies will need to refine our understanding of the histologic patterns of eosinophilia, the impact of eosinophil-specific mediators on epithelial dysfunction, and the expression of epithelial chemokines that drive mucosal eosinophilia. Answers to these questions will provide the groundwork for new diagnostic techniques and therapeutic interventions.

REFERENCES

1. DeBrosse CW, Case JW, Putnam PE, et al. Quantity and distribution of eosinophils in the gastrointestinal tract of children. Pediatr Dev Pathol 2006;9:210.
2. Lowichik A, Weinberg AG. A quantitative evaluation of mucosal eosinophils in the pediatric gastrointestinal tract. Mod Pathol 1996;9:110.
3. Hogan SP, Rosenberg HF, Moqbel R, et al. Eosinophils: biological properties and role in health and disease. Clin Exp Allergy 2008;38:709.
4. Rothenberg ME, Hogan SP. The eosinophil. Annu Rev Immunol 2006;24:147.
5. Woodruff SA, Fillon S, Robinson ZD, et al. JPGN, in press.
6. Forbes E, Hulett M, Ahrens R, et al. ICAM-1-dependent pathways regulate colonic eosinophilic inflammation. J Leukoc Biol 2006;80:330.
7. Kita H. The eosinophil: a cytokine-producing cell? J Allergy Clin Immunol 1996;97: 889.
8. Rosenberg HF, Phipps S, Foster PS. Eosinophil trafficking in allergy and asthma. J Allergy Clin Immunol 2007;119:1303.

9. Foley SC, Prefontaine D, Hamid Q. Images in allergy and immunology: role of eosinophils in airway remodeling. J Allergy Clin Immunol 2007;119:1563.

10. Furuta GT, Nieuwenhuis EE, Karhausen J, et al. Eosinophils alter colonic epithelial barrier function: role for major basic protein. Am J Physiol Gastrointest Liver Physiol 2005;289:G890.

11. Mukkada V, Colgan SP, Furuta GT. Eosinophils enhance epithelial barrier function. J Pediatr Gastroenterol Nutr 2007;45:S12.

12. Garcia-Zepeda EA, Rothenberg ME, Ownbey RT, et al. Human eotaxin is a specific chemoattractant for eosinophil cells and provides a new mechanism to explain tissue eosinophilia. Nat Med 1996;2:449.

13. Kay AB, Phipps S, Robinson DS. A role for eosinophils in airway remodelling in asthma. Trends Immunol 2004;25:477.

14. Broide DH. Immunologic and inflammatory mechanisms that drive asthma progression to remodeling. J Allergy Clin Immunol 2008;121:560.

15. Chehade M, Sampson HA, Morotti RA, et al. Esophageal subepithelial fibrosis in children with eosinophilic esophagitis. J Pediatr Gastroenterol Nutr 2007;45:319.

16. Straumann A, Rossi L, Simon HU, et al. Fragility of the esophageal mucosa: a pathognomonic endoscopic sign of primary eosinophilic esophagitis? Gastrointest Endosc 2003;57:407.

17. Gleich GJ. Mechanisms of eosinophil-associated inflammation. J Allergy Clin Immunol 2000;105:651.

18. Wardlaw AJ, Dunnette S, Gleich GJ, et al. Eosinophils and mast cells in bronchoalveolar lavage in subjects with mild asthma. Relationship to bronchial hyperreactivity. Am Rev Respir Dis 1988;137:62.

19. Choe MM, Sporn PH, Swartz MA. An in vitro airway wall model of remodeling. Am J Physiol Lung Cell Mol Physiol 2003;285:L427.

20. Pegorier S, Wagner LA, Gleich GJ, et al. Eosinophil-derived cationic proteins activate the synthesis of remodeling factors by airway epithelial cells. J Immunol 2006;177:4861.

21. Gomes I, Mathur SK, Espenshade BM, et al. Eosinophil-fibroblast interactions induce fibroblast IL-6 secretion and extracellular matrix gene expression: implications in fibrogenesis. J Allergy Clin Immunol 2005;116:796.

22. Kiehl P, Falkenberg K, Vogelbruch M, et al. Tissue eosinophilia in acute and chronic atopic dermatitis: a morphometric approach using quantitative image analysis of immunostaining. Br J Dermatol 2001;145:720.

23. Spergel JM, Mizoguchi E, Oettgen H, et al. Roles of TH1 and TH2 cytokines in a murine model of allergic dermatitis. J Clin Invest 1999;103:1103.

24. Ohno I, Ohtani H, Nitta Y, et al. Eosinophils as a source of matrix metalloproteinase-9 in asthmatic airway inflammation. Am J Respir Cell Mol Biol 1997;16:212.

25. Okada S, Kita H, George TJ, et al. Migration of eosinophils through basement membrane components in vitro: role of matrix metalloproteinase-9. Am J Respir Cell Mol Biol 1997;17:519.

26. Schwingshackl A, Duszyk M, Brown N, et al. Human eosinophils release matrix metalloproteinase-9 on stimulation with TNF-alpha. J Allergy Clin Immunol 1999;104:983.

27. Han Z, Junxu J, Zhong N. Expression of matrix metalloproteinases MMP-9 within the airways in asthma. Respir Med 2003;97:563.

28. Ding GQ, Zheng CQ, Bagga SS. Up-regulation of the mucosal epidermal growth factor receptor gene in chronic rhinosinusitis and nasal polyposis. Arch Otolaryngol Head Neck Surg 2007;133:1097.

29. Burgel PR, Lazarus SC, Tam DC, et al. Human eosinophils induce mucin production in airway epithelial cells via epidermal growth factor receptor activation. J Immunol 2001;167:5948.

30. Hur GY, Lee SY, Lee SH, et al. Potential use of an anticancer drug gefinitib, an EGFR inhibitor, on allergic airway inflammation. Exp Mol Med 2007;39:367.

31. Shen HH, Xu F, Zhang GS, et al. CCR3 monoclonal antibody inhibits airway eosinophilic inflammation and mucus overproduction in a mouse model of asthma. Acta Pharmacol Sin 2006;27:1594.

32. Ngo P, Furuta GT, Antonioli DA, et al. Eosinophils in the esophagus—peptic or allergic eosinophilic esophagitis? Case series of three patients with esophageal eosinophilia. Am J Gastroenterol 2006;101:1666.

33. Spechler SJ, Genta RM, Souza RF. Thoughts on the complex relationship between gastroesophageal reflux disease and eosinophilic esophagitis. Am J Gastroenterol 2007;102:1301.

34. Mishra A, Wang M, Pemmaraju VR, et al. Esophageal remodeling develops as a consequence of tissue specific IL-5-induced eosinophilia. Gastroenterology 2008;134:204.

35. Hahn C, Islamian AP, Renz H, et al. Airway epithelial cells produce neurotrophins and promote the survival of eosinophils during allergic airway inflammation. J Allergy Clin Immunol 2006;117:787.

36. Mishra A, Rothenberg ME. Intratracheal IL-13 induces eosinophilic esophagitis by an IL-5, eotaxin-1, and STAT6-dependent mechanism. Gastroenterology 2003;125:1419.

Role of Tolerance in the Development of Eosinophilic Gastrointestinal Diseases

Pooja Varshney, MD, A. Wesley Burks, MD*

KEYWORDS

- Eosinophilic esophagitis • Eosinophilic gastroenteritis
- Oral tolerance • Food allergy

Although the precise link is not completely understood, eosinophilic gastrointestinal diseases (EGIDs) have been shown to be highly associated with atopy. Oral tolerance describes the specific suppression of immune responses to an antigen by prior administration of the antigen by the oral route. Like other allergic gastrointestinal diseases, EGIDs may result from a loss of oral tolerance or a failure in the induction of tolerance. Allergy may be a stimulus for the recruitment of eosinophils to the gastrointestinal tract or may lead to the failure of key regulatory T cells, leading to the loss of immunologic tolerance. Bypassing mechanisms of high-dose tolerance, which include induction of lymphocyte anergy or deletion, may also facilitate the development of EGIDs and other forms of food allergy. Further study to clarify the role of tolerance in the development of EGIDs can help identify potential prevention strategies and therapeutic targets.

EOSINOPHILIC GASTROINTESTINAL DISEASES IN THE SPECTRUM OF FOOD HYPERSENSITIVITY

Gastrointestinal manifestations of food hypersensitivity may range from oropharyngeal pruritus to profuse vomiting and diarrhea and anaphylaxis. Likewise, there is a spectrum of immunologic mechanisms underlying the various forms of food hypersensitivity, from immediate-type IgE-mediated processes to cell-mediated allergy. EGIDs are an increasingly recognized category of disorders characterized by infiltration of the esophageal, gastric, and intestinal walls with eosinophils. Unlike classic IgE-mediated food allergy, eosinophilic esophagitis (EoE) and allergic eosinophilic

Division of Allergy and Immunology, Department of Pediatrics, Duke University Medical Center, Box 2898, Durham, NC 27710, USA
* Corresponding author.
E-mail address: wesley.burks@duke.edu (A.W. Burks).

Immunol Allergy Clin N Am 29 (2009) 179–187
doi:10.1016/j.iac.2008.10.001   immunology.theclinics.com

gastroenteritis generally have an insidious onset and result in a range of symptoms, from dysphagia and food impaction to reflux, vomiting, and failure to thrive.

Although dissimilar in their clinical presentations, EGIDs and other forms of food allergy likely have common pathophysiologic mechanisms. Genetic predisposition, allergen sensitization, and environmental factors play important roles in the pathogenesis of these diseases. Although the precise link is not completely understood, EoE has been shown to be highly associated with atopic disease. Sensitization to both food and environmental allergens has been demonstrated in patients with EoE.[1] Studies have shown that a significant proportion of patients with EGIDs have evidence of allergic disease by history or skin testing.[2] In one series of 13 patients, 77% had a history of an allergic disorder (asthma, allergic rhinitis, urticaria, atopic dermatitis, food allergy, or drug allergy) or positive radioallergosorbent testing or skin prick testing.[3] Another study of 21 children revealed that 68% of subjects had a positive result to foods on skin or radioallergosorbent testing.[4]

The mucosal accumulation of eosinophils in the gastrointestinal tract suggests a Th2-mediated process.[1] Murine studies have shown impaired induction of esophageal eosinophilia in response to allergen in mice who are genetically deficient in signal transducer and activator of transcription 6, interleukin (IL)-13, IL-4, and IL-5, providing evidence that allergen-induced EoE is dependent on classic Th2 cytokine signaling.[5] Like other Th2-dependent disease processes, EGIDs likely represent the interplay of extrinsic allergic triggers and intrinsic Th2 cytokines in genetically predisposed individuals.[1] Eosinophils, occasionally discounted as mere markers of disease, likely make important contributions to disease pathogenesis.[1] Eosinophils contain granule proteins, such as major basic proteins 1 and 2, eosinophilic cationic protein, eosinophil-derived neurotoxin, and eosinophil peroxidase, which have a range of proinflammatory properties. Mast cells and lymphocytes also contribute to the development of disease. (See the articles by authors elsewhere in this issue.)

FUNDAMENTALS OF TOLERANCE

The role of food antigen sensitization is being recognized as a key player in the development of eosinophilic disease. A fundamental principle underlying the development of food allergy is the concept of tolerance. Oral tolerance is used to describe the specific suppression of cellular or humoral responses to an antigen by prior administration of the antigen by the oral route.[6] The lumen of the gastrointestinal tract, the largest immunologic organ in the body, is continually exposed to an array of dietary proteins. Despite the large daily dietary antigen load, most ingested proteins do not provoke local or systemic immune responses. Oral tolerance presumably evolved as an analog of self-tolerance to prevent hypersensitivity reactions to food proteins and bacterial antigens present in the mucosal microbiota.[7] It is a natural immunologic process driven by exogenous antigens, ultimately allowing them to gain access to the body without activating a potentially damaging immune response.

In the mid-twentieth century, Chase[6] established that oral feeding of an antigen induces T cell–mediated inhibition of subsequent immune responses, or oral tolerance (**Fig. 1**). He contrasted the induction of oral tolerance from the generation of strong cell-mediated and humoral responses that follows subcutaneous immunization and booster administration of an antigen. Further experiments demonstrated that the transfer of T cells from antigen-fed "tolerant" mice to naive mice also resulted in reduced in vitro immune responses to subcutaneous immunization.

Antigen exposure in the gut results in several major immunologic responses. The local production and release of noninflammatory secretory IgA antibody is the initial

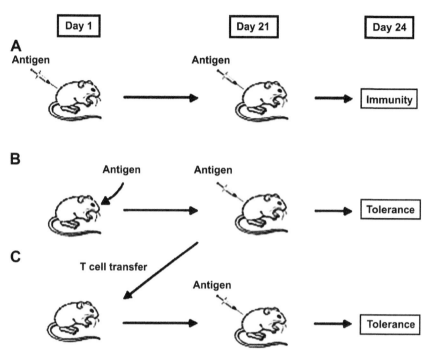

| Day 1 | Day 21 | Day 24 |

Fig. 1. Induction of oral tolerance. (*A*) Mice immunized subcutaneously and then boosted subcutaneously with an antigen show strong in vitro cell-mediated and antibody responses to the antigen. (*B*) When mice are first fed the antigen orally and then immunized subcutaneously, in vitro immune responses to the antigen are greatly reduced. (*C*) Transferring T cells from mice that were fed antigen to naive mice results in reduced in vitro immune responses to subsequent subcutaneous immunization. This shows that oral feeding of an antigen can induce a T cell–mediated active inhibitory immune response. (*Adapted from* Chehade M, Mayer L. Oral tolerance and its relation to food hypersensitivities. J Allergy Clin Immunol 2005;115:4; with permission.)

response that occurs in the gastrointestinal mucosa. Antigens stimulate B lymphocytes in the organized mucosal lymphoid tissue. These effector B cells migrate to distant mucosal and glandular sites and differentiate into polymeric-IgA-producing plasma cells.[8] Secretory IgA is transported to the lumen of the gastrointestinal tract and crosslinks microorganisms, thereby blocking the contact of antigens with epithelial surfaces and preventing invasion and infection.[8] Subsequent priming of the systemic immune system leads to antibody production and activation of cellular immunity that protect against the invading antigen on subsequent exposures.[7]

In contrast, exposure to dietary antigens and commensal bacteria leads to a state of local and immunologic tolerance that prevents the activation of potentially harmful immunologic responses on future encounters with these antigens. Food proteins also play a critical role in stimulating maturation of both the local and systemic immune system. Mice reared on a balanced diet containing amino acids but no intact food proteins have poorly developed gut-associated lymphoid tissue and reduced numbers of intraepithelial lymphocytes and secretory IgA levels, parameters that resemble suckling mice. They also have low levels of circulating IgG and IgA and a predominantly Th2 cytokine profile.[9]

MECHANISMS OF ORAL TOLERANCE

The journey for a dietary protein involves multiple steps before tolerance or hypersensitivity is established. Ingested dietary proteins are degraded by gastric acid and luminal digestive enzymes; this process often results in the destruction of immunogenic epitopes.[7] Amino acid chains less than 8 amino acids long are nonreactive with structures responsible for antigen recognition and are immunologically ignored.[10] Failure of the enzymatic digestion process can disrupt tolerance, leading to hypersensitivity in animal and human models.[11] Human studies have correlated the suppression of gastric acid by proton pump inhibitors with induction of food allergy.[12] A peptic digest of bovine serum albumin is tolerogenic when injected into the mouse ileum, but untreated bovine serum albumin is immunogenic when administered in the same manner.[13] Interestingly, an elemental diet has been shown to result in striking clinical and histologic improvement in children and adolescents with EoE.[14]

After undergoing modification in the lumen, antigens are sampled by the gut immune system in several different ways (**Fig. 2**).[15] Dendritic cells, potent antigen-presenting cells, extend processes into the gut lumen to sample antigens. M cells overlying Peyer's patches take up particulate antigens and deliver them to subepithelial dendritic cells. Soluble antigens may cross the epithelium by transcellular or paracellular routes to the lamina propria, where they encounter T cells or macrophages. Intestinal epithelial cells are nonprofessional antigen-presenting cells that can endocytose soluble dietary antigens that have escaped proteolysis and present them to primed T cells.

FACTORS INFLUENCING DEVELOPMENT OF TOLERANCE

There are two primary effector mechanisms for inducing oral tolerance: activation of regulatory T cells and clonal anergy or deletion.[7] The dose of the antigen is the principal factor determining which process takes place (**Fig. 3**).[16] Low doses of antigen induce tolerance by regulatory T cells that mediate immune suppression through secretion of down-regulatory cytokines, such as transforming growth factor (TGF)-β, IL-10, and IL-4. These antigen-specific regulatory cells migrate to lymphoid organs, where they suppress the generation of effector cells, and to target organs, where they inhibit disease by releasing non–antigen-specific cytokines.[17] High-dose tolerance results in anergy or deletion of T cells through T-cell receptor cross-linking in the absence of costimulatory signals or in the presence of inhibitory ligands.[15] It is important to note, however, that low- and high-dose tolerance may not be mutually exclusive and may actually have overlapping effects.[17]

Regulatory T cells are CD4+CD25+ cells that mediate suppression of CD4+CD25− cells through cell-cell interaction involving surface-bound TGF-β,[18] although their suppressor function has also been shown to occur independently of TGF-β.[19] A breakdown in regulatory T-cell activity likely contributes to the development of food allergy. A study of subjects with gastrointestinal milk hypersensitivity examined the cytokine profiles of milk-specific lymphocytes from the duodenal lamina propria. Cells were cultured in vitro in the presence of milk, revealing a clear Th2 cytokine profile. Following restimulation with milk protein, cells released Th2-associated cytokines but failed to release significant amounts of TGF-β and IL-10, key regulatory cytokines important in the development of oral tolerance.[20]

CD4+CD25+ regulatory T cells express the transcription factor forkhead box P3 (FOXP3),[21] which is thought to inhibit Th1 and Th2 responses.[22] Disruptions in the gene encoding FOXP3 can lead to immune dysregulation, as seen in IPEX syndrome, a fatal disorder characterized by autoaggressive lymphocyte clones,

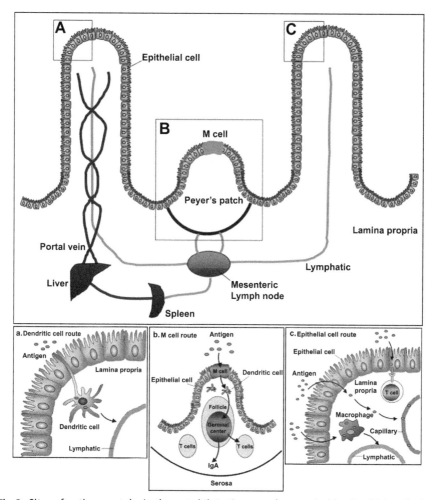

Fig. 2. Sites of antigen uptake in the gut. (*A*) Antigen can be sampled by dendritic cells that extend processes into the lumen. (*B*) M cells overlying Peyer's patches take up particulate antigens and then deliver them to dendritic cells in the subepithelial region and then to underlying B-cell follicles, where IgA commitment occurs. (*C*) Soluble antigens can cross the epithelium through transcellular or paracellular routes to then encounter T cells or macrophages in the lamina propria. (*Adapted from* Chehade M, Mayer L. Oral tolerance and its relation to food hypersensitivities. J Allergy Clin Immunol 2005;115:5; with permission.)

polyendocrinopathy, enteropathy, and X-linked transmission.[23] Recently, a mutation in a noncoding region of FOXP3 that impairs mRNA splicing has been shown to result in a distinct form of IPEX syndrome that combines autoimmune and allergic manifestations including severe enteropathy, food allergies, atopic dermatitis, elevated serum IgE, and eosinophilia.[24]

Furthermore, the appearance of circulating CD4$^+$CD25$^+$ T cells has been associated with the development of tolerance in children with milk allergy. T-cell responses were studied in subjects with non–IgE-mediated milk allergy. Children who achieved milk tolerance had higher numbers of circulating CD4$^+$CD25$^+$ T cells and lower in vitro

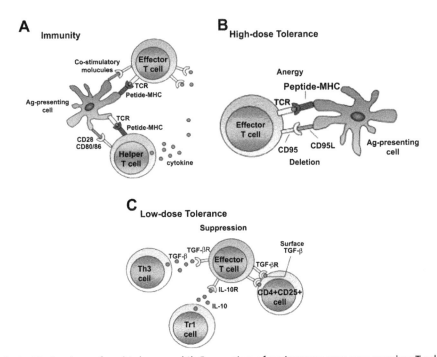

Fig. 3. Mechanisms of oral tolerance. (*A*) Generation of an immune response requires T-cell receptor ligation with peptide-MHC complexes in the presence of appropriate costimulatory molecules (CD80 and CD86) and cytokines. (*B*) High-dose tolerance is induced by T-cell receptor cross-linking in the absence of costimulation or in the presence of inhibitory ligands (CD95 and CD95 ligand), leading to anergy or deletion, respectively. (*C*) Low doses of oral antigen lead to the activation of regulatory CD4+ CD25+ T cells, which suppress immune responses through soluble or cell surface–associated cytokines (IL-10 and TGF-β). L, Ligand; R, receptor. (*Adapted from* Chehade M, Mayer L. Oral tolerance and its relation to food hypersensitivities. J Allergy Clin Immunol 2005;115:7; with permission.)

proliferative responses to bovine β-lactoglobulin in peripheral blood mononuclear cells than those who maintained clinically active allergy.[25] Depletion of CD25[+] cells from peripheral blood mononuclear cells of tolerant children led to a fivefold increase in in vitro proliferation against β-lactoglobulin.

Whereas low-dose tolerance is induced by regulatory T-cell activity, high-dose tolerance is mediated by lymphocyte anergy or clonal deletion (see **Fig. 3**). Anergy can occur through T-cell receptor ligation in the absence of costimulatory signals provided by soluble cytokines, such as IL-2, or through interaction between receptors on T cells (CD28) and counterreceptors on antigen-presenting cells (CD80 and CD86).[26] High antigen doses induce deletion by means of FAS-mediated apoptosis,[27] which can be blocked by the proinflammatory cytokine IL-12.[28]

Aside from antigen dose, several other factors contribute to the development of oral tolerance, including antigen properties, route of exposure, age of the host, and genetic factors. Soluble antigens tend to be more tolerogenic than particulate antigens, although most food allergens are soluble proteins.[7] Solubility can change during food preparation, and a contributing factor to food allergen stability is heat resistance. For example, peanut protein becomes less soluble with progressive roasting, which increases the capacity of peanut-specific IgE binding to the protein.[29] Innate immunostimulatory properties of certain dietary proteins may also play a role in inducing food allergy.[7] The mammalian immune system recognizes microbial proteins in association with pathogen-associated molecular patterns that induce either Th1 or Th2 responses. Similarly, other motifs on nonmammalian proteins may be recognized and result in activation of a Th2 response in susceptible individuals.[30] The route of allergen exposure also plays a role in the development of tolerance. Food antigen exposure by means other than ingestion may cause hypersensitivity; epicutaneous and epidermal exposure to peanut has been shown to prevent oral tolerance and enhance allergic EoE, emphasizing a connection between the development of inflammation in extraintestinal organs and the esophagus.[5,31]

Genetics of the host contributes to the development of oral tolerance or food hypersensitivity and has also been associated with EGIDs, which show a clear male predilection[2] and strong familial clustering.[1] In a murine study of peanut allergen gene immunization, the magnitude of tolerance achieved was highly variable in the different strains of mice.[32] Differential susceptibility to food allergy may be related to the dominant response (Th1 versus Th2) present in different mice strains.[7] Another host factor that has been found to play an important role in oral tolerance is the age of the subject. Feeding a weight-related dose of ovalbumin to mice within the first week of life results in priming of both humoral and cell-mediated immune responses, in contrast to the profound tolerance found in adult animals when treated in the same way.[33]

SUMMARY

Allergy has been implicated in the etiology of EGIDs based on patient characteristics, diagnostic evidence of allergen sensitization, and in vivo and in vitro immunologic findings.[34] Like other forms of food allergy, EGIDs are increasing in prevalence. A recent study reported a fourfold increase in the prevalence of pediatric EoE over the 2000 to 2003 time period.[2] Nonetheless, the incidence of food allergy is remarkably low considering the complexities of the gut-associated lymphoid system, where tolerance is the norm. Like other allergic gastrointestinal diseases, EGIDs may result from a breakdown in oral tolerance mechanisms or a failure of induction of oral tolerance.[15] The precise role of food, cutaneous, or airborne allergen sensitization in the development of EGIDs has yet to be elucidated. Allergy may be a stimulus for the recruitment of eosinophils to the gastrointestinal tract or may lead to the failure of key regulatory $CD4^+CD25^+$ T cells leading to the loss of immunologic tolerance.[35] Bypassing mechanisms of high-dose tolerance, which includes induction of lymphocyte anergy or deletion, may also facilitate the development of EGIDs and other forms of food allergy. Further study to clarify the role of tolerance in the development of EGIDs can help identify potential prevention strategies and therapeutic targets.

REFERENCES

1. Blanchard C, Rothenberg ME. Basic pathogenesis of eosinophilic esophagitis. Gastrointest Endosc Clin N Am 2008;18(1):133–43, x.
2. Noel RJ, Putnam PE, Rothenberg ME. Eosinophilic esophagitis. N Engl J Med 2004;351(9):940–1.
3. Vitellas KM, Bennett WF, Bova JG, et al. Idiopathic eosinophilic esophagitis. Radiology 1993;186(3):789–93.
4. Orenstein SR, Shalaby TM, Di Lorenzo C, et al. The spectrum of pediatric eosinophilic esophagitis beyond infancy: a clinical series of 30 children. Am J Gastroenterol 2000;95(6):1422–30.

5. Akei HS, Mishra A, Blanchard C, et al. Epicutaneous antigen exposure primes for experimental eosinophilic esophagitis in mice. Gastroenterology 2005;129(3): 985–94.

6. Chase M. Inhibition of experimental drug allergy by prior feeding of the sensitizing agent. Proc Soc Exp Biol Med 1946;61:257–9.

7. Burks AW, Laubach S, Jones SM. Oral tolerance, food allergy, and immunotherapy: implications for future treatment. J Allergy Clin Immunol 2008;121(6):1344–50.

8. Kraehenbuhl JP, Neutra MR. Transepithelial transport and mucosal defense II: secretion of IgA. Trends Cell Biol 1992;2(6):170–4.

9. Menezes Jda S, Mucida DS, Cara DC, et al. Stimulation by food proteins plays a critical role in the maturation of the immune system. Int Immunol 2003;15(3):447–55.

10. Aalberse RC. Structural biology of allergens. J Allergy Clin Immunol 2000;106(2): 228–38.

11. Untersmayr E, Jensen-Jarolim E. The role of protein digestibility and antacids on food allergy outcomes. J Allergy Clin Immunol 2008;121(6):1301–8 [quiz: 1309–10].

12. Untersmayr E, Bakos N, Scholl I, et al. Anti-ulcer drugs promote IgE formation toward dietary antigens in adult patients. FASEB J 2005;19(6):656–8.

13. Michael J. The role of digestive enzymes in orally induced immune tolerance. Immunol Invest 1989;18:1049–54.

14. Markowitz JE, Spergel JM, Ruchelli E, et al. Elemental diet is an effective treatment for eosinophilic esophagitis in children and adolescents. Am J Gastroenterol 2003; 98(4):777–82.

15. Chehade M, Mayer L. Oral tolerance and its relation to food hypersensitivities. J Allergy Clin Immunol 2005;115(1):3–12 [quiz: 13].

16. Friedman A, Weiner HL. Induction of anergy or active suppression following oral tolerance is determined by antigen dosage. Proc Natl Acad Sci USA 1994;91(14): 6688–92.

17. Faria AM, Weiner HL. Oral tolerance. Immunol Rev 2005;206:232–59.

18. Nakamura K, Kitani A, Strober W. Cell contact-dependent immunosuppression by CD4(+)CD25(+) regulatory T cells is mediated by cell surface-bound transforming growth factor beta. J Exp Med 2001;194(5):629–44.

19. Piccirillo CA, Letterio JJ, Thornton AM, et al. CD4(+)CD25(+) regulatory T cells can mediate suppressor function in the absence of transforming growth factor beta1 production and responsiveness. J Exp Med 2002;196(2):237–46.

20. Beyer K, Castro R, Birnbaum A, et al. Human milk-specific mucosal lymphocytes of the gastrointestinal tract display a TH2 cytokine profile. J Allergy Clin Immunol 2002;109(4):707–13.

21. Fontenot JD, Gavin MA, Rudensky AY. Foxp3 programs the development and function of CD4+CD25+ regulatory T cells. Nat Immunol 2003;4(4):330–6.

22. Ostroukhova M, Seguin-Devaux C, Oriss TB, et al. Tolerance induced by inhaled antigen involves CD4(+) T cells expressing membrane-bound TGF-beta and FOXP3. J Clin Invest 2004;114(1):28–38.

23. Ochs HD, Gambineri E, Torgerson TR. IPEX, FOXP3 and regulatory T-cells: a model for autoimmunity. Immunol Res 2007;38(1–3):112–21.

24. Torgerson TR, Linane A, Moes N, et al. Severe food allergy as a variant of IPEX syndrome caused by a deletion in a noncoding region of the FOXP3 gene. Gastroenterology 2007;132(5):1705–17.

25. Karlsson MR, Rugtveit J, Brandtzaeg P. Allergen-responsive CD4+CD25+ regulatory T cells in children who have outgrown cow's milk allergy. J Exp Med 2004; 199(12):1679–88.

26. Appleman LJ, Boussiotis VA. T cell anergy and costimulation. Immunol Rev 2003; 192:161–80.
27. Chen Y, Inobe J, Marks R, et al. Peripheral deletion of antigen-reactive T cells in oral tolerance. Nature 1995;376(6536):177–80.
28. Marth T, Zeitz Z, Ludviksson B, et al. Murine model of oral tolerance: induction of Fas-mediated apoptosis by blockade of interleukin-12. Ann N Y Acad Sci 1998; 859:290–4.
29. Kopper RA, Odum NJ, Sen M, et al. Peanut protein allergens: the effect of roasting on solubility and allergenicity. Int Arch Allergy Immunol 2005;136(1):16–22.
30. Shreffler WG, Castro RR, Kucuk ZY, et al. The major glycoprotein allergen from *Arachis hypogaea*, Ara h 1, is a ligand of dendritic cell-specific ICAM-grabbing nonintegrin and acts as a Th2 adjuvant in vitro. J Immunol 2006;177(6):3677–85.
31. Strid J, Hourihane J, Kimber I, et al. Epicutaneous exposure to peanut protein prevents oral tolerance and enhances allergic sensitization. Clin Exp Allergy 2005;35(6):757–66.
32. Li X, Huang CK, Schofield BH, et al. Strain-dependent induction of allergic sensitization caused by peanut allergen DNA immunization in mice. J Immunol 1999; 162(5):3045–52.
33. Strobel S, Ferguson A. Immune responses to fed protein antigens in mice. Systemic tolerance or priming is related to age at which antigen is first encountered. Pediatr Res 1984;18(7):588–94.
34. Furuta GT, Liacouras CA, Collins MH, et al. Eosinophilic esophagitis in children and adults: a systematic review and consensus recommendations for diagnosis and treatment. Gastroenterology 2007;133(4):1342–63.
35. Seibold F. Food-induced immune responses as origin of bowel disease? Digestion 2005;71(4):251–60.

Exploring the Role of Mast Cells in Eosinophilic Esophagitis

Barry K. Wershil, MD

KEYWORDS

• Mast cells • Eosinophils • Esophagitis • Mediators

For most of the last 125 years, since its identification, the mast cell has been narrowly viewed in the context of immediate-type hypersensitivity, as seen in allergic reactions and parasite infections. Over the last decade, it has become increasingly clear that mast cells are involved in a wide variety of important biologic processes, including innate immunity and host defense, adaptive immunity, nonimmunologic inflammation, tissue remodeling, and homeostasis. Moreover, several lines of evidence suggest that, under certain circumstances, mast cells act to limit inflammation and tissue damage.[1] Thus, traditional dogma about the proinflammatory role of mast cells must now be reconsidered to take into account the versatility and complexity of the cell's biologic potential.[2]

This article considers the role of mast cells in eosinophilic esophagitis (EoE). The biologic diversity of the cell is discussed and the evidence implicating mast cells in this condition is reviewed. The evidence to date is still indirect and inconclusive, but several mechanisms by which mast cells could potentially contribute to the pathogenesis of EoE are explored.

THE MAST CELL

Mast cells are found in virtually all vascularized tissues and are particularly abundant at host–environment interfaces, such as the skin or mucosal surfaces like the gastrointestinal tract. They are derived from hematopoietic progenitor cells in the bone marrow but their maturation and differentiation occur in tissues under the influence of several growth factors, such as interleukin (IL)-3, -4, -6, -9, -10, nerve growth factor, and prostaglandin E_2 (in the gastrointestinal tract). However, a critical cytokine in the growth, differentiation, survival, and function of mast cells is stem cell factor, derived from stromal cells and other sources.[3]

Mast cells do not represent a homogenous population of cells but rather, have morphologic, biochemical, and functional differences based on the factors seen in the microenvironment. Human mast cells are classified into two types based on their

Division of Pediatric Gastroenterology, Hepatology, and Nutrition, Children's Memorial Hospital, 2300 Children's Plaza, Box 65, Chicago, IL 60614, USA
E-mail address: bwershil@childrensmemorial.org

Immunol Allergy Clin N Am 29 (2009) 189–195
doi:10.1016/j.iac.2008.09.006   immunology.theclinics.com
0889-8561/08/$ – see front matter © 2009 Elsevier Inc. All rights reserved.

protease content: tryptase-containing mast cells (MC_T), and mast cells with tryptase and chymase within the cytoplasmic granules (MC_{TC}).[4] Human MC_T are located predominantly in mucosal tissues, such as the intestine and respiratory tract, whereas human MC_{TC} are mainly found in connective tissues such as the skin but are also in the submucosa and muscularis propria of the intestinal tract. Mast cells are a significant component of the gastrointestinal tract, making up as much as 1% of cells in the submucosa and 2% to 3% of the cells in the lamina propria.[5]

Mast cells are normally found in the mucosa and submucosa of the esophagus, but rarely in the muscularis.[6] The expansion of mast cells into the muscularis has been reported in esophageal leiomyomatosis, in conjunction with diffuse eosinophilic infiltration.[7] But our understanding of the numbers and distribution of mast cells in EoE has been limited by several factors. The esophagus has long been thought to be little more than a conduit for food, with little interest from an immunologic perspective, until recently. As a result, we still have only a rudimentary understanding of the immunology of this portion of the gastrointestinal tract. Most of what we know comes from biopsies obtained at the time of endoscopy, which are typically superficial and therefore do not give us a complete picture. With regard to the mast cells in the human esophagus, the subsets of cell types have not been described in detail either, but the assumption is that, because the esophagus is composed of squamous epithelium, MC_{TC} type mast cells would be predominant.

Mast cell activation with the release of mediators can occur through several mechanisms (**Box 1**). The most extensively studied is antigen cross linking of IgE antibodies on the surface of the mast cell, leading to degranulation and mediator release. Although this mechanism may be relevant in some cases of EoE, it is probably a minority. But many alternative pathways can induce mast cell mediators independent of IgE. These include stem cell factor, complement fragments (C3a and C5a), neuropeptides, adenosine, and cell wall components of bacteria (see **Box 1**). Particularly relevant to EoE is the ability of eosinophil-derived proteins to induce mast cell degranulation. Other mechanisms that can induce mast cell mediator release in the gastrointestinal tract include acid reflux[8] and bile acids.[9] Thus, several classic immunologic and alternative mechanisms may be involved in the activation of esophageal mast cells during inflammation.

At one time, it was thought that mast cell activation/mediator production was synonymous with degranulation. However, it is now clear that the production of mediators is specific to the eliciting stimulus and may be independent of the process of degranulation. A now well-studied example is the interaction of bacterial lipopolysaccharide and other components of bacteria with Toll-like receptors expressed on the mast cell.[10] These interactions result in cytokine production (eg, tumor necrosis factor-alpha [TNF-α] and IL-6) in the absence of degranulation. This dissociation of mast cell mediator release and degranulation makes it difficult to assess mast cell participation in any condition solely on a histologic evaluation of mast cell degranulation. Equally important is the evolving concept that without knowledge of the activating stimulus, the finding of mast cell degranulation alone does not provide insight into the specific mediators being produced.

Mast cells contain, and can synthesize, various biologically potent mediators, as depicted in **Fig. 1**. Within the cytoplasmic granules of the mast cell are a panel of preformed mediators, including histamine, neutral proteases, TNF-α, and others.[11] Mast cells can also produce newly synthesized mediators, such as leukotrienes, platelet-activating factor, and a host of cytokines and chemokines (see **Fig. 1**). Cytokines such as IL-5 and IL-13 are particularly important because they have been implicated in the etiopathogenesis of EoE.[12]

Box 1
Relevant potential pathways involved in the activation and release of mediators from mast cells in eosinophilic esophagitis

Antibody receptors

IgE

IgG_1

Superantigens

Cytokines/mediators

Stem cell factor

Tryptase

IL-1, IL-12

Adenosine

Prostaglandin E_2

Tumor necrosis factor

Granule-associated products of eosinophils

Major basic protein

Eosinophil cationic protein

Fragments of complement activation

C3a, C5a

C3b, C4b

Endogenous peptides

Neuropeptides: substance P, calcitonin gene-related peptide, neurotensin, vasoactive intestinal polypeptide

Nerve growth factor

Endothelin-1

Antimicrobial peptides (source: neutrophils)

Bacterial products

Lipopolysaccharide

Peptidoglycan

CpG-DNA

This list of mast cell activating agents is incomplete. The particular agents involved and their precise contribution in EoE is unknown. The response of mast cells to each agent may differ, depending on the species (rodent versus human) and mast cell population (mucosal versus connective tissue) examined. See Ref.[26] for a more comprehensive review of this topic.

The production of these mediators by mast cells can have several direct or indirect effects (ie, they may interact directly with eosinophils or resident cells to elicit a response, or indirectly by recruiting additional immune cells into the esophagus).

EVIDENCE OF MAST CELL PARTICIPATION IN EOSINOPHILIC ESOPHAGITIS

Much of the data implicating mast cells in the pathogenesis of EoE is indirect and inferential. An increased number of mast cells have been noted in esophageal biopsies

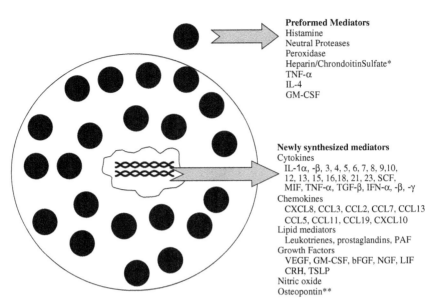

Fig. 1. Mast cell activation can lead to release of preformed mediators contained within cytoplasmic granules or newly synthesized mediators. *Matrix proteoglycan differs in connective tissue and mucosal mast cell populations. **To date, osteopontin has only been identified as a product of murine connective tissue-type mast cells. bFGF, basic fibroblast growth factor; CRH, corticotropin-releasing hormone; GM-CSF, granulocyte-macrophage colony-stimulating factor; IFN, interferon; LIF, leukemia inhibitory factor; MIF, macrophage inhibitory factor; NGF, nerve growth factor; PAF, platelet-activating factor; SCF, stem cell factor; TGF, transforming growth factor; TSLP, thymic stromal lymphopoietin; VEGF, vascular endothelial growth factor.

from patients who had EoE,[13–17] with as many as 20 times the normal number of mast cells found in the mucosal layer of the esophagus.[17] An increase in mast cell numbers correlates with the degree of esophageal eosinophilia and the number of mast cells diminishes with effective treatment.[17–19] However, studies differ in being able to find evidence of mast cell degranulation.[14,15] Elevated levels of mast cell–specific/associated genes have been reported,[14] including a 13-fold and 6-fold increase in the genes carboxypeptidase A3 and tryptase, respectively, and a 4-fold increase in the gene for the high affinity receptor for IgE, $Fc_\varepsilon RI$.[14]

The significance of these findings remains to be determined but taken together, they suggest that mast cells are an active cellular component of the pathology associated with EoE.

POTENTIAL MECHANISMS OF MAST CELL INVOLVEMENT IN EOSINOPHILIC ESOPHAGITIS

Mast cells can contribute to the pathogenesis of EoE through several possible mechanisms.

Mast cells can have several direct and indirect interactions with eosinophils. They may be involved in eosinophil activation or survival through the production of IL-4, -5, granulocyte-macrophage colony-stimulating factor (GM-CSF), IL-13, and eotaxin-1. Mast cell release of tryptase may also activate eosinophils by way of protease-activated receptor 2 (PAR_2) expressed on their cell surface, which can induce eosinophil granule protein release, superoxide generation, and cytokine secretion.[20] Mast cells can promote eosinophil recruitment by their ability to synthesize and release eosinophil-selective chemokines and leukotrienes (see **Fig. 1**). The release of mast cell-granule–associated proteoglycans, like heparin from connective tissue mast cells, can potentiate the action of chemokines such as eotaxin, an eosinophil-specific chemokine.[21] Some of the cationic proteins contained by eosinophils, particularly eosinophil-derived major basic protein, can induce mast cell degranulation and TNF-α production,[7] which represents a potential positive feedback loop augmenting the inflammatory response.

The release of mediators, such as histamine, leukotrienes, TNF-α, and eosinophil chemoattractants, can act to augment edema, inflammatory cell recruitment, and smooth muscle contractility, and enhance adaptive immune responses. Mast cells are also a source of transforming growth factor-beta (TGF-β) and IL-5, which have been implicated in various conditions associated with tissue fibrosis, including EoE.[22] The effect of mast cell mediator production could be to augment inflammation, alter esophageal motility, and promote stricture formation.

However, some aspects of mast cell involvement in EoE may act to limit the inflammatory response. Several products of mast cells, such as TGF-β, histamine, IL-4, and IL-10 can have anti-inflammatory effects or the potential to down-regulate aspects of acquired immune responses. Mast cells can also produce mediators that degrade proinflammatory molecules. For example, mast cell tryptase can cleave and inactivate calcitonin gene-related peptide, and some mast cell proteases can degrade endothelin-1.

In patients who have esophageal achalasia, a primary motility disorder, mast cell numbers expand in the esophagus and the mast cells seem to associate with the interstitial cells of Cajal (ICC),[23] which are important in motor activity in the gastrointestinal tract. This association appears to correlate with survival of the ICC,[23] implying

---

Box 2
Theoretic consideration of mast cell functions in eosinophilic esophagitis (effector and immunomodulatory roles)

Proinflammatory

Alter vascular endothelium (eg, histamine, leukotrienes, tryptase, vascular endothelial growth factor, platelet-activating factor, nitric oxide, corticotropin-releasing hormone)

Recruit eosinophils and other immune cells (eg, chemokines, IL-8, TNF-α, leukotrienes)

Promote proliferation of eosinophils and other immune cells (eg, IL-5, GM-CSF, IL-3, and other growth factors)

Activate eosinophils (eg, tryptase activation of PAR_2 receptors)

Promote tissue remodeling/fibrosis (eg, TGF-β, tryptase, IL-5)

Promote T helper-1 response (eg, histamine, osteopontin)

Anti-inflammatory

Promote clearance of pathogens by phagocytosis, secretion of antimicrobial peptides

Degrade potential toxic endogenous peptides (eg, protease inactivation of endothelin-1)

Release anti-inflammatory peptides (eg, somatostatin)

Suppress adaptive immune responses (eg, IL-10)

Promote antigenic tolerance (eg, IL-10)

Suppress T helper-1 and T helper-2 cell activation (eg, histamine)

These roles include direct and indirect action of mast cell mediators on immune targets and on "nonimmune" cells, such as vascular endothelial cells, fibroblasts, nerve cells, and muscle cells.

a protective function for mast cells with regards to enteric nerves. This protective function of the mast cell for ICCs has also been suggested in Crohn's disease.[24]

It can also be argued that the proinflammatory and anti-inflammatory actions of mast cells are not mutually exclusive. Inflammation is a dynamic process composed of phases, including initiation, augmentation, and resolution. It is certainly possible that mast cells could make a proinflammatory contribution during the initiation and augmentation phases and play an anti-inflammatory role in the resolution phase (**Box 2**).

SUMMARY

Current evidence suggests that mast cells are involved in EoE, and several potential mechanisms were suggested for how mast cells might contribute to this condition. However, the precise role of the mast cell in EoE remains unknown. Further research will be necessary to define the mast cell populations in EoE, the relevant biologic triggers inducing mast cell activation, the specific "panel" of mediators produced, and the net contribution of mast cells to the pathophysiology of this condition. This research will require intense basic investigation, which should be facilitated by animal models, particularly mast cell–deficient mice, in which it is possible to isolate the mast cell as an experimental variable.[25] Although a proinflammatory component to the involvement of mast cells in EoE appears to exist, it will be important to keep an open mind and explore all possibilities.

REFERENCES

1. Galli SJ, Grimbaldeston M, Tsai M. Immunomodulatory mast cells: negative, as well as positive, regulators of immunity. Nat Rev Immunol 2008;8(6):478–86.
2. Leslie M. Mast cells show their might. Science 2007;317(5838):614–6.
3. Galli SJ, Zsebo KM, Geissler EN. The kit ligand, stem cell factor. Adv Immunol 1994;55:1–96.
4. Irani AA, Schechter NM, Craig SS, et al. Two types of human mast cells that have distinct neutral protease compositions. Proc Natl Acad Sci U S A 1986;83(12): 4464–8.
5. Bischoff SC, Wedemeyer J, Herrmann A, et al. Quantitative assessment of intestinal eosinophils and mast cells in inflammatory bowel disease. Histopathology 1996;28(1):1–13.
6. Tung HN, Schulze-Delrieu K, Shirazi S. Infiltration of hypertrophic esophageal smooth muscle by mast cells and basophils. J Submiscrosc Cytol Pathol 1993; 25:93–102.
7. Nicholson AG, Li D, Pastorino U, et al. Full thickness eosinophilia in oesophageal leiomyomatosis and idiopathic eosinophilic oesophagitis. A common allergic inflammatory profile? J Pathol 1997;183(2):233–6.
8. Paterson WG. Role of mast cell-derived mediators in acid-induced shortening of the esophagus. Am J Phys 1998;274(2 Pt 1):G385–8.
9. Quist RG, Ton-Nu HT, Lillienau J, et al. Activation of mast cells by bile acids. Gastroenterology 1991;101(2):446–56.
10. Marshall JS. Mast-cell responses to pathogens. Nat Rev Immunol 2004;4(10): 787–99.
11. Galli SJ, Kalesnikoff J, Grimbaldeston MA, et al. Mast cells as "tunable" effector and immunoregulatory cells: recent advances. Annu Rev Immunol 2005;23:749–86.
12. Blanchard C, Rothenberg ME. Basic pathogenesis of eosinophilic esophagitis. Gastrointest Endosc Clin N Am 2008;18(1):133–43, x.

13. Straumann A, Bauer M, Fischer B, et al. Idiopathic eosinophilic esophagitis is associated with a TH2-type allergic inflammatory response. J Allergy Clin Immunol 2001;108(6):954–61.
14. Blanchard C, Wang N, Stringer KF, et al. Eotaxin-3 and a uniquely conserved gene-expression profile in eosinophilic esophagitis. J Clin Invest 2006;116(2): 536–47.
15. Kirsch R, Bokhary R, Marcon MA, et al. Activated mucosal mast cells differentiate eosinophilic (allergic) esophagitis from gastroesophageal reflux disease. J Pediatr Gastroenterol Nutr 2007;44(1):20–6.
16. Gupta SK, Fitzgerald JF, Kondratyuk T, et al. Cytokine expression in normal and inflamed esophageal mucosa: a study into the pathogenesis of allergic eosinophilic esophagitis. J Pediatr Gastroenterol Nutr 2006;42(1):22–6.
17. Lucendo AJ, Navarro M, Comas C, et al. Immunophenotypic characterization and quantification of the epithelial inflammatory infiltrate in eosinophilic esophagitis through stereology: an analysis of the cellular mechanisms of the disease and the immunologic capacity of the esophagus. Am J Surg Pathol 2007;31(4): 598–606.
18. Chehade M, Sampson HA, Morotti RA, et al. Esophageal subepithelial fibrosis in children with eosinophilic esophagitis. J Pediatr Gastroenterol Nutr 2007;45(3): 319–28.
19. Konikoff MR, Noel RJ, Blanchard C, et al. A randomized, double-blind, placebo-controlled trial of fluticasone propionate for pediatric eosinophilic esophagitis. Gastroenterology 2006;131(5):1381–91.
20. Shpacovitch V, Feld M, Hollenberg MD, et al. Role of protease-activated receptors in inflammatory responses, innate and adaptive immunity. J Leukoc Biol 2008;83(6):1309–22.
21. Ellyard JI, Simson L, Bezos A, et al. Eotaxin selectively binds heparin. An interaction that protects eotaxin from proteolysis and potentiates chemotactic activity in vivo. J Biol Chem 2007;282(20):15238–47.
22. Mishra A, Wang M, Pemmaraju VR, et al. Esophageal remodeling develops as a consequence of tissue specific IL-5-induced eosinophilia. Gastroenterology 2008;134(1):204–14.
23. Zarate N, Wang XY, Tougas G, et al. Intramuscular interstitial cells of Cajal associated with mast cells survive nitrergic nerves in achalasia. Neurogastroenterol Motil 2006;18(7):556–68.
24. Wang XY, Zarate N, Soderholm JD, et al. Ultrastructural injury to interstitial cells of Cajal and communication with mast cells in Crohn's disease. Neurogastroenterol Motil 2007;19(5):349–64.
25. Tsai M, Grimbaldeston MA, Yu M, et al. Using mast cell knock-in mice to analyze the roles of mast cells in allergic responses in vivo. Chem Immunol Allergy 2005; 87:179–97.
26. Metz M, Grimbaldeston MA, Nakae S, et al. Mast cells in the promotion and limitation of chronic inflammation. Immunol Rev 2007;217:304–28.

Relationships Between Eosinophilic Inflammation, Tissue Remodeling, and Fibrosis in Eosinophilic Esophagitis

Seema S. Aceves, MD, PhD[a,b,c], Steven J. Ackerman, PhD[d,e],*

KEYWORDS

- Eosinophilic esophagitis • Eosinophils • Inflammation
- Remodeling • Fibrosis • Angiogenesis
- Transforming growth factor-β

Eosinophilic esophagitis (EE) is a disease of increasing prevalence and detection.[1–4] Its pathogenesis relies in part on an allergic immune reaction that can involve both IgE and T-cell mediated hypersensitivity to inhaled aeroallergens and ingested food allergens. The clinical manifestations of EE include vomiting, abdominal pain, regurgitation, heartburn, and failure to thrive, especially in young children. In adolescents and

This work was supported by grants from the National Institutes of Health, R21AI079925 (SJA); an American Gastroenterological Association (AGA) Translational Research Award (SJA); an American Partnership for Eosinophilic Diseases (APFED) HOPE Research Award (SSA); an American Academy of Allergy, Asthma, Immunology Junior Women in Allergy grant (SSA); and a gift from the Campaign Urging Research on Eosinophilic Diseases (CURED) (SJA).

a Division of Allergy and Immunology, Rady Children's Hospital, 3020 Children's Way, MC 5114, San Diego, CA 92123–6791, USA
b Department of Pediatrics, Division of Allergy and Immunology, 9500 Gilman Drive, MC-0635, University of California, La Jolla, CA 92093, USA
c Department of Medicine, Division of Allergy and Immunology, 9500 Gilman Drive, MC-0635, University of California, La Jolla, CA 92093, USA
d Department of Biochemistry and Molecular Genetics (M/C 669), 900 South Ashland Avenue, Room 2074, Molecular Biology Research Building, The University of Illinois at Chicago College of Medicine, Chicago, IL 60607-7170, USA
e Department of Medicine, 900 South Ashland Avenue, University of Illinois at Chicago, Chicago, IL 60607-7170, USA
* Corresponding author. Department of Biochemistry and Molecular Genetics (M/C 669), 900 South Ashland Avenue, Room 2074, Molecular Biology Research Building, The University of Illinois at Chicago College of Medicine, Chicago, IL 60607.
E-mail address: 7170.sackerma@uic.edu (S.J. Ackerman).

adults, the symptoms can progress to odynophagia and dysphagia that can be associated with the clinical complications of food impactions with or without concurrent esophageal strictures.[5–7] EE seems to be a chronic disease with persistent dysphagia when left untreated in adults.[8] In children, the disease remits with therapies, including systemic or topical esophageal corticosteroids, and elimination or elemental diets, but recurs in most patients when the therapeutic intervention is removed.[9]

The histopathologic changes that occur in EE traverse the depths of the esophageal wall.[10,11] The mucosa becomes infiltrated with eosinophils, mast cells, and T cells, and active proliferation of the epithelium leads to the histologic finding of basal zone hyperplasia.[12,13] The submucosal lamina propria also becomes infiltrated by inflammatory cells and demonstrates increased collagen deposition that provides an extracellular matrix for the capture of cells and their cytokine, interleukin (IL), and chemokine[14–17] products. The muscularis mucosa and the circular and longitudinal muscle layers have reported abnormalities with hypertrophy and dysfunction.[10] In combination, the multiple facets of esophageal remodeling and subepithelial fibrosis that occur during the instigation and propagation of EE could explain many of the clinical symptoms. This article reviews the known aspects of esophageal remodeling, the basic molecular mechanisms used by eosinophils to promote tissue remodeling and fibrosis, and the clinical correlates of esophageal remodeling in EE.

Based on the paradigms of other eosinophil-mediated diseases, the role of tissue remodeling in the pathogenesis and clinical manifestations of EE is beginning to be investigated (**Fig. 1**). Tissue remodeling in response to Th2 and eosinophil-associated diseases was first characterized in the hypereosinophilic syndrome and asthma.[18–21] In hypereosinophilic syndrome, eosinophil activation and degranulation causes target organ fibrosis. Significant patient mortality and morbidity is related to the development of endomyocardial fibrosis and subsequent cardiac failure associated with eosinophilic infiltration.[21,22] Another Th2- and eosinophil-associated disease, asthma, is characterized by tissue remodeling consisting of airway epithelial cell transformation to mucous production, smooth muscle hyperplasia and hypertrophy, subepithelial fibrosis, and angiogenesis.[19] These histologic and structural changes cause clinical disease manifestations of bronchial hyperreactivity, airway edema, and mucous plugging with subsequent airway lumen narrowing. In a subset of patients, this airways obstruction becomes irreversible. Although the role of the eosinophil in hypereosinophilic syndrome is clear, its role in asthma is beginning to be resolved.[18,23]

Murine models of asthma have demonstrated a significant contribution of the eosinophil to disease pathogenesis. Double transgenic mice with airway eotaxin-2 and systemic IL-5 have severe asthma and collagen deposition that is significantly diminished if the animals lack eosinophils.[20,24] The best human correlate to absent eosinophils is treatment with anti–IL-5 antibodies. Through the reduction in IL-5, the major eosinophilopoietic stimulus is lost. As compared with control patients, asthmatics treated with a humanized, monoclonal anti–IL-5 antibody demonstrate decreased levels of extracellular matrix proteins, such as lumican, tenascin, and procollagen III.[25] Studies on the role of tissue remodeling in eosinophilic gastrointestinal diseases are beginning to evolve and are delineated next.

CLINICAL IMPLICATIONS OF TISSUE REMODELING
Epithelial Changes in Relation to Fibrosis

The nonkeratinized squamous epithelial cells of the esophagus are important mediators of inflammation in EE. When in a Th2 milieu, the esophageal epithelium becomes an immunologically active tissue that expresses chemotactic factors for eosinophils,

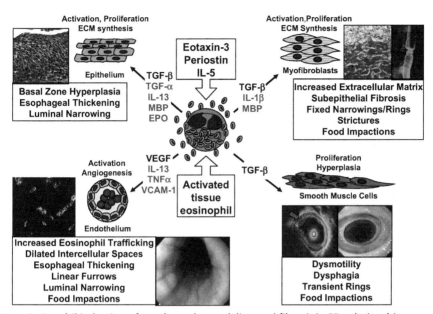

Fig. 1. Eosinophil induction of esophageal remodeling and fibrosis in EE: relationships to endoscopic and histologic pathologies. Eosinophil activation during recruitment to the esophagus occurs in response to eotaxin-3, periostin, IL-5, and interactions with vascular endothelium, epithelium, and fibroblasts, leading to their expression of fibrogenic factors, such as TGF-β. Eosinophil-expressed TGF-β and granule proteins (MBP, EPO) induce epithelial basal zone hyperplasia, contributing to esophageal thickening and luminal narrowing. Eosinophil-derived TGF-β induces fibroblast activation, with transdifferentiation to myofibroblasts and consequent overproduction of ECM leading to subepithelial fibrosis, fixed narrowings and rings, strictures, and food impactions. Alternatively, TGF-β expressed by eosinophils or MBP-EPO damaged epithelium itself may induce epithelial to mesenchymal (myofibroblast) transition (EMT) contributing to subepithelial fibrosis. Eosinophil-expressed TGF-β may induce smooth muscle cell hypertrophy and hyperplasia leading to thickening of the esophageal muscularis propria, contributing to dysmotility, dysphagia, transient rings, and nonstricture food impactions. Eosinophil expression of vascular endothelial growth factor (VEGF) likely supports increased angiogenic responses of vascular endothelium with vascular cell adhesion molecule-1 (VCAM-1) activation by IL-13 and TNF-α, contributing to increased eosinophil trafficking, dilated intercellular spaces, esophageal thickening, furrowing, luminal narrowing, and nonstricture food impactions. (*Adapted from* Teitelbaum JE, Fox VL, Twarog FJ, et al. Eosinophilic esophagitis in children: immunopathological analysis and response to fluticasone propionate. Gastroenterology 2002;122:1221; Straumann A, Spichtin HP, Grize L, et al. Natural history of primary eosinophilic esophagitis: a follow-up of 30 adult patients for up to 11.5 years. Gastroenterology 2003;125(6):1665; Fox VL, Nurko S, Teitelbaum JE, et al. High-resolution EUS in children with eosinophilic "allergic" esophagitis. Gastrointest Endosc 2003;57:31, 33; Aceves SS, Newbury RO, Dohil R, et al. Esophageal remodeling in pediatric eosinophilic esophagitis. J Allergy Clin Immunol 2007;119:210; Wikimedia Commons; with permission. Endoscopic view of trachealization in eosinophilic esophagitis courtesy of A. F. Kagalwalla, MD, Chicago, IL.)

including eotaxin-3 and periostin.[26,27] In addition, both an aeroallergen-driven murine model of EE and human biopsy specimens demonstrate the induction of mucin genes, such as muc-5, in the epithelium.[28]

The Th2 cytokine, IL-13, is pivotal for airway remodeling. Studies in murine asthma models overexpressing airway epithelial IL-13 demonstrate robust tissue fibrosis and airway mucous production.[29,30] IL-13 also seems to be an important inflammatory mediator in EE with IL-13 mRNA levels induced 16-fold in epithelial biopsies from pediatric EE patients as compared with normal controls.[31] Esophageal epithelial cells increase their production of eotaxin-3 in a signal transducer activation transcription-6 (STAT6)-dependent manner when cultured with IL-13, providing a potential positive feedback loop for eosinophil recruitment.[16,31] The increased bulk of epithelial cells in EE patients, reflected in the histologic finding of basal zone hyperplasia and the endoscopic finding of epithelial mucosal thickening with luminal narrowing, may further enhance eosinophil recruitment and, hence, eosinophil-mediated esophageal remodeling and fibrosis (see **Fig. 1**). Although the eosinophil can be a significant cellular source of IL-13 in other disease states,[32] the source of IL-13 in EE remains to be clearly identified.

Clinical Implications of Smooth Muscle Hyperplasia

Dysphagia, in part a reflection of esophageal dysmotility, is a cardinal and distinguishing clinical feature in both pediatric and adult EE.[2,33–35] Pediatric studies[5] have shown that EE patients complain of dysphagia at significantly higher rates than their normal, allergic, or gastroesophageal reflux disease counterparts.[33,36,37] Whereas young children with EE have vomiting, heartburn, and poor growth, older children and adults often complain of persistent or recurrent dysphagia.[8,38] In one adult series, 10% of patients who complained of solid food dysphagia met histologic criteria (defined as >20 eosinophils per hpf) for EE, and adults with EE are 2.6 times more likely to complain of dysphagia.[39]

Studies of esophageal dysmotility in EE have occurred exclusively in adult patients. To date, 61 adult patients have had published motility studies.[40] Of these patients, 60% had abnormal motility, mainly categorized as spastic or hypercontractile.[40,41] More recently, Hariprasad and colleagues[42] have reported that the longitudinal muscle contractions in EE patients are abnormal, whereas circular muscle contractions are normal, leading to the dissociation of coordinated muscle contraction. The eosinophil, with granule products such as major basic protein-1 (MBP-1), which are known to alter smooth muscle contractility through inhibition of M2 muscarinic receptors,[43] may contribute to the motor dysfunction of the esophagus, and topical steroid therapy with resultant resolution of eosinophilia is associated with the resolution of esophageal dysmotility.[40]

Muscular hypertrophy and hyperplasia may exacerbate the contractile abnormalities seen in EE. Although analyses of the smooth muscle in EE are limited to date, endoscopic ultrasound studies in pediatric EE patients have demonstrated thickening through the entire esophagus wall, including the mucosa and submucosa and the muscularis propria.[10] Esophageal involvement in eosinophilic gastroenteritis is also reportedly associated with smooth muscle hypertrophy and infiltration of the muscularis propria with eosinophils.[11] Lastly, an EE model using inhaled *Aspergillus* demonstrates an increase in muscularis mucosa thickness.[28] Taken together, these data demonstrate that aeroallergen-driven EE can cause muscle hypertrophy and hyperplasia with eosinophilic inflammation. Resultant discordant hypercontractility, likely driven in part by eosinophil granule products, such as MBP-1, could explain the endoscopic finding of transient concentric rings and the clinical symptom of food impaction without strictures (see **Fig. 1**).

Pathogenic Mechanisms of Eosinophil–Smooth Muscle Interactions

Evidence for the pathophysiologic participation of eosinophils in smooth muscle hypertrophy and hyperplasia, contraction, and hyperreactivity to cholinergic agents comes from in vitro, animal model, and human studies of eosinophil-derived transforming growth factor (TGF)-β and the eosinophil granule cationic proteins, particularly MBP-1, on airway bronchial smooth muscle in asthma. In chronic murine allergic asthma models, eosinophil-deficient mice show significant decreases in airway smooth muscle hyperplasia in association with decreased numbers of TGF-β–positive cells, primarily eosinophils, and myofibroblasts in the airways.[24,44,45] Likewise, treatment of mild to moderate asthmatics with anti–IL-5 antibody (Mepolizumab) significantly decreases the numbers of TGF-β–positive cells, primarily eosinophils, in the airways, with concomitant decreases in airways remodeling in terms of the deposition of extracellular matrix proteins and numbers of myofibroblasts.[19,25]

A connection between eosinophils and smooth muscle contractility was initially demonstrated by the ability of eosinophil granule cationic proteins, such as MBP-1, directly to induce airway smooth muscle contraction, bronchoconstriction, and airways hyperreactivity in rat,[46,47] guinea pig,[48] and primate[49] asthma models. The mechanism by which eosinophils increase (airway) smooth muscle contractility and hyperresponsiveness to cholinergic stimulation was initially highlighted by studies demonstrating that MBP-1 is a potent antagonist of inhibitory M2 muscarinic receptors.[50] Studies in the guinea pig asthma model followed showing that parasympathetic neurons in the airways secrete eotaxin, which recruits eosinophils to the nerves, resulting in eosinophil secretion of MBP-1 and inhibition of M2 muscarinic receptors, leading to airways hyperreactivity.[43] Importantly, pretreatment of allergen-challenged guinea pigs with a neutralizing antibody to eosinophil MBP was shown to prevent airway hyperresponsiveness by protecting neuronal M2 muscarinic receptors.[51] Hyperreactivity to histamine in this model was vagally mediated and dependent on MBP.[52] Loss of M2 receptor function leads to increased acetylcholine release from cholinergic nerves, providing a mechanism for the vagally mediated airway hyperreactivity seen in this model.[53] Studies also showed that eosinophils localize to the airway nerves of sensitized animals after antigen challenge, and that inhibiting this localization with an antibody to IL-5[54] or the eosinophil adhesion molecule very late activation-4 (VLA-4),[55,56] or with an eotaxin receptor (CCR3) antagonist,[57] prevents airway hyperreactivity subsequent to the loss of inhibitory M2 muscarinic receptor function. Although this mechanism remains to be confirmed in human asthma, loss of function of lung neuronal M2 muscarinic receptors may also occur, and neurons in human airways have been shown to secrete eotaxin[57] and to be infiltrated by eosinophils in fatal human asthma.[58] The rapid reappearance of both eosinophils and concentric rings (trachealization) in the esophagus of some EE patients within 2 to 3 days of reintroducing an offending food allergen into their diet is entirely consistent with eosinophil-mediated effects on smooth muscle or neurons through these types of mechanisms.[59] Whether eosinophils contribute to the discordant hypercontractility of esophageal smooth muscle directly in EE, or whether eosinophil-neuronal cell interactions contribute to the endoscopic finding of trachealization and clinical symptoms of food impaction in the absence of strictures remains to be determined.

Clinical Implications of Fibrosis

Fibrosis is defined histologically by increased collagen content of the subepithelial tissue. Although the exact collagen subtypes that are elevated in esophageal remodeling in EE remain to be elucidated, both adult and pediatric patients have increased subepithelial fibrosis.[7,14,15] Fibrosis likely contributes to multiple clinical aspects of EE, including dysphagia symptoms, disease chronicity, and stricture formation.

Among pediatric EE patients with increased subepithelial fibrosis, 42% complain of dysphagia, often with concurrent food impaction.[15] Pediatric EE patients with long-standing or stricture-associated disease have increased subepithelial collagen deposition as compared with their normal or gastroesophageal reflux disease counterparts. It is likely that both TGF-β and the eosinophil play important roles in the mechanism of fibrosis in EE because pediatric EE patients have increased numbers of TGF-β₁–producing cells and increased activation of the TGF-β signaling pathway as reflected by the increased numbers of cells expressing the nuclear phosphorylated Smad2/3 complex.[14] The eosinophil is one cellular source of TGF-β in EE; patients and animals that lack eosinophils have diminished subepithelial fibrosis in response to aeroallergen challenge.[14,28]

IL-5 is a master regulator of eosinophilopoesis, trafficking, survival, and activation. Biopsies from both adult and pediatric EE patients demonstrate elevated IL-5 levels[60] and murine allergen-driven EE requires IL-5.[28] IL-5, together with the eotaxins, activates eosinophils to release their inflammatory products. IL-5–deficient EE mice lack esophageal subepithelial fibrosis,[28] and patients with both asthma and atopic dermatitis have decreased tissue remodeling of the airways and skin, respectively, when treated with a humanized monoclonal antibody that blocks IL-5.[25,61] Adult EE patients treated with anti–IL-5 (Mepolizumab) have been reported to have decreased dysphagia and improvement in EE-associated strictures following therapy in a small open-label study,[62] suggesting the role of eosinophils or IL-5 in the pathogenesis of human esophageal narrowing. In contrast, a recent placebo-controlled study of anti–IL-5 in adult EE patients showed approximately 55% decreases in esophageal eosinophils without improvements in clinical disease.[63] It is possible that, as suggested by studies with topical corticosteroids and food elimination or elemental diets, esophageal eosinophils may need to be reduced to near normal levels (ie, essentially no eosinophils) to reverse clinical symptoms, and anti–IL-5 alone may not be sufficient to induce significant clinical and pathologic remissions. Current clinical trials ongoing in EE should contribute to the understanding of the role of IL-5 and the eosinophil in esophageal remodeling and fibrosis.

Pathogenic Mechanisms of Eosinophil-Mediated Fibrosis

In addition to EE,[10,64] eosinophils are considered a major effector cell of tissue fibrosis[65] in a variety of eosinophil-associated allergic diseases and hypereosinophilic syndromes including asthma,[66,67] eosinophil myalgia syndrome,[68] eosinophilic endomyocardial fibrosis,[22] idiopathic pulmonary fibrosis,[69] and scleroderma.[68] Eosinophils are implicated in fibrogenesis through these clinical disease associations; their elaboration of fibrogenic growth factors, such as TGF-β,[70,71] PDGF-BB,[72] IL-1β;[73] and secretion of their granule cationic proteins, particularly MBP[74] and eosinophil peroxidase.[75] The association of degranulating eosinophils and deposition of their granule cationic proteins in tissues with pathologic fibrosis is a recurrent finding in a broad group of eosinophilic illnesses including EE.[5] Eosinophils have been identified as the major TGF-β–producing cell in the lungs of asthmatics[67] and in the esophagus in pediatric EE.[14]

Both human and animal model studies provide compelling evidence for eosinophils as effectors of tissue remodeling and fibrosis. Reduction in bronchial eosinophils induced by treatment of asthmatics with anti–IL-5 antibody (Mepolizumab) decreases the expression of ECM proteins in the reticular basement membrane,[25] and anti–IL-5 similarly decreases both eosinophils and deposition of ECM proteins in allergen-induced late-phase skin reactions in atopic subjects.[61] Direct evidence for eosinophil induction of remodeling and fibrosis comes from studies in eosinophil-deficient mice, demonstrating their essential role in the development of airway remodeling, including mucus (goblet) cell metaplasia, smooth muscle cell hyperplasia, and subepithelial fibrosis.[20,44,45]

Multiple growth factors and cytokines expressed by eosinophils[76] are implicated in tissue remodeling and fibrosis. TGF-β, the most widely studied and potently fibrogenic, regulates the expression of the profibrogenic cytokine IL-6; the myofibroblast marker α-smooth muscle actin (α-SMA); and other ECM proteins, such as the collagens. TGF-β expression is correlated with bronchial airway fibrosis and asthma severity,[77] and it's overexpression in the lung in rodent animal models induces pulmonary fibrosis.[70]

Eosinophil-fibroblast interactions have been implicated in the generation of sub epithelial fibrosis and airway remodeling characteristic of human asthma in murine allergic asthma models.[78,79] Mechanistic assessments of eosinophil-fibroblast interactions that may lead to fibrosis, however, are still limited. Rochester and colleagues[74] reported that eosinophil granule MBP synergizes with TGF-β or IL-1β primed lung fibroblasts to induce significant increases in gene transcription and secretion of the IL-6 family of inflammatory and fibrogenic cytokines, including IL-6 and IL-11. TGF-β–induced fibroblast secretion of IL-6 is implicated in the overproduction of collagens, tissue inhibitor of metalloproteinases, and glycosaminoglycans in fibrogenesis.[80,81] Eosinophil-lung fibroblast coculture in the presence of IL-5 induces fibroblasts to transdifferentiate into myofibroblasts with increased expression of α-SMA and ECM proteins.[82] Eosinophils may indirectly impact fibroblast phenotype and fibrogenesis through activation of the epithelial-mesenchymal trophic unit[83] (eg, through secretion of MBP and eosinophil peroxidase) (see **Fig. 1**).[75] Alternatively, eosinophils may induce fibrogenesis through TGF-β induction of the epithelial to mesenchymal transition, as is shown to occur in the kidney[84] and lung.[85]

Subepithelial fibrosis, a component of airway remodeling in asthma pathogenesis, is initiated by insults that include Th2-mediated allergic responses. Eosinophilic inflammation is thought to drive the differentiation of airway fibroblasts to myofibroblasts as characterized by the expression of myofibroblast-specific markers, such as α-SMA; the deposition of ECM proteins, such as collagens; fibronectin; and other ECM constituents, such as tenascin and lumican.[25,83] Eosinophils recruited to the lung in asthma likely interact with fibroblasts beneath the reticular basement membrane, become activated to release their fibrogenic growth factors, such as TGF-β, driving fibroblasts to differentiate into myofibroblasts, which then deposit pathologic amounts of collagens and other ECM proteins contributing to airway subepithelial fibrosis.[19] A report showing correlations between pulmonary expression of eotaxin-1, expression of eotaxin-1 receptor (CCR3), TGF-β_1, and pulmonary fibrosis in a bleomycin mouse model supports this general mechanism.[86]

Studies of eosinophil-mediated tissue remodeling and fibrosis in EE are still limited to date, principally because of the difficulties inherent in obtaining sufficient biopsies containing esophageal lamina propria below the stiffened hyperplastic epithelium. For this reason, evidence for progressive remodeling and fibrosis of the esophagus has been derived principally from endoscopic and radiologic features of the disease.[7] The recent study by Aceves and colleagues,[14] however, demonstrated that pediatric EE esophageal biopsies showed increased levels of subepithelial fibrosis and increased expression of TGF-β_1 by eosinophils and its signaling molecule phospho-SMAD2/3 compared with gastroesophageal reflux disease and normal controls. Beyond this report, the mechanisms regulating esophageal remodeling and fibrosis in chronic EE have not been systematically studied to define the changes in epithelial cell and fibroblast phenotype, the role of eosinophil-fibroblast interactions, or the contribution of epithelial to mesenchymal transition to this process.

Finally, recent genome-wide expression profiling studies of EE esophageal tissue that identified increased expression of eotaxin-3 as the principal mediator of eosinophil recruitment,[27] interestingly did not identify many genes known to participate in tissue remodeling and fibrosis, perhaps because the biopsy specimens analyzed were sufficiently superficial to include mainly hyperplastic epithelium and not subepithelial fibrotic tissue. One of the identified genes, however, periostin, expressed predominantly in collagen-rich fibrous connective tissues subject to mechanical stresses and in wound healing, has been reported to participate in the development of subepithelial fibrosis in bronchial asthma downstream of the IL-4 and IL-13 signals.[87] Primary esophageal fibroblasts have recently been shown to release periostin when cultured with IL-13 and TGF-β.[26] Periostin, found mainly in the vascular papillae (projections of subepithelial lamina propria into the epithelium) in the esophagus, could contribute to eosinophil trafficking by increasing eosinophil adhesion to fibronectin.[26] Eosinophil-derived TGF-β, through induction of fibroblast periostin expression, might provide an amplification loop for eosinophilic inflammation and its consequent induction of the remodeling and fibrosis characteristic of EE.

Clinical Implications of Angiogenesis

Angiogenesis, the formation of new blood vessels, has a number of implications in inflammatory diseases, such as EE. Increased vasculature increases the density of conduits for inflammatory cell trafficking, propagating inflammation. In addition, ILs and histamine can modulate vascular permeability and lead to enhanced tissue edema. One of the histologic features of EE is dilated intercellular spaces,[88] which may be a reflection of increased tissue edema and, ultimately, increased mucosal and submucosal thickness when compared with control patients.[89,90] Linear furrowing, caused by a thickened esophagus folding on itself, could be an endoscopic finding related to esophageal edema. Ultimately, an edematous esophagus decreases luminal size and predisposes to clinical complications, such as food impaction.

Pediatric EE patients have an increased vascular density as compared with their age-matched counterparts with either a normal esophagus or esophagitis associated with gastroesophageal reflux disease.[14] Blood vessels from EE patients also demonstrate an activated endothelial phenotype with increased expression of vascular cell adhesion molecule-1(VCAM-1).[14] VCAM-1 interactions with the cognate ligand VLA-4 molecule allows leukocytes, particularly eosinophils, selectively to traffic to Th2 activated tissues. Interestingly, IL-13 and tumor necrosis factor-α can induce vascular endothelial VCAM-1 expression, and both are present at elevated levels in the esophageal mucosa in patients EE.[17,31]

Recent EE animal model studies demonstrate that IL-13 also increases vessel density in EE in a manner dependent on IL-13 interaction with IL-13Rα2.[91] Mice with increased expression of airway Clara cell CC-10–driven IL-13 have increased esophageal vascular density and increased esophageal circumference,[91] consistent with the linear furrowing and luminal narrowing seen in the human disease; this IL-13 effect is dependent on an intact IL-13Rα.[91] Because pediatric EE patients demonstrate an elevated expression of IL-13 mRNA,[31] IL-13 is also implicated in the generation of new blood vessels in the human disease. Animal models have also shown that the induction of EE by IL-13 is dependent on both IL-5 and STAT6,[16,31] and therapy with either IL-5 or IL-13 blocking agents[62,92] may remediate not only esophageal fibrosis, but also the increased angiogenesis associated with EE.[14]

PATHOGENIC MECHANISMS OF EOSINOPHIL-INDUCED ANGIOGENESIS

Eosinophils express a number of angiogenic factors, not the least of which is vascular endothelial growth factor (VEGF),[93] and they are implicated in the increased angiogenesis seen in many eosinophil-associated allergic inflammatory diseases, such as asthma.[94–96] The expression of VEGF, basic fibroblast growth factor, angiogenin, and the VEGF receptors (flt-1 and flk-1) is increased in asthmatic airways, and the numbers of cells including eosinophils expressing these factors and receptors is correlated with measurements of increased lung vascularity.[97,98] Increased expression of VEGF has been demonstrated in the induced sputum of asthmatic children, supporting the concept that it participates in the pathophysiology of augmented angiogenesis seen in bronchial asthma.[99]

Eosinophils, through expression of VEGF, have been shown experimentally by Puxeddu and colleagues[96] to induce new vessel formation in chick embryo models. Blood eosinophil extracts were found to induce rat aortic endothelial cell proliferation in vitro, rat aorta sprouting ex vivo, and angiogenesis in the chick embryo chorioallantoic membrane in vivo.[100] These proangiogenic effects were mediated principally by eosinophil-expressed VEGF, because they could significantly be inhibited by neutralizing antibodies to VEGF.[100] Intact eosinophils were found to induce VEGF mRNA expression and increased VEGF receptor density expression on endothelial cells, to enhance endothelial cell proliferation, and to augment angiogenic responses in aorta rings and chorioallantoic membranes.[100] Eosinophils are capable of inducing angiogenesis, in part by their secretion of preformed VEGF.[96] Whether eosinophils, through their expression of angiogenic factors, such as VEGF (see **Fig. 1**), contribute to increased vascularization and activated VCAM-1–positive vascular endothelium in the esophagus, as shown in children with EE,[14] remains to be determined.

THERAPEUTICS AND TISSUE REMODELING

Currently, there are no large clinical trials that demonstrate the efficacy of EE therapies on reducing tissue remodeling and fibrosis. One case report demonstrates that inhaled budesonide in a patient with stricture-associated EE and concurrent asthma was associated with decreased subepithelial fibrosis following 2 months of therapy.[101] Current observations demonstrate that a subset of children with EE have reversal of deep tissue remodeling following topical esophageal corticosteroid therapy (Aceves and Broide, unpublished data, 2008). Successful EE therapy with swallowed fluticasone results in the normalization of an EE-specific transcriptome, including IL-13.[31] As such, topical corticosteroids could diminish esophageal remodeling by their effects on the esophageal levels of ILs, such as IL-13. Anti–IL-5 therapy has also been reported to result in the improvement of EE-associated strictures and esophageal narrowing and improvement of basal zone hyperplasia and eosinophilic inflammation in an open-label trial in a small number of patients.[62] In contrast, a second placebo-controlled study in adults with severe EE concluded that anti–IL-5 therapy, although effective in reducing the numbers of esophageal eosinophils on average by approximately 55% (but not less than 10 eosinophils per hpf), showed little efficacy in reducing patients' clinical symptom scores.[63] Whether this is sufficient to result in histologic remission of the remodeling and fibrosis of the subepithelial tissue in EE remains to be determined. Of note, this finding is reminiscent of the first studies of anti–IL-5 therapy in asthmatic subjects, in which reductions of pulmonary tissue eosinophils by approximately 55% did not significantly impact pulmonary function or airway hyperreactivity,[102,103] but did significantly reduce the deposition of ECM proteins in the bronchial subepithelial basement membrane of mild atopic asthmatics.[25] These results suggest that an additional therapy (eg, one targeting eosinophil recruitment through antagonism of eotaxin-3 or its receptor on eosinophils [CCR3]) may need to be combined with anti–IL-5 to achieve a therapeutic reduction in eosinophils with complete endoscopic and histologic remission of esophageal remodeling in EE.

SUMMARY

The central role of the eosinophil in esophageal remodeling and subepithelial fibrosis, and the relationships of this remodeling to the clinical signs, symptoms, and pathogenesis of EE, are now beginning to be defined at the cellular and molecular levels, but clearly warrant further study. The natural history of EE, the time frame from disease onset to the development of epithelial hyperplasia, thickening of the muscularis propria and esophageal wall, and subepithelial deposition of collagens and other ECM constituents that contribute to esophageal remodeling and fibrosis in EE, however, are still not well defined. Also unclear are the relationships of esophageal remodeling to disease severity and duration, and to what extent esophageal remodeling and fibrosis are reversible with treatments that significantly reduce tissue eosinophils in the esophagus. Better understanding of the mechanisms by which eosinophils promote tissue remodeling and fibrogenesis in the esophagus should contribute to the development of novel therapeutic approaches for blocking eosinophil recruitment to the esophagus or reversing the debilitating consequences of esophageal remodeling in EE, and the tissue remodeling and fibrosis seen in many other eosinophil-associated allergic diseases and hypereosinophilic syndromes.

REFERENCES

1. Chehade M, Sampson HA. Epidemiology and etiology of eosinophilic esophagitis. Gastrointest Endosc Clin N Am 2008;18:33–44, viii.
2. Potter JW, Saeian K, Staff D, et al. Eosinophilic esophagitis in adults: an emerging problem with unique esophageal features. Gastrointest Endosc 2004;59:355–61.
3. Straumann A, Simon HU. Eosinophilic esophagitis: escalating epidemiology? J Allergy Clin Immunol 2005;115:418–9.
4. Vanderheyden AD, Petras RE, DeYoung BR, et al. Emerging eosinophilic (allergic) esophagitis: increased incidence or increased recognition? Arch Pathol Lab Med 2007;131:777–9.
5. Liacouras CA, Bonis P, Putnam PE, et al. Summary of the first international gastrointestinal research symposium. J Pediatr Gastroenterol Nutr 2007;45:370–91.
6. Noel RJ, Putnam PE, Rothenberg ME. Eosinophilic esophagitis. N Engl J Med 2004;351:940–1.
7. Straumann A, Spichtin HP, Grize L, et al. Natural history of primary eosinophilic esophagitis: a follow-up of 30 adult patients for up to 11.5 years. Gastroenterology 2003;125:1660–9.
8. Straumann A. The natural history and complications of eosinophilic esophagitis. Gastrointest Endosc Clin N Am 2008;18:99–118, ix.
9. Assa'ad AH, Putnam PE, Collins MH, et al. Pediatric patients with eosinophilic esophagitis: an 8-year follow-up. J Allergy Clin Immunol 2007;119:731–8.
10. Fox VL, Nurko S, Teitelbaum JE, et al. High-resolution EUS in children with eosinophilic allergic esophagitis. Gastrointest Endosc 2003;57:30–6.
11. Stevoff C, Rao S, Parsons W, et al. EUS and histopathologic correlates in eosinophilic esophagitis. Gastrointest Endosc 2001;54:373–7.
12. Furuta GT, Liacouras CA, Collins MH, et al. Eosinophilic esophagitis in children and adults: a systematic review and consensus recommendations for diagnosis and treatment. Gastroenterology 2007;133:1342–63.
13. Noel RJ, Putnam PE, Collins MH, et al. Clinical and immunopathologic effects of swallowed fluticasone for eosinophilic esophagitis. Clin Gastroenterol Hepatol 2004;2:568–75.

14. Aceves SS, Newbury RO, Dohil R, et al. Esophageal remodeling in pediatric eosinophilic esophagitis. J Allergy Clin Immunol 2007;119:206–12.
15. Chehade M, Sampson HA, Morotti RA, et al. Esophageal subepithelial fibrosis in children with eosinophilic esophagitis. J Pediatr Gastroenterol Nutr 2007;45: 319–28.
16. Mishra A, Rothenberg ME. Intratracheal IL-13 induces eosinophilic esophagitis by an IL-5, eotaxin-1, and STAT6-dependent mechanism. Gastroenterology 2003;125:1419–27.
17. Straumann A, Kristl J, Conus S, et al. Cytokine expression in healthy and inflamed mucosa: probing the role of eosinophils in the digestive tract. Inflamm Bowel Dis 2005;11:720–6.
18. Jacobsen EA, Ochkur SI, Lee NA, et al. Eosinophils and asthma. Curr Allergy Asthma Rep 2007;7:18–26.
19. Kay AB, Phipps S, Robinson DS. A role for eosinophils in airway remodelling in asthma. Trends Immunol 2004;25:477–82.
20. Lee JJ, Dimina D, Macias MP, et al. Defining a link with asthma in mice congenitally deficient in eosinophils. Science 2004;305:1773–6.
21. Tai PC, Ackerman SJ, Spry CJ, et al. Deposits of eosinophil granule proteins in cardiac tissues of patients with eosinophilic endomyocardial disease. Lancet 1987;1:643–7.
22. Spry CJ. The pathogenesis of endomyocardial fibrosis: the role of the eosinophil. Springer Semin Immunopathol 1989;11:471–7.
23. Jacobsen EA, Ochkur SI, Pero RS, et al. Allergic pulmonary inflammation in mice is dependent on eosinophil-induced recruitment of effector T cells. J Exp Med 2008;205:699–710.
24. Ochkur SI, Jacobsen EA, Protheroe CA, et al. Coexpression of IL-5 and eotaxin-2 in mice creates an eosinophil-dependent model of respiratory inflammation with characteristics of severe asthma. J Immunol 2007;178:7879–89.
25. Flood-Page P, Menzies-Gow A, Phipps S, et al. Anti-IL-5 treatment reduces deposition of ECM proteins in the bronchial subepithelial basement membrane of mild atopic asthmatics. J Clin Invest 2003;112:1029–36.
26. Blanchard C, Mingler MK, McBride M, et al. Periostin facilitates eosinophil tissue infiltration in allergic lung and esophageal responses. Mucosal Immunol 2008;1: 289–96.
27. Blanchard C, Wang N, Stringer KF, et al. Eotaxin-3 and a uniquely conserved gene-expression profile in eosinophilic esophagitis. J Clin Invest 2006;116:536–47.
28. Mishra A, Wang M, Pemmaraju VR, et al. Esophageal remodeling develops as a consequence of tissue specific IL-5-induced eosinophilia. Gastroenterology 2008;134:204–14.
29. Fulkerson PC, Fischetti CA, Rothenberg ME. Eosinophils and CCR3 regulate interleukin-13 transgene-induced pulmonary remodeling. Am J Pathol 2006;169: 2117–26.
30. Zhu Z, Homer RJ, Wang Z, et al. Pulmonary expression of interleukin-13 causes inflammation, mucus hypersecretion, subepithelial fibrosis, physiologic abnormalities, and eotaxin production. J Clin Invest 1999;103:779–88.
31. Blanchard C, Mingler MK, Vicario M, et al. IL-13 involvement in eosinophilic esophagitis: transcriptome analysis and reversibility with glucocorticoids. J Allergy Clin Immunol 2007;120:1292–300.
32. Schmid-Grendelmeier P, Altznauer F, Fischer B, et al. Eosinophils express functional IL-13 in eosinophilic inflammatory diseases. J Immunol 2002;169: 1021–7.

33. Aceves SS, Newbury RO, Dohil R, et al. Distinguishing eosinophilic esophagitis in pediatric patients: clinical, endoscopic, and histologic features of an emerging disorder. J Clin Gastroenterol 2007;41:252–6.

34. Kapel RC, Miller JK, Torres C, et al. Eosinophilic esophagitis: a prevalent disease in the United States that affects all age groups. Gastroenterology 2008; 134:1316–21.

35. Parfitt JR, Gregor JC, Suskin NG, et al. Eosinophilic esophagitis in adults: distinguishing features from gastroesophageal reflux disease: a study of 41 patients. Mod Pathol 2006;19:90–6.

36. Aceves SS, Arii B, Dohil M, et al. Prospective analysis of an abdominal symptom scoring system tool's efficacy in the clinical distinction of pediatric eosinophilic esophagitis from gastroesophageal reflux disease. J Allergy Clin Immunol 2008;121:S70.

37. Aceves SS, Furuta GT, Spechler SJ. Integrated approach to treatment of children and adults with eosinophilic esophagitis. Gastrointest Endosc Clin N Am 2008;18:195–217, xi.

38. Noel RJ, Tipnis NA. Eosinophilic esophagitis: a mimic of GERD. Int J Pediatr Otorhinolaryngol 2006;70:1147–53.

39. Prasad GA, Talley NJ, Romero Y, et al. Prevalence and predictive factors of eosinophilic esophagitis in patients presenting with dysphagia: a prospective study. Am J Gastroenterol 2007;102:2627–32.

40. Lucendo AJ, Pascual-Turrion JM, Navarro M, et al. Endoscopic, bioptic, and manometric findings in eosinophilic esophagitis before and after steroid therapy: a case series. Endoscopy 2007;39:765–71.

41. Remedios M, Campbell C, Jones DM, et al. Eosinophilic esophagitis in adults: clinical, endoscopic, histologic findings, and response to treatment with fluticasone propionate. Gastrointest Endosc 2006;63:3–12.

42. Korsapati HR, Dohil R, Quinn AM, et al. Normal circular muscle but dysfunctional longitudinal muscle in eosinophilic esophagitis. Gastroenterology 2008;134:A-59.

43. Jacoby DB, Costello RM, Fryer AD. Eosinophil recruitment to the airway nerves. J Allergy Clin Immunol 2001;107:211–8.

44. Cho JY, Miller M, Baek KJ, et al. Inhibition of airway remodeling in IL-5-deficient mice. J Clin Invest 2004;113:551–60.

45. Humbles AA, Lloyd CM, McMillan SJ, et al. A critical role for eosinophils in allergic airways remodeling. Science 2004;305:1776–9.

46. Coyle AJ, Ackerman SJ, Burch R, et al. Human eosinophil-granule major basic protein and synthetic polycations induce airway hyperresponsiveness in vivo dependent on bradykinin generation. J Clin Invest 1995;95:1735–40.

47. Coyle AJ, Ackerman SJ, Irvin CG. Cationic proteins induce airway hyperresponsiveness dependent on charge interactions. Am Rev Respir Dis 1993;147:896–900.

48. Desai SN, Van G, Robson J, et al. Human eosinophil major basic protein augments bronchoconstriction induced by intravenous agonists in guinea pigs. Agents Actions 1993;39(Spec No):C132–5.

49. Gundel RH, Letts LG, Gleich GJ. Human eosinophil major basic protein induces airway constriction and airway hyperresponsiveness in primates. J Clin Invest 1991;87:1470–3.

50. Jacoby DB, Gleich GJ, Fryer AD. Human eosinophil major basic protein is an endogenous allosteric antagonist at the inhibitory muscarinic M2 receptor. J Clin Invest 1993;91:1314–8.

51. Evans CM, Fryer AD, Jacoby DB, et al. Pretreatment with antibody to eosinophil major basic protein prevents hyperresponsiveness by protecting neuronal M2

muscarinic receptors in antigen-challenged guinea pigs. J Clin Invest 1997;100: 2254–62.

52. Costello RW, Evans CM, Yost BL, et al. Antigen-induced hyperreactivity to histamine: role of the vagus nerves and eosinophils. Am J Physiol 1999;276:L709–14.
53. Costello RW, Jacoby DB, Gleich GJ, et al. Eosinophils and airway nerves in asthma. Histol Histopathol 2000;15:861–8.
54. Elbon CL, Jacoby DB, Fryer AD. Pretreatment with an antibody to interleukin-5 prevents loss of pulmonary M2 muscarinic receptor function in antigen-challenged guinea pigs. Am J Respir Cell Mol Biol 1995;12:320–8.
55. Fryer AD, Costello RW, Yost BL, et al. Antibody to VLA-4, but not to L-selectin, protects neuronal M2 muscarinic receptors in antigen-challenged guinea pig airways. J Clin Invest 1997;99:2036–44.
56. Yost BL, Gleich GJ, Jacoby DB, et al. The changing role of eosinophils in longterm hyperreactivity following a single ozone exposure. Am J Physiol Lung Cell Mol Physiol 2005;289:L627–35.
57. Fryer AD, Stein LH, Nie Z, et al. Neuronal eotaxin and the effects of CCR3 antagonist on airway hyperreactivity and M2 receptor dysfunction. J Clin Invest 2006; 116:228–36.
58. Costello RW, Schofield BH, Kephart GM, et al. Localization of eosinophils to airway nerves and effect on neuronal M2 muscarinic receptor function. Am J Physiol 1997;273:L93–103.
59. Gonsalves N, Yang G-Y, Doerfler B, et al. A prospective clinical trial of six food elimination diet and reintroduction of causative agents in adults with eosinophilic esophagitis. Gastroenterology 2008;134:A104.
60. Straumann A, Bauer M, Fischer B, et al. Idiopathic eosinophilic esophagitis is associated with a T(H)2-type allergic inflammatory response. J Allergy Clin Immunol 2001;108:954–61.
61. Phipps S, Flood-Page P, Menzies-Gow A, et al. Intravenous anti-IL-5 monoclonal antibody reduces eosinophils and tenascin deposition in allergen-challenged human atopic skin. J Invest Dermatol 2004;122:1406–12.
62. Stein ML, Collins MH, Villanueva JM, et al. Anti-IL-5 (mepolizumab) therapy for eosinophilic esophagitis. J Allergy Clin Immunol 2006;118:1312–9.
63. Straumann A, Conus S, Kita H, et al. Mepolizumab, a humanized antibody to IL-5, for severe eosinophilic esophagitis in adults: a randomized, placebo-controlled double-blind trial. J Allergy Clin Immunol 2008;121:S44.
64. Rothenberg ME. Eosinophilic gastrointestinal disorders (EGID). J Allergy Clin Immunol 2004;113:11–28 [quiz 29].
65. Gharaee-Kermani M, Phan SH. The role of eosinophils in pulmonary fibrosis. Int J Mol Med 1998;1:43–53.
66. Kay AB. The role of eosinophils in the pathogenesis of asthma. Trends Mol Med 2005;11:148–52.
67. Minshall EM, Leung DY, Martin RJ, et al. Eosinophil-associated TGF-beta1 mRNA expression and airways fibrosis in bronchial asthma. Am J Respir Cell Mol Biol 1997;17:326–33.
68. Varga J, Kahari VM. Eosinophilia-myalgia syndrome, eosinophilic fasciitis, and related fibrosing disorders. Curr Opin Rheumatol 1997;9:562–70.
69. Gharaee-Kermani M, Phan SH. Molecular mechanisms of and possible treatment strategies for idiopathic pulmonary fibrosis. Curr Pharm Des 2005;11:3943–71.
70. Gauldie J, Sime PJ, Xing Z, et al. Transforming growth factor-beta gene transfer to the lung induces myofibroblast presence and pulmonary fibrosis. Curr Top Pathol 1999;93:35–45.

71. Ohno I, Nitta Y, Yamauchi K, et al. Transforming growth factor beta 1 (TGF-beta 1) gene expression by eosinophils in asthmatic airway inflammation. Am J Respir Cell Mol Biol 1996;15:404–9.

72. Ohno I, Nitta Y, Yamauchi K, et al. Eosinophils as a potential source of platelet-derived growth factor B-chain (PDGF-B) in nasal polyposis and bronchial asthma. Am J Respir Cell Mol Biol 1995;13:639–47.

73. Gomes I, Mathur SK, Espenshade BM, et al. Eosinophil-fibroblast interactions induce fibroblast IL-6 secretion and extracellular matrix gene expression: implications in fibrogenesis. J Allergy Clin Immunol 2005;116:796–804.

74. Rochester CL, Ackerman SJ, Zheng T, et al. Eosinophil-fibroblast interactions: granule major basic protein interacts with IL-1 and transforming growth factor-beta in the stimulation of lung fibroblast IL-6-type cytokine production. J Immunol 1996;156:4449–56.

75. Pegorier S, Wagner LA, Gleich GJ, et al. Eosinophil-derived cationic proteins activate the synthesis of remodeling factors by airway epithelial cells. J Immunol 2006;177:4861–9.

76. Lacy P, Moqbel R. Eosinophil cytokines. Chem Immunol 2000;76:134–55.

77. Minshall EM, Cameron L, Lavigne F, et al. Eotaxin mRNA and protein expression in chronic sinusitis and allergen-induced nasal responses in seasonal allergic rhinitis. Am J Respir Cell Mol Biol 1997;17:683–90.

78. Hoshino M, Nakamura Y, Sim J, et al. Bronchial subepithelial fibrosis and expression of matrix metalloproteinase-9 in asthmatic airway inflammation. J Allergy Clin Immunol 1998;102:783–8.

79. Hoshino M, Nakamura Y, Sim JJ. Expression of growth factors and remodelling of the airway wall in bronchial asthma. Thorax 1998;53:21–7.

80. Eickelberg O, Pansky A, Mussmann R, et al. Transforming growth factor-beta1 induces interleukin-6 expression via activating protein-1 consisting of JunD homodimers in primary human lung fibroblasts. J Biol Chem 1999;274:12933–8.

81. Varga J, Jimenez SA. Modulation of collagen gene expression: its relation to fibrosis in systemic sclerosis and other disorders. Ann Intern Med. 1995;122:60–2.

82. Phipps S, Ying S, Wangoo A, et al. The relationship between allergen-induced tissue eosinophilia and markers of repair and remodeling in human atopic skin. J Immunol 2002;169:4604–12.

83. Phipps S, Benyahia F, Ou TT, et al. Acute allergen-induced airway remodeling in atopic asthma. Am J Respir Cell Mol Biol 2004;31:626–32.

84. Zeisberg M, Kalluri R. Fibroblasts emerge via epithelial-mesenchymal transition in chronic kidney fibrosis. Front Biosci 2008;13:6991–8.

85. Kim KK, Kugler MC, Wolters PJ, et al. Alveolar epithelial cell mesenchymal transition develops in vivo during pulmonary fibrosis and is regulated by the extracellular matrix. Proc Natl Acad Sci U S A 2006;103:13180–5.

86. Huaux F, Gharaee-Kermani M, Liu T, et al. Role of Eotaxin-1 (CCL11) and CC chemokine receptor 3 (CCR3) in bleomycin-induced lung injury and fibrosis. Am J Pathol 2005;167:1485–96.

87. Takayama G, Arima K, Kanaji T, et al. Periostin: a novel component of subepithelial fibrosis of bronchial asthma downstream of IL-4 and IL-13 signals. J Allergy Clin Immunol 2006;118:98–104.

88. Ravelli AM, Villanacci V, Ruzzenenti N, et al. Dilated intercellular spaces: a major morphological feature of esophagitis. J Pediatr Gastroenterol Nutr 2006;42:510–5.

89. Fox VL. Eosinophilic esophagitis: endoscopic findings. Gastrointest Endosc Clin N Am 2008;18:45–57, viii.

90. Mueller S, Aigner T, Neureiter D, et al. Eosinophil infiltration and degranulation in oesophageal mucosa from adult patients with eosinophilic oesophagitis: a retrospective and comparative study on pathological biopsy. J Clin Pathol 2006;59: 1175–80.

91. Zuo L, Mingler M, Blanchard C, et al. IL-13 transgene induced experimental eosinophilic esophagitis is associated with increased esophageal circumference and extensive angiogenesis. J Allergy Clin Immunol 2008;121:S72.

92. Blanchard C, Mishra A, Saito-Akei H, et al. Inhibition of human interleukin-13-induced respiratory and oesophageal inflammation by anti-human-interleukin-13 antibody (CAT-354). Clin Exp Allergy 2005;35:1096–103.

93. Horiuchi T, Weller PF. Expression of vascular endothelial growth factor by human eosinophils: upregulation by granulocyte macrophage colony-stimulating factor and interleukin-5. Am J Respir Cell Mol Biol 1997;17:70–7.

94. Aceves SS, Broide DH. Airway fibrosis and angiogenesis due to eosinophil trafficking in chronic asthma. Curr Mol Med 2008;8:350–8.

95. Broide DH. Immunologic and inflammatory mechanisms that drive asthma progression to remodeling. J Allergy Clin Immunol 2008;121:560–70 [quiz 571–2].

96. Puxeddu I, Ribatti D, Crivellato E, et al. Mast cells and eosinophils: a novel link between inflammation and angiogenesis in allergic diseases. J Allergy Clin Immunol 2005;116:531–6.

97. Hoshino M, Nakamura Y, Hamid QA. Gene expression of vascular endothelial growth factor and its receptors and angiogenesis in bronchial asthma. J Allergy Clin Immunol 2001;107:1034–8.

98. Hoshino M, Takahashi M, Aoike N. Expression of vascular endothelial growth factor, basic fibroblast growth factor, and angiogenin immunoreactivity in asthmatic airways and its relationship to angiogenesis. J Allergy Clin Immunol 2001;107:295–301.

99. Hossny E, El-Awady H, Bakr S, et al. Vascular endothelial growth factor overexpression in induced sputum of children with bronchial asthma. Pediatr Allergy Immunol 2008, in press.

100. Puxeddu I, Alian A, Piliponsky AM, et al. Human peripheral blood eosinophils induce angiogenesis. Int J Biochem Cell Biol 2005;37:628–36.

101. Maples KM, Henderson SC, Graham M, et al. Treatment of eosinophilic esophagitis with inhaled budesonide in a 7-year-old boy with concomitant persistent asthma: resolution of esophageal submucosal fibrosis and eosinophilic infiltration. Ann Allergy Asthma Immunol 2007;99:572–4.

102. Flood-Page PT, Menzies-Gow AN, Kay AB, et al. Eosinophil's role remains uncertain as anti-interleukin-5 only partially depletes numbers in asthmatic airway. Am J Respir Crit Care Med 2003;167:199–204.

103. Leckie MJ, ten Brinke A, Khan J, et al. Effects of an interleukin-5 blocking monoclonal antibody on eosinophils, airway hyper-responsiveness, and the late asthmatic response. Lancet 2000;356:2144–8.

Index

Note: Page numbers of article titles are in **boldface** type.

Immunol Allergy Clin N Am 29 (2009) 213–222
doi:10.1016/S0889-8561(08)00124-0
0889-8561/08/$ – see front matter © 2009 Elsevier Inc. All rights reserved.

immunology.theclinics.com

Moving?

Make sure your subscription moves with you!

To notify us of your new address, find your **Clinics Account Number** (located on your mailing label above your name), and contact customer service at:

E-mail: elspcs@elsevier.com

800-654-2452 (subscribers in the U.S. & Canada)
314-453-7041 (subscribers outside of the U.S. & Canada)

Fax number: 314-523-5170

Elsevier Periodicals Customer Service
11830 Westline Industrial Drive
St. Louis, MO 63146

*To ensure uninterrupted delivery of your subscription, please notify us at least 4 weeks in advance of move.

Printed and bound by CPI Group (UK) Ltd, Croydon, CR0 4YY

03/10/2024

01040443-0005